Social Occupational Therapy: Theoretical and Practical Designs

Roseli Esquerdo Lopes, MSc, PhD
Professor
Occupational Therapy Department
Federal University of São Carlos (UFSCar)
Metuia Network – Social Occupational Therapy
São Carlos, São Paulo, Brazil

Ana Paula Serrata Malfitano MSc, PhD
Associate Professor
Occupational Therapy Department
Federal University of São Carlos (UFSCar)
Metuia Network – Social Occupational Therapy
São Carlos, São Paulo, Brazil

ELSEVIER

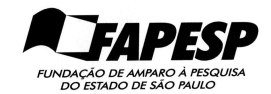

FUNDAÇÃO DE AMPARO À PESQUISA
DO ESTADO DE SÃO PAULO

Elsevier
1600 John F. Kennedy Blvd.
Ste 1800
Philadelphia, PA 19103-2899

SOCIAL OCCUPATIONAL THERAPY: THEORETICAL AND PRACTICAL DESIGNS   ISBN: 978-0-323-69549-7

International Standard Book Number: 978-0-323-69549-7

Content Strategist: Lauren Willis
Content Development Specialist: Kevin Travers
Publishing Services Manager: Deepthi Unni
Project Manager: Srividhya Vidhyashankar
Design Direction: Margaret Reid
Cover by External Designer: Ana Lua Contatore
Content Development Manager: Meghan Andress

Printed in United States of America

Last digit is the print number: 9   8   7   6   5   4   3   2   1

Working together to grow libraries in developing countries

www.elsevier.com • www.bookaid.org

Social Occupational Therapy:
Theoretical and Practical Designs

Changing the world is as difficult as possible
(Mudar o mundo é tão difícil quanto possível)
Paulo Freire

(Freire, P. (2000). Pedagogia da indignação: cartas pedagógicas e outros escritos [Indignation pedagogy: pedagogical letters and others written]. São Paulo: Editora UNESP).

ACKNOWLEDGEMENTS

The book organizers acknowledge the occupational therapists who supported the English language review process of the chapters of this book. They are:

Amelia Di Tommaso
Anne Kinsella
Antoine Bailliard
Ben Sellar
Clare Hocking
Dikaios Sakellariou
Elizabeth Townsend
Gail Whiteford
Geyla Frank
Lilian Magalhães
Lisette Farias Vera
Lynn Shaw
Matthew Molineux
Natalia Rivas Quarneti
Nerida Hyett
Nicholas Pollard
Niki Kiepek
Pamela Block
Roshan Galvaan
Sarah Kantartzis

Cover
Ana Lua Contatore

Translation-funding

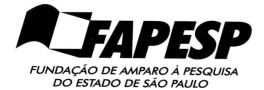

FUNDAÇÃO DE AMPARO À PESQUISA
DO ESTADO DE SÃO PAULO

FAPESP - São Paulo Research Foundation
Grant 2019/02674-5

CONTRIBUTORS

Marta Carvalho de Almeida, MSc, PhD
Assistant Professor
Department of Physiotherapy,
Communication Science & Disorders
and Occupational Therapy
University of São Paulo
Metuia Network – Social
Occupational Therapy
São Paulo, SP
Brazil

Giovanna Bardi, MSc, PhD
Assistant Professor
Occupational Therapy Department
Federal University of Espírito Santo
Metuia Network – Social
Occupational Therapy
Vitória, ES
Brazil

Rafael Garcia Barreiro, MSc, PhD
Assistant Professor
Brasiília University
Metuia Network – Social
Occupational Therapy
Brasília, DF
Brazil

Denise Dias Barros, MSc, PhD
Assistant Professor
University of São Paulo
Metuia Network – Social
Occupational Therapy
São Paulo, SP
Brazil

Sandra Benites, PhD
Guarani Teacher
Indigenous School
Paraty, RJ
National Museum
Federal University of Rio de Janeiro
Rio de Janeiro, RJ
Brazil

Patrícia Leme de Oliveira Borba, MSc, PhD
Assistant Professor
Health, Education and Society
Department
Federal University of São Paulo
Metuia Network – Social
Occupational Therapy
Santos, SP
Brazil

Mayra Cappellaro, MSc
Occupacional Therapist
Ludens Clinics
Campinas, SP
Brazil

Luciana Assis Costa, MSc, PhD
Associate Professor
Occupationial Therapy Department
Federal University of Minas Gerais,
Belo Horizonte, MG
Brazil

Samira Lima da Costa, MSc, PhD
Associate Professor
Occupational Therapy Department
Federal University of Rio de Janeiro
Rio de Janeiro, RJ
Brazil

Patricia Silva Dorneles, MSc, PhD
Assistant Professor
Occupational Therapy Department
Federal University of Rio de Janeiro
Rio de Janeiro, RJ
Brazil

Regina Celia Fiorati, MSc, PhD
Assistant Professor
Department of Health Science
University of São Paulo
Ribeirão Preto, SP
Brazil

Hetty Fransen-Jaïbi, MSc
Senior Lecturer
Division of Occupational Therapy
University Tunis El Manar, Tunis
Tunisia

Sandra Maria Galheigo, MSc, PhD
Assistant Professor
Department of Physiotherapy,
Communication Science & Disorders
and Occupational Therapy
University of São Paulo
São Paulo, SP
Brazil

Debora Galvani, MSc, PhD
Assistant Professor
Health, Education and Society
Departament
Federal University of São Paulo
Metuia Network – Social
Occupational Therapy
Santos, SP
Brazil

Maria Isabel Garcez Ghirardi, MSc, PhD
Occupational Therapist
University of São Paulo,
São Paulo, SP
Brazil

Sarah Kantartzis, MSc
Senior Lecturer
Occupational Therapy Department
Queen Margaret University,
Edinburgh
United Kingdom

Roseli Esquerdo Lopes, MSc, PhD
Professor
Occupational Therapy Department
Federal University of São Carlos
Metuia Network – Social
Occupational Therapy
São Carlos, São Carlos, SP
Brazil

Maria Daniela Corrêa de Macedo, MSc, PhD
Assistant Professor
Occupational Therapy Department
Federal University of Espírito Santo
Metuia Network – Social
Occupational Therapy
Vitória, ES
Brazil

Ana Paula Serrata Malfitano, MSc, PhD
Associate Professor
Occupational Therapy Department
Federal University of São Carlos
Metuia Network – Social
Occupational Therapy
São Carlos, SP
Brazil

Gustavo Artur Monzeli MSc, PhD
Assistant Professor
Occupational Therapy Department
Federal University of Paraíba
Metuia Network – Social
Occupational Therapy
João Pessoa, PB
Brazil

Aline Cristina Morais, MSc
Occupational Therapist
Municipal Secretary of Social
Services
Franca, SP
Brazil

Livia Celegati Pan, MSc, PhD
Assistant Professor
Occupational Therapy Department
Federal University of São Carlos
Metuia Network – Social
Occupational Therapy
São Carlos, SP
Brazil

Beatriz Prado Pereira, MSc, PhD
Assistant Professor
Occupational Therapy Department
Federal University of Paraíba
Metuia Network – Social
Occupational Therapy
João Pessoa, PB
Brazil

Paulo Estevão Pereira MSc
Brazilian Company of Hospital
Services
Rehabilitation Unit
Federal University of Triângulo
Mineiro
Uberaba, MG
Brazil

Nick Pollard, MA, MSc, PhD
Senior Lecturer
Occupational Therapy and
Vocational Rehabilitation
Department
Sheffield Hallam University
Sheffield
United Kingdom

Debbie Laliberte Rudman, MSc, PhD
Professor
Occupational Therapy Department
University of Western Ontario,
London, Ontario
Canada

Carolina Donato da Silva, MSc
Occupation Therapist
Albert Einstein Israelite Hospital
São Paulo, SP
Brazil

Carla Regina Silva, MSc, PhD
Assistant Professor
Occupational Therapy Department
Federal University of São Carlos
São Carlos, SP
Brazil

Marina Jorge da Silva, MSc, PhD
Assistant Professor
Occupational Therapy Department
Federal University of São Carlos
Metuia Network – Social
Occupational Therapy
São Carlos, SP
Brazil

Carla Regina Silva Soares, MSc
Occupational Therapist
Department of Physiotherapy,
Communication Science & Disorders
and Occupational Therapy,
University of São Paulo
Metuia Network – Social
Occupational Therapy
São Paulo, SP
Brazil

Letícia Brandão de Souza
Occupational Therapist
São Carlos, SP
Brazil

Elizabeth Ann Townsend, MA, PhD
Professor Emerita
Occupational Therapy Department
Dalhousie University
Halifax, Nova Scotia
Canada
Adjunct Professor
Faculty of Education
University of Prince Edward Island
Charlottetown, PEI
Canada

Inés Viana-Moldes, MSc, PhD
Associate Professor
Health Sciences Department
University of A Coruña
A Coruña
Spain

As men [and women] relate to the world by responding to the challenges of the environment, they begin to dynamize, to master, and to humanize reality.
(Freire, 1989, p. 5)

In *Education for Critical Consciousness,* Paulo Freire (1989) challenges us "to dynamize, to master, and to humanize reality" by directing our attention to "the environment." *Social Occupational Therapy* takes up that challenge, inspired by creative thinking, actions, and nonmedical funding. With examples from Brazil, the book asserts a radical call for occupational therapists around the world to practice in social contexts with funding beyond health services. The key strategy is to develop practices with populations, communities, and groups more than with individuals.

The phrase "social occupational therapy" is fairly new, although I see ALL occupational therapy practices as inherently social. We cannot practice any occupational therapy effectively in any country without knowing the environment in which people work, play, plan, grow, and adapt to life challenges. Where people cannot participate in society or have nothing meaningful to do, for example, this book shows how occupational therapists can address social problems, especially where there is funding support beyond health services.

The inherent social nature of occupational therapy has drawn me to support this book with great enthusiasm. I love the 10 stories that point to the social relevance of global life issues and practical occupational therapy actions that can be adapted in any country. *Social Occupational Therapy* is a bold text, prompting education for critical consciousness for occupational therapists to learn from Brazil how to be a creative, highly practical profession. How lovely it is for Brazil to lead the way. The examples show how occupational therapists anywhere can advance the humanizing reality of everyday life. Readers will find an integration of theoretical designs and practical actions that demonstrate how funding and partners outside health services enable us to work with poor youth, territorial work, public schools, the "Estatuto da Criança e do Adolescente" (Brazilian law about children and adolescents), youth, and conflicts with the law, drugs, gender, and sexuality.

One reason that I'm strongly attracted to this book is because it challenges the Western medicalization of occupational therapy. *Social Occupational Therapy* provides students, educators, occupational therapy practitioners, and researchers anywhere with an educational resource for practices that do not rely on medical funding. Medical knowledge is integrated with social, economic, political science, and other knowledge to guide occupational therapists as leaders and partners taking action on social challenges. Instead of illustrating practices that aim mainly to restore the mind and body in health care systems, *Social Occupational Therapy* focuses on the environment as an integrated force in everyday life. Here, the environment is not viewed as an abstract idea or an inanimate object. Rather, the stories here show how the real lives of poor youth, children in conflict with the law, and issues of sexuality, for example, are shaped by and shape the environment. Readers will see in the 10 stories how the environment is embedded in everyday life and is simultaneously social, cultural, economic, political, geographic, and historical. The examples will help readers to think about ways of helping people to develop their capabilities instead of being frozen, seemingly unable to act in everyday life. In other words, *Social Occupational Therapy* takes an activist view of occupational therapists as leaders and partners who engage people in changing their lives.

The ideals and practices described in *Social Occupational Therapy* revive early aims in the founding of this profession virtually everywhere in the world. Occupational therapy education and practices have arisen typically where there have been veterans of war or people struggling to live with chronic disease or disability resulting, for instance, from polio. Some early occupational therapy practices were highly social, such as establishing children's early development programs, setting up vocational training for adults with disabilities, and advocating for services when older people are isolated with too little support. To me, the authors of *Social Occupational Therapy* are capturing not only the historical promise but also the untapped future for occupational therapists.

The focus on social occupational therapy reminds me of stories that inflamed my imagination when I started my career as an occupational therapist more than 50 years ago. I was drawn unconsciously to work with populations, communities, and groups, not only with individuals. And I was driven to explore solutions where people's daily lives were deprived, alienated, marginalized, oppressed, or otherwise restricted in a range of social contexts—what we now call occupational injustice. I feel that this book advances my dream for a profession that has so much more to offer than we have seen in the world to date.

I applaud the authors for their celebration of what I see as the heart and history and future of occupational therapy. May readers use this book to bring forth the social theories and practices that make occupational therapy uniquely relevant to today's societies everywhere!

Elizabeth Townsend

REFERENCE

Freire, P. (1989). *Education for critical consciousness.* New York, NY: Continuum.

Gathering the theoretical assumptions and practical propositions arising from social occupational therapy in Brazil has significant value to us because it represents our collective work since the late 1990s, when a specific context motivated occupational therapists, academics, professionals, and researchers to address issues arising from the "social question." This material was originally published in Portuguese by the Federal University of Sao Carlos Publisher (EdUFSCar) with support from the São Paulo Research Foundation (FAPESP) in 2016. The first version of the book consisted of reflections from occupational therapy researchers and professionals representing various higher education institutions in Brazil, as well as former master's and doctoral students in the "Social Networks and Vulnerabilities" line of research of the graduate studies program in occupational therapy at the Federal University of São Carlos (PPGTO/UFSCar), a pioneering program in Latin America. This English edition broadens the symbolic value of this work by expanding the dialogue around occupational therapy, sending it worldwide.

The Brazilian account begins in the mid-1950s, when occupational therapy courses were first created in the states of Rio de Janeiro and São Paulo. These courses were directed at the education of "rehabilitation professionals," especially physical and occupational therapists, based on agreements with the United Nations (UN) and UNICEF. These courses adhered to the framework of health rehabilitation in a broad sense, although they were quite focused on rehabilitation after work-related injuries, understood from the perspective of physical disability. A psychiatric dimension was also included, and both types of rehabilitation aimed to restore people to life in occupations (Lopes, 1990; Soares, 1991). This rehabilitation-oriented axis was (and remains) important and controversial for Brazilian occupational therapists, their identity, and professional practice, which sometimes focuses on the function itself, sometimes on the occupational function and/or occupational performance (Barros, Galheigo, & Lopes, 2007).

It is difficult to reconstruct the history of occupational therapy in Brazil prior to the 1980s, the time of its professionalization, which effectively occurred in the late 1970s. For most occupational therapists at that time, it was essential to develop a local point of reference, that is, to consider the demands and realities surrounding them in their Brazilian context. As a consequence, a specific occupational therapy was designed, with its own vocabulary, based on practices that addressed those particular demands and realities. This situation directed the professional paths of occupational therapy beyond functional rehabilitation and the pursuit of therapeutic activity (Lopes, 2004; Nascimento, 1990).

The expansion of the professional field initially arose from discussions about the limitations of the biomedical perspective in occupational therapy; although its relevance in the profession is acknowledged, this perspective is incapable of representing occupational therapy in its totality. This issue was a subject of discussion in the late 1970s and early 1980s, with advocacy for an occupational therapy that was politically committed to its target population (Lopes, 1990). The debate was influenced by authors such as Antonio Gramsci (1988), Franco Basaglia (1979), Franco Basaglia and Franca Basaglia (1977), and Paulo Freire (1970), among others, who encouraged questioning of the social function of professionals, pointing out the relevance of the contexts and the presence or absence of rights, justice, and social injustice as elements inherent to occupational therapy practice. Since then, Brazilian occupational therapy has recognized that "the social" should be present in the practice of all occupational therapists and that it should occupy different levels of centrality depending on each particular set of actions.

In the context of the "Global North,"[1] where the voices that dominated (and still dominate) occupational therapy worldwide originated, such discussions pervaded what was termed the "renaissance of the paradigm of occupation" (Kielhofner, 1992). For some of these voices, the central concern lay in the need for occupational therapy (and occupational therapists) to address the occupations performed by people, encompassing their social perspectives (Townsend, 1993), and not "only" their duties and/or performances. Whiteford, Townsend, and Hocking (2000), who drew on postmodernism as a theoretical framework, discussed the relevance of this idea on the grounds that it contributes to approaching the relations of power, diversity, and institutional issues, which are part of occupational therapy practice. They associated the renaissance of occupation as the profession's central concept with the history of occupational science and its commitment to challenging forms of capitalist hegemony that generate inequalities or, in their words, "occupational deprivation." In addition, discussion about the contexts of

---

[1]The "Global North" refers to a group of capitalist countries that dominates the world economic order, which includes the sociocultural dimension (Lewis, Dwyer, Hodkinson, & Waite, 2015).

injustice and their influence on people's occupations was highlighted, leading to proposal of the term "occupational justice" (Wilcock & Townsend, 2000), which has influenced diverse practices among occupational therapists (Malfitano, Souza, Townsend, & Lopes, 2019). Therefore, while the occupational paradigm was central to discussions about occupational therapy practice in the Global North, for some researchers, it also represented tensions and demands to be explained critically.

Thus, it should be noted that the moment, the period, the paths, and the theoretical influences shaping discussion about the identity of occupational therapy in both Brazil and the Global North were diverse, albeit addressing similar concerns about the need for the field to go beyond biomedical intervention models. However, when we analyze the Brazilian context, it is worth pointing out the specificity of occupational therapy vocabulary to its local historicity. The literature clearly shows that the return to the use of the term "occupation" in occupational therapy in the Global North was marked by the broadening of a critical perspective for the profession (Whiteford et al., 2000). In contrast, critical perspectives followed other paths in Brazil, where the word "occupation" retained its pejorative sense. On the one hand, it was associated with the notion of work (for which it is a synonym), and its practitioners were therefore tasked with rehabilitating/enabling people with formal or informal work-related disabilities or injuries (Soares, 1991). On the other hand, it was associated with alienation, especially with processes related to "moral treatment" in psychiatric institutions like asylums, where occupational therapists were responsible for keeping patients occupied without disturbing the institutional order (Nascimento, 1991). This understanding of occupational therapy remains prevalent when it is understood as an approach for difficulties and resistance that are encountered in the context of a "total institution" (Goffman, 1961).

Therefore, the word "occupation" has not undergone its "renaissance" in the historical development of Brazilian occupational therapy; on the contrary, it has been linked to negativity or coercion, associating professionals with processes that alienate people. Thus, the word assumes a pejorative meaning among Brazilian occupational therapists, notably those who struggled to separate their professional practices from alienation processes, seeking, in contrast, means of mediating emancipatory actions. For this reason, some aversion to the term "occupation" was, and still is, quite present.

Nevertheless, it is necessary to consider the language barrier that shut out Brazilian occupational therapy from the debates occurring in Anglo-Saxon countries in the early 2000s. This fact, on one hand, led to a lack of participation because English was not the language being used by occupational therapy in this process[2] and, on the other hand, fostered a uniquely Brazilian path in the local history of the profession, especially for those occupational therapists linked to a critical perspective. Along the way, the word "activity" predominated among occupational therapists in Brazil (Magalhães & Galheigo, 2010). More recently, the term *cotidiano* (which translates into "everyday life," although not having the same meaning) has been used in theoretical publications and professional practices in Brazil (Galheigo, 2020). In this context, the chapters that compose this book make little use of the term "occupation," with "everyday life" (*cotidiano*) being more frequent.

Recently, the word "occupation" has become more widespread in Brazilian occupational therapy. It is hypothesized that its increased use is attributable to a greater dialogue between Brazilian occupational therapy researchers and researchers around the world, which has occurred because of the greater academic institutionalization of this field in Brazil and the consequent demands and interests involving the internationalization and circulation of national knowledge production. However, some Brazilian researchers still have reservations on the grounds of the importance of maintaining the historicity and relevance of local developments and the necessary concern for academic dialogues not becoming new colonizing processes within this area of knowledge, through the de-historicized and decontextualized assumptions of some concepts.

In Brazil, in addition to the debate around the health–disease dichotomy and the unsustainable individual-society, individual–nature, and individual–culture dichotomies, occupational therapy has moved toward discussing professional practice specifically intended to address social needs. These needs cannot, or should not, be tied to theoretical and therapeutic principles applicable in health contexts. To approach specifically social needs, some Brazilian occupational therapists designed and developed what we call "social occupational therapy." Social occupational therapy refers to politically and ethically framed professional actions that target individuals, groups, or systems to enable justice and social rights for people in disadvantageous social conditions (Barros, Ghirardi, & Lopes, 2005).

Brazilian social occupational therapy developed from two complementary theoretical perspectives. The first had the analysis of social processes as a parameter, especially from the late 1970s to the mid-1980s, a time of heightened unrest regarding the demands of the social question in Brazil. This process arose from the capital–labor relations, as well as from the construction of the public sphere mobilized by civil society, during a period of political opening and

---

[2]According to the British Council (2014), 5.1% of the Brazilian population over 16 years old has some knowledge of English.

democratization of Brazil, in the struggle to end the dictatorship imposed by a military *coup d'état* in 1964. The Brazilian state, which was in a process of transformation rooted in the struggle arising from social movements, was founded on democratic and legal perspectives, within the limits of capitalism. This process, which involved review of professional postulates, reached different segments of society, including occupational therapists. Professionals' responsibilities in shaping social values were discussed, as well as how to consciously exercise a political role within their practice, deciding between consensus and dissent, and also participating politically in the struggle for hegemony (Gramsci, 1988; Lopes, 1993/1996). This review of professional practice fostered questions, propositions, and a theoretical perspective that underpinned social occupational therapy (Barros, Ghirardi, & Lopes, 2002).

The second perspective stemmed from the questioning of medical-psychological knowledge. Its reductionist ways of understanding and dealing with phenomena that were categorized within the "health–disease" dichotomy was problematized, based on the disciplinization and institutionalization of social problems—that is, because they are bounded by certain dominant values aimed at controlling and suppressing the freedom of people, both individual and collective (Barros, Ghirardi, & Lopes, 1999). There was discussion about how much the medical/psychological/clinical disciplines were impregnated with these values, with strong influence from psychiatry, as well as various psychological approaches, which offered a series of propositions that shaped professionals' actions. Therefore, it was necessary to adopt concepts relating to the dynamics of social negotiations, to incorporate relevant sociological and anthropological theories into occupational therapy, and to invest in individual and collective actions that were informed by transdisciplinary, interprofessional, and intersectoral perspectives. In short, there was a need to define what was meant by "action" in the social field and in social occupational therapy (Barros et al., 2007).

Thus, there was opportunity for dialogue on the creation, proposal, and analysis of practice in the social field. This began to be carried out with a sense of urgency in Brazil in the late 1990s, specifically from 1998, when occupational therapy academics in the state of São Paulo created the Metuia Project, actually named by Metuia Network – Social Occupational Therapy.[3] Since then, reflections, debates, proposals, and social appeals related to inequalities have been intense.

A great deal of this work, within the realms of both teaching and research, served as a foundation for the creation of the "Social Networks and Vulnerabilities" line of research, integrating and supporting the first *stricto sensu* graduate studies program in occupational therapy in South America in 2009. This was the PPGTO/UFSCar, which had master's and doctoral courses implemented in 2010 and 2015, respectively. The objects of study in this line of research are occupational therapy interventions with socially vulnerable populations and the development of social technologies of inclusion, participation, and autonomy, which intersect with social themes such as poverty, social policies, urban occupation and mobility/circulation, cultural identity, access to social services (health, education, culture, social assistance, justice, etc.), and entry into the labor market, among others. This research program has been developing studies focusing on socially vulnerable children and adolescents, contemporary youth, homeless populations, the inclusion and social participation of people with disabilities and mental disorders, and the generation of income and value in relation to the world of work.

After more than 15 years of activity at the METUIA Laboratory in the Department of Occupational Therapy at UFSCar, we felt an obligation to organize the knowledge we were producing, in the form of a book, to stimulate dialogue at a national level. The book materialized in 2016. Now, after more than 20 years of university teaching, research, and extension activities at the METUIA/UFSCar Laboratory, and as a result of our efforts to bring Brazilian social occupational therapy into dialogue with other occupational therapies worldwide, we were urged to expand the circulation of our book by translating it. This is how this project arose[4] and developed, with the hope of contributing to ongoing reflections on critical perspectives in occupational therapy worldwide, from the Brazilian theoretical and practical experiences, specifically those that have been configured based on social occupational therapy. Twenty-six Brazilian occupational therapists, all involved in teaching and research in social occupational therapy, have contributed to this book. For this edition, we also invited five colleagues of different nationalities to grow this "conversation" with us, in addition to the foreword by Elizabeth Townsend (already present in the Portuguese edition of 2016).

This translation work has not been simple. It not only involves a literal translation of the text from Portuguese to English but also gives rise to different cultural forms of verbal and written expression of arguments and rationalities, providing them with consistency in another language. Therefore, it is important to say that the book is not "easy" to read in its English version because, although we have

---

[3]*Metuia* is a word from the native Brazilian language of the *Bororo* ethnic group that means friend, companion.

[4]We would like to thank Elizabeth Townsend for strongly encouraging us to believe in the viability of this project. Her determination and encouragement have helped us achieve this publication.

conducted a careful process aimed at better translations, we have chosen to maintain some words, some rationalities, and the historicity of Brazilian occupational therapy (specifically social occupational therapy), believing that they are essential elements of the theoretical and methodological frameworks herein presented.

This process included authors reviewing and updating the Portuguese versions of their chapters, translation into English by a Brazilian professional, linguistic revision by a native English-speaking professional, review by occupational therapy researchers domiciled and/or with professional experience in English-speaking countries to suggest modifications to better enable understanding, and then a final proofreading of the chapters prior to being sent to the publisher. We would like to thank the translation and proofreading professionals who have helped us considerably and who, although working in the field of language, are now much more knowledgeable about social occupational therapy. We are also very grateful to the occupational therapy researchers (whose names are listed as collaborators to this book) for their availability and generosity in reading the texts and thus assisting us in achieving a greater understanding of our work. Finally, we have added two chapters written by colleagues of other nationalities, demonstrating our ongoing dialogue. However, despite this process, we recognize that there are limitations to communication, which may generate difficulties in understanding. We therefore count on the willingness of the readers interested in accompanying us on this journey to enter into dialogue with us and the ideas discussed.

To support this dialogical reading and facilitate understanding, we would like to introduce some frequently used words. The first point refers to the aforementioned discussion of the term "occupation," its historicity, the reasons for its limited use in Brazil, and the preference for the word "cotidiano." Cotidiano was translated herein as "everyday life," based on the work of Agnes Heller, a Hungarian philosopher who focused on defining this term based on dialectical historical materialism in a study with the English title *Everyday Life* (Heller, 1984). The concept of *cotidiano* has been adopted by occupational therapists in Brazil since the 1990s, based on critique of practices that narrowly focus on an individual's life and take an instrumental and technical perspective, ignoring other aspects of life. Studies addressing *cotidiano* incorporate "subjectivity, culture, history and social power as elements that influence the understanding of the phenomenon; they definitely break with any more positivist reading" (Galheigo, 2003, p. 107). From our perspective, there is a dialogue between what we understand here as "everyday life" and the notion of "occupation" used in the Anglo-Saxon literature (Dickie, Cutchin, & Humphry, 2006; Fogelberg & Frauwirth, 2010; Laliberte Rudman, 2013,

2018; Ramugondo & Kronenberg, 2015; Whiteford, Jones, Rahal, & Suleman, 2018). Thus, references to everyday life in this book encompass a broad understanding of the social, historical, economic, and cultural contexts of the individuals and groups that occupational therapists work with[5] and the forms of individual and collective participation they engage in.

Another word that is difficult to translate is "*sujeito*," which has been translated as "people." In Portuguese, there are two ways of speaking of individuals: a word that is strongly concerned with individual aspects (*indivíduo*) and another that encompasses an association of individual and collective issues (*sujeito*). However, in the context of social occupational therapy, we are concerned with both individual and collective issues. Trying to approach this meaning, we have used *people*. Such debate is supported by theoretical contributions drawn from different lines of research (Spink, 2011), but this is not our focus here. In this book, due to the impossibility of using the second definition (individual and collective *subjects/people*), which frequently appears in the original version of the texts, the expression "individuals and/or people" is used in some passages in an attempt to include the collective dimensions in themes and/or practices in occupational therapy. This demarcation is relevant to us to the extent that social occupational therapy includes the inseparability of micro- and macro-social dimensions as one of its assumptions. In other words, it would be contradictory to speak of individuals when we focus, centrally, on economic inequalities and the consequent impediments those inequalities pose to participation in social life. Therefore, the collective dimension of social life is embedded in the references made here to individuals and/or people.

Some terms in this book are seldom used in the English language or are used differently: for example, "territory" and "life sharing." The word "territory" is associated with the place, the community in which actions are carried out, as opposed to closed institutional settings. According to Santos (1979, 2007), a Brazilian geographer and intellectual, the concept of territory is hybrid and is understood as the "used territory," which means a geographical space shaped by historicity, social and material relations, and the use that people make of it in their everyday lives. As for "community," according to the theoretical proposition of

---

[5]We present here an informal conversation we had the opportunity to have with Ann Wilcock in 2019, when she told us about the relevance of discussions coming from occupational therapy in South America and the need to further discuss our vocabulary and possibilities for understanding occupational therapy practices critically and with social responsibility. Specifically, she referred to *cotidiano* and the possibilities of incorporating these elements into occupational therapy.

community psychology, it is defined as a historical social group under constant transformation and evolution, interconnected by a sense of belonging and social identity, with common interests, needs, and sometimes organization (Montero, 2004). Therefore, territorial (and community) work in social occupational therapy refers to practices conducted in the streets, in people's homes, in the community, at school, in health and social assistance services, and in other real life spaces of people. Hence, territorial practice necessarily includes that the professional be available in places that have meaning for people, in the territories where their lives are constituted.

When in the territory, one of the goals of occupational therapists working from a social occupational therapy perspective is to develop spaces for life sharing, which requires facilitating different actions, both individual and collective. Life sharing occurs through relationships between individuals and is necessary to staying together, as long as the people involved have a shared regard for each other, contextualizing the historical moment and their choices for the production and reproduction of social life. According to Freire (1988), living together is a collective learning process that should involve aspects of social consciousness. Therefore, the work of occupational therapists aims to foster spaces where experiences and ways of being are shared, where solidarity can be woven into life. The development of *social occupational therapy workshops* has had this objective of bringing people together and discussing projects, weaving solidarity through activities in a joint and shared way. Inspired by the Brazilian poet Mário Quintana (2006), we can speak of the art of creating life-sharing spaces: "The art of living is simply the art of life sharing.... I said it simply? But it's so hard!" (*A arte de viver é simplesmente a arte de conviver... simplesmente, disse eu? Mas como é difícil!*). Certainly, there are other terms used in this book that may cause some surprise to the readers; however, we have highlighted those identified by our collaborators as the most difficult to understand, hoping that they can be read beyond their literal translation.

The scientific outputs contained in this book bear the marks of the present time, and one of those is the diversity of theoretical influences permeating the field. The 27 chapters presented here in two sections are a sample of the thematic and epistemological pluralism that currently characterizes research in social occupational therapy. Section I, entitled "Conceptual Outlines: Colors and Textures," is composed of 15 chapters arrayed along an axis encompassing different theoretical perceptions and practical formulations.

Roseli Esquerdo Lopes, in Chapter 1, "Citizenship, Rights, and Social Occupational Therapy," presents her thoughts derived from a lecture given during her application for the position of full professor at the Occupational Therapy Department at UFSCar, in the subarea of social occupational therapy. She articulates concepts that were central to her academic trajectory, detailing the unfolding, in concrete reality, of what is understood as social needs, professional actions, and the role of occupational therapists. From the fundamentals of "citizenship and rights," she, in an academic partnership with colleagues in the area, seeks to support what is defined as "social occupational therapy."

In Chapter 2, "Social Occupational Therapy in Brazil: A Historical Synthesis of the Constitution of a Field of Knowledge and Practice," Sandra Maria Galheigo highlights some historical notes on the constitution of social occupational therapy, examining its emergence in Brazil in the 1970s. Arguing that this is knowledge of the "South," with local theoretical-epistemological roots, she claims that social occupational therapy supports its ethical-political commitment through sensitively listening to the individuals and collectives with whom it develops projects and by adopting a critical perspective of social and political contexts. At the intersection of sensitivity, ethics, and politics, permeated by a critical approach, she writes in dialogue with Lopes' text, defending autonomy, citizenship, and law, searching for new strategies to construct and/or strengthen the collectives.

Maria Isabel Garcez Ghirardi, with coauthors Ana Paula Serrata Malfitano and Roseli Esquerdo Lopes, in Chapter 3, "Occupational Therapy and Socioeconomic Processes," defends the fundamentals of social occupational therapy, which are anchored in collective actions aimed at creating conditions of democratic intensification and social integration in response to the problems exposed by the thinning of the social fabric. In contrast to clinical and individual practices, they emphasize that collective doing is an essential element of social occupational–therapeutic action. Based on a university extension project and research experience developed with the support of an economic enterprise working with the homeless population, the authors illustrate the challenges of creating instruments that assist with social participation and activate trust in themselves and others, by constructing a place of collective belonging that values know-how regarding economically relevant productions in the market of goods and cultural values.

Denise Dias Barros and Debora Galvani, in Chapter 4, "Occupational Therapy: Social, Cultural? Diverse and Multiple!" describe an array of experiences developed between social and cultural issues, weaving a mosaic of populations, approaches, and discussions that demand that social occupational therapists deal sensitively with various populations who are frequently othered. With contributions from anthropology and urban sociology, they highlight the need for reflection on methodologies in social occupational therapy, designing a plurality of theoretical-methodological perspectives for the construction of actions and social technologies.

Ana Paula Serrata Malfitano, in Chapter 5, "Social Context and Social Action: Generalizations and Specificities in Occupational Therapy," brings to the debate a question that is always present in occupational therapy: is the social in everything? In agreement with Sandra Galheigo, who claims that the bases of social occupational therapy are unambiguous, she discusses the social context as an overarching element that should be present in every occupational-therapeutic practice. Based on this recognition, the author describes the specificities of developing a social occupational therapy under the principle of social law, committed to expanding access to social goods for all through technical, ethical, and political work.

According to Luciana Assis Costa, it is not possible to separate social occupational therapy from the transformations of Brazil's political regime and corporate organization, which resulted from the democratic opening. In the course of that process, the issue of social inequality and poverty was placed on the political agenda as a problem of the state and law. The expansion of occupational therapy practice to deal with social problems emerged in the paradox constituted by the process of reinstating democracy. On one hand, it celebrates the extension of citizenship rights, especially in the political and social spheres of life; on the other hand, it faces a developmental trajectory of the state with strong liberal traits, marked by a historical social debt, sustained by extreme inequality and poverty. In Chapter 6, "Occupational Therapy in the Context of Social Protection Expansion," Costa discusses the sociopolitical conjuncture in which the problem of poverty and social exclusion is shaped, to consider the possible contributions of occupational therapy to this area.

The proposal to synthesize our knowledge of occupational therapy practice in Brazilian social assistance opens a wide range of possibilities, considering the challenge of qualifying the debate and preparing professional interventions in this field. There are many possible ways. In Chapter 7, "Occupational Therapy and Social Assistance: Building a Critical Thinking About the Field," authored by Marta Carvalho de Almeida and Carla Regina Silva Soares, the direction chosen prioritizes the gathering of themes that enable a foray into some social processes that affect professional practice in the social field. The authors privilege a narrative path that understands social assistance as a set of actions supporting the general plan of the political and historical development of social interventions. That narrative makes it opportune to discuss the emergence and development of social policies in the context of capitalist socioeconomic formations, marked by the contradictions of this production mode. Occupational therapy, a profession that also emerged within these contradictions, is approached

as a profession shaped by capitalist policies to address problems that have been produced historically, often by capitalist policies. In this macro-social path, the authors also present this process in Brazil, which culminated in recognition of occupational therapy as one of the professions qualified to work in the social assistance sector. This process has been of great relevance in encouraging occupational therapists to work in spaces beyond the health and education sector, bringing other challenges.

Regina Célia Fiorati presents a dialogue between Jürgen Habermas' theoretical framework and social occupational therapy in Chapter 8, "The Theory of Communicative Action: A Theoretical-Methodological Contribution to Social Occupational Therapy." The author conceives possibilities grounded in the concepts of communicative action, dialogicity, intersubjectivity, democracy, and emancipation as, for instance, in the promotion of service networks, named "decision-making forums." She highlights that social occupational therapy presents a basis for the development of technologies that focus on the expansion of democratic spaces for individuals, groups, and communities.

In Chapter 9, Patrícia Dorneles and Roseli Esquerdo Lopes propose "Citizenship and Cultural Diversity in Management of Cultural Policies." For these authors, cultural diversity and cultural citizenship are diffuse emerging concepts that intersect with the agendas of current policies in this sector in Brazil. Cultural policies that are presented as democratic are charged with responsibility for interrupting processes of exclusion caused by traditional Eurocentric and elitist views of art and culture, as well as assimilationist political practices associated with neoliberal globalization. With a view to fostering and ensuring respect for people of all cultures and, horizontally, the broad concept of cultural diversity and the more localized concept of cultural citizenship, commitments and efforts to reorganize investment and promotion proposals in the field have been initiated by public cultural managers at different levels. The authors try to contextualize the theme of cultural public policies within citizenship and cultural diversity, reflecting on the possibilities of occupational therapy practice in the area of culture. The paths for such action have been associated with social occupational therapy and its current paradigms.

Continuing with the theme of culture, along with the different theoretical currents related to the concept of tradition, Samira Lima da Costa, Maria Daniela Corrêa de Macedo, and Sandra Benites-Guarani Nhandewa work on this concept from the perspective of collective meaning built in time and space and legitimized by a particular group. The authors understand that, in tradition, there is always something that changes and something that remains, so what changes supports the maintenance of what remains within a code of meaning for a given collective. In Chapter 10, "Traditional

Peoples and Communities: Traditional Occupation as a Theme of Social Occupational Therapy," they consider occupation as the various everyday actions that people perform individually and collectively. The authors propose a reading of traditional occupation as an object of interest in social occupational therapy. Traditional occupation is presented as a relevant element in the organization of the lives of collectives known as traditional peoples and communities, in their relationships with each other, work, and nature.

Roseli Esquerdo Lopes, Carla Regina Silva, and Patrícia Leme de Oliveira Borba contextualize relevant experiences in social occupational therapy when working with youth: the school space and, especially, the public school. They understand public school as a privileged setting for occupational therapy practice. It is a setting that, in Brazil and many other parts of the world, has begun the 21st century demanding contributions from different professions, including occupational therapy, since one of its basic dilemmas has not been solved: how to be a school for the masses while responding effectively to collective and individual demands. Moreover, how can education concerned with human emancipation be promoted, that is, with the priority of developing the intellectual and cultural autonomy of the people? Despite all the historical and contemporary dilemmas inherent in the educational setting, it should be affirmed and reaffirmed that the public school is an indispensable part of society and a priority partner, because it is where the vast majority of children and adolescents are. Public school is the focus of these considerations in Chapter 11, "School and Youth: Contributions of Social Occupational Therapy," in which the authors consider the essential elements of actions based on social occupational therapy developed within this institutional structure.

Staying on the theme of school, Patrícia Leme de Oliveira Borba, Beatriz Prado Pereira, and Roseli Esquerdo Lopes present a study conducted with three adolescents whose offences were the result of unruly acts occurring within a public school. Their experience reveals the existence of complex relationships and the fragility of possible supports at a certain time in their lives, both within the school itself and in the juvenile justice system. Informed by the assumptions of social occupational therapy and Freire's concept of education for freedom, in Chapter 12, "Social Occupational Therapy, Offenses, and School: Complex Plots in Fragile Relations," some possible contributions to occupational therapy are outlined in the dialogue between the social assistance and education sectors. There is a focus on conducting individual and territorial follow-ups with students facing vulnerability and difficulties around staying in school.

In Brazil, since the 1990s, public policies have been developed in response to international conventions on ways to tackle child labor, with actions involving different social sectors and movements; the executive, legislative, and judiciary powers; and participation of the national, state, and municipal management levels. In Chapter 13, "Social Occupational Therapy and the Eradication of Child Labor in Brazil: The Challenge of Articulating Social Protection and Autonomy," Carla Regina Silva Soares and Marta Carvalho de Almeida highlight those policies linked to the National Program to Eradicate Child Labor. In 2005, this program was integrated into the Unified Social Assistance System (SUAS), in which occupational therapists work. These professionals have been striving to contribute to the development of strategies and the implementation of actions that promote the social protection of children and adolescents who are experiencing, or have experienced, early work situations, in conjunction with those aimed at family autonomy and emancipation. They seek to enhance the ability of families and communities to achieve, produce, and sustain a decent everyday life, as well as to promote the rights of children and adolescents.

Finally, there are two chapters written by authors who have become important interlocutors for social occupational therapy. Debbie Laliberte Rudman, in Chapter 14, "Informing Social Occupational Therapy: Unpacking the 'Social' Using Critical Social Theory," addresses the relevance of a dialogue between occupational therapy and critical social theories. She points out the existence of an ethical imperative in contemporary times through the development of professional practices that combat individualism and question the possibilities for social transformation, moving toward an occupation-based social transformation. It is in this context that the author contextualizes social occupational therapy, placing us in dialogue with other initiatives that function under such perspectives in occupational therapy internationally.

To close this section, Nick Pollard, Inés Viana-Moldes, Hetty Fransen-Jaïbi, and Sarah Kantartzis, who are members of the citizenship project group of the European Network of Occupational Therapy in Higher Education (ENOTHE), present Chapter 15, "Occupational Therapy on the Move: On Contextualizing Citizenships and Epistimicide," closely dialoguing with the frameworks that inform social occupational therapy's production, such as the concept of citizenship. By advocating multiple perspectives that cross Anglo-Saxon barriers, the authors defend territoriality and the need for locally rooted knowledge, as we believe Brazilian occupational therapy has been doing. In the necessary debate on citizenship, capitalism, and processes of colonialism, they advocate the link between occupational therapy and citizenship as an ethical and moral responsibility.

Section II "Sketches and Scenarios," presents contemporary themes that have challenged social occupational therapy. To this end, it draws on experiences of teaching, research, and projects developed by the university in partnership with the community, government, and/or nongovernmental organizations, called university extension projects. These are experiences developed by the METUIA/UFSCar Laboratory team. Twelve chapters examine themes of youth poverty, community and territorial work, public school, the Statute of the Child and Adolescent, offending, drugs, the Internet, and gender and sexuality, to discuss social relevance, academic knowledge, and professional practice.

This section begins with Chapter 16, which synthesizes what we have so far proposed as "resources and technologies in social occupational therapy: actions with poor urban youth," co-authored by Carla Silva and Patrícia Borba. This chapter points out that the importance of social technologies and the work of social occupational therapists do not lie in their mere existence but in the fact that the existence of social technologies is a means for professionals to help tackle the harmful consequences that stem from social inequities.

In the context of social occupational therapy experiences in education, four chapters are presented, addressing public school, education, and the issue of rights in occupational-therapeutic practice. Lívia Celegati Pan highlights the importance of the autonomous and political organization of young students in public schools as a theme for social occupational therapy. Letícia Brandão de Souza and Aline Cristina de Morais create occupational-therapeutic strategies for children to learn the rights they are guaranteed by law. Carla Regina Silva points out the gap between youth and education through a life story that demonstrates the nonplace. Patrícia Leme de Oliveira Borba and Beatriz Prado Pereira work with young offenders to present their life paths and the marks that are left by the juvenile justice system.

The next two chapters address the contemporary issue of drugs from a social perspective. Paulo Estevão Pereira and Giovanna Bardi discuss the social rights of youth, specifically the rights to circulate and live together in different spaces in cities and the right to access assistance and personal and social support.

Support and care can help people overcome invisibilities, as in the story of Carla, reported by Mayra Cappellaro, while professional actions that fail to produce this support and care can reproduce violence that leaves marks and create the invisibilization of individuals and their bodies, as in the reflections shared by Gustavo Artur Monzeli. In contrast, the excessive visibility of the online world is discussed by Rafael Garcia Barreiro as a contemporary problem that should be of concern to occupational therapists when working with youth.

Constructing and enforcing rights, support, and assistance, opening the streets and spaces of the city to the beings and doings of our youth also means advancing the experiences of community and territorial work, as is

pointed out in two chapters. Marina Jorge Silva shares an experience of social occupational therapy in a public square, and Carolina Donato da Silva and Letícia Brandão de Souza reflect on an experience related to a community organization to plant trees, a process that strengthened ties.

With this selection of texts, drawn from the reflections and individual research of academics or in partnership with colleagues and alumni, we composed and formatted this book, hoping that it will be a contribution and a stimulus for further and necessary research. We hope that this work can broaden the dialogue around the diversity of occupational therapy worldwide, based on Brazilian experiences in social occupational therapy and its commitment to social change, a change that could produce more participation, with more freedom, autonomy, and solidarity.

Ana Paula Serrata Malfitano
and Roseli Esquerdo Lopes

REFERENCES

Barros, D. D., Ghirardi, M. I. G., & Lopes, R. E. (1999). Terapia ocupacional e sociedade [Occupational therapy and society]. *Revista de Terapia Ocupacional da Universidade de São Paulo, 10*(2–3), 71–76.

Barros, D. D., Ghirardi, M. I. G., & Lopes, R. E. (2002). Terapia ocupacional social [Social occupational therapy]. *Revista de Terapia Ocupacional da Universidade de São Paulo, 13*(3), 95–103.

Barros, D. D., Ghirardi, M. I. G., & Lopes, R. E. (2005). Social occupational therapy: A socio-historical perspective. In F. Kronenberg, S. S. Algado, & N. Pollard (Eds.), *Occupational therapy without borders: Learning from the spirit of survivors* (pp. 140–151). London, UK: Elsevier Science/Churchill Livingstone.

Barros, D. D., Lopes, R. E., & Galheigo, S. M. (2007). Terapia ocupacional social: concepções e perspectivas [Social occupational therapy: Conceptions and perspectives]. In A. Cavalcanti & C. Galvão (Org.), *Terapia ocupacional: fundamentação e prática* [Occupational therapy: Fundamentals and practice] (pp. 347–353). Rio de Janeiro, Brazil: Guanabara Koogan.

Basaglia, F., & Basaglia, F. (1977). *O. Los crímenes de la paz: investigación sobre los intelectuales y los técnicos como servidores de la oppression* [The crimes of peace: Research on intellectuals and professionals as servants of oppression]. Cidade do México, México: Siglo XXI.

Basaglia, F. (1979). *O homem no pelourinho* [The man in the pillory]. São Paulo, Brazil: Tradução IPSO – Instituto de Psiquiatria Social.

British Council. (2014). *Learning English in Brazil: Understanding the aims and expectations of the Brazilian emerging middle classes.* São Paulo, Brazil: British Council.

Dickie, V., Cutchin, M. P., & Humphry, R. (2006). Occupation as transactional experience: A critique of individualism in occupational science. *Journal of Occupational Science, 13*(1), 83–93. doi:10.1080/14427591.2006.9686573

Fogelberg, D., & Frauwirth, S. (2010). A complexity science approach to occupation: Moving beyond the individual. *Journal of Occupational Science, 17*(3), 131–139. doi:10.1080/14427591.2010.9686687

Freire, P. (1970). *Pedagogy of the oppressed.* New York, NY: Herder and Herder.

Freire, P. (1988). *Pedagogy of freedom: Ethics, democracy, and civic courage.* New York, NY: Rowan & Little field Publishers.

Galheigo, S. (2020). Terapia ocupacional, cotidiano e a textura da vida: aportes teórico-conceituais para a construção de perspectivas críticas e emancipatória. [Occupational therapy, everyday life, and the texture of life: Theoretical-conceptual contributions for the construction of critical and emancipatory perspectives]. *Brazilian Journal of Occupational Therapy, 28*(1), 5–25. https://doi.org/10.4322/2526-8910.ctoao2590

Galheigo, S. M. (2003). O cotidiano na terapia ocupacional: cultura, subjetividade e contexto histórico-social. [The concept of daily life in occupational therapy: Culture, subjectivity and the social and historical context]. *Revista de Terapia Ocupacional da Universidade de São Paulo, 14*(3), 104–109. doi:10.11606/issn.2238-6149.v14i3p104-109

Goffman, E. (1961). *Asylums: Essays on the social situation of mental patients and other inmates.* New York, NY: Anchor Books Doubleday & Company.

Gramsci, A. (1988). *Os intelectuais e a organização da cultura* [Intellectuals and the organization of the culture] (6th ed.). Rio de Janeiro, Brazil: Civilização Brasileira.

Heller, A. (1984). *Everyday life.* London, UK: Routledge & Kegan Paul.

Kielhofner, G. (1992). *Conceptual foundations of occupational therapy.* Philadelphia, PA: F. A. Davis.

Laliberte Rudman, D. (2013). Enacting the critical potential of occupational science: Problematizing the "individualizing of occupation." *Journal of Occupational Science, 20*(4), 298–313. doi:10.1080/14427591.2013.803434

Laliberte Rudman, D. (2018). Occupational therapy and occupational science: Building critical and transformative alliances. *Brazilian Journal of Occupational Therapy, 26*(1), 241–249. doi:10.4322/2526-8910.ctoEN1246

Lewis, H., Dwyer, P., Hodkinson, S., & Waite, L. (2015). Hyperprecarious lives: Migrants, work and forced labour in the Global North. *Progress in Human Geography, 39*(5), 580–600. doi:10.1177/0309132514548303

Lopes, R. E. (1990). Currículo mínimo para terapia ocupacional: uma questão técnico-ideológica [Minimum curriculum for occupational therapy: A technical-ideological issue]. *Revista de Terapia Ocupacional da Universidade de São Paulo, 1*(1), 33–41.

Lopes, R. E. (1993/1996). A direção que construímos: algumas reflexões sobre a formação do terapeuta ocupacional [The direction we have built: Some reflections on occupational therapist education]. *Revista de Terapia Ocupacional da Universidade de São Paulo, 4/7,* 27–35.

Lopes, R. E. (2004). Terapia ocupacional em São Paulo – um percurso singular e geral [Occupational therapy in São Paulo - a general and singular way]. *Cadernos de Terapia Ocupacional da UFSCar, 12*(2), 75–88.

Magalhães, L., & Galheigo, S. M. (2010). Enabling international communication among Brazilian occupational therapists: Seeking consensus on occupational terminology. *Occupational Therapy International, 17*(3), 113–124.

Malfitano, A. P. S., de Souza, R. G. D M., Townsend, E. A., & Lopes, R. E. (2019). Do occupational justice concepts inform occupational therapists' practice? A scoping review. *Canadian Journal of Occupational Therapy, 86*(4), 299–312. doi:10.1177/0008417419833409.

Montero, M. (2004). *Introducción a la Psicología Comunitaria. Desarrollo, conceptos y procesos* [Introduction to communitary psychology: Development, concepts and processes]. Buenos Aires, Argentina: Editorial Paidós.

Nascimento, B. A. (1990). O mito da atividade terapêutica [The myth of therapeutic activity]. *Revista de Terapia Ocupacional da Universidade de São Paulo, 1*(1),17–21.

Nascimento, B. A. (1991). *Loucura, trabalho e ordem: O uso do trabalho em instituições psiquiátricas* [Madness, work and order: The use of work in psychiatric institutions] (Dissertação de Mestrado). Pontifícia Universidade Católica de São Paulo, Programa de Pós-Graduação em Ciências Sociais, São Paulo, Brasil.

Quintana, M. (2006). *Poesia completa* [Complete poetry]. Rio de Janeiro, Brazil: Editora Nova Aguiar.

Ramugondo, E. L., & Kronenberg, F. (2015). Explaining collective occupations from a human relations perspective: Bridging the individual-collective dichotomy. *Journal of Occupational Science, 22*(1), 3–16. doi:10.1080/14427591.2013.781920

Santos, M. (1979). *The shared space: The two circuits of the urban economy and its spatial repercussions.* London, UK: Methuen.

Santos, M. (2007). *O Espaço Cidadão* [The citizen space]. São Paulo, Brazil: Edusp.

Spink, M.J.P. (2011). Pessoa, indivíduo e sujeito: notas sobre efeitos discursivos de opções conceituais [Person, individual and subject: notes about discursive effects on conceptual options]. In M.J.P. Spink, P. Figueiredo, & J. Brasilino (Eds.), Psicologia social e pessoalidade [Social psychology and personality] (pp. 1–22). Rio de Janeiro: Centro Edelstein de Pesquisas Sociais; ABRAPSO.

Soares, L. B. T. (1991). *Terapia ocupacional. Lógica do capital ou do trabalho?* [Occupational therapy: logic of capital or work?]. São Paulo: Hucitec.

Townsend, E. (1993). Occupational therapy's social vision. *Canadian Journal of Occupational Therapy, 60*(4), 174–184. https://doi.org/10.1177/000841749306000403

Whiteford, G., Townsend, E., & Hocking, C. (2000). Reflections on a renaissance of occupation. *Canadian Journal of Occupational Therapy, 67*(1), 61–69. https://doi.org/10.1177/000841740006700109

Whiteford, G., Jones, K., Rahal, C., & Suleman, A. (2018). The participatory occupational justice framework as a tool for change: Three contrasting case narratives. *Journal of Occupational Science, 25*(4), 497–508. doi:10.1080/14427591.2018.1504607

Wilcock, A. A., & Townsend, E. (2000). Occupational terminology interactive dialogue. *Journal of Occupational Science, 7,* 84–86. doi:10.1080/14427591.2000.9686470

1

Citizenship, Rights, and Social Occupational Therapy[1]

Roseli Esquerdo Lopes

INTRODUCTION

This chapter proposes an articulation of the nexus between "citizenship," "rights," and "social occupational therapy." This is a central reflection that I have considered in the trajectory of my work, driven from the unfolding, in concrete reality, of what is covered by "social needs," "technical actions," and the role of occupational therapists in the social field. Based on the foundations of "citizenship and rights," I have sought to establish, in academic partnership with some colleagues, a definition for "social occupational therapy." In this context, I wish to introduce to the dialogue the searches and encounters that have enabled me to understand the propositions of occupational therapy and that have contributed to the design of social occupational therapy.

Why Citizenship, Rights, and Social Occupational Therapy Should Be Articulated

What is the social function of occupational therapists? This question, which had been ubiquitous since the end of the 1970s for those of us involved in the processes of professional education and in the practice spaces of Brazil, is based on the critique of the need for social adaptation,

without questioning the social structure and its inequalities. The implied aim at the root of this question is to insert and reintegrate individuals into their environments without questioning the reasons for their exclusion or their resistance to reinsertion. Failure in reintegration attempts was almost always attributed to the specific difficulties faced by individuals, their chronicity, and the attitudes of their families and only sometimes to society itself and its rejection of these individuals, its dismissal of their remaining capacities, and its failure to provide them with the necessary opportunities (Galheigo, 1997). The understanding of structural issues as the causative agents of this failure began to be included in conversation between occupational therapists in this period.

I decided to study occupational therapy in 1976 and joined the course at the University of Sao Paulo (USP) in 1977, integrating into what Elio Gaspari, in the fourth volume of his tome about the military dictatorship in Brazil, *A ditadura encurralada* (which roughly translates to *The Endangered Dictatorship*), calls "the generation of struggle for democratic freedom." This excerpt from the book is illustrative of what I experienced:

> *The demonstrations gathered two types of students. In the first category, there were the leaders of organizations set up in universities and a few hundred followers. . . . In the second category, there was the crowd, composed of youths who had incorporated some of the 1968 ideals into their customs. In less than a decade, women had taken a part in politics and the labor market. They all shared with the Trotskyists the cultural refinement and horror of the dictatorship and*

[1]This paper was part of the Academic Test of the Public Contest for the Position of Full Professor in Occupational Therapy, Social Occupational Therapy subarea, Department of Occupational Therapy, Centre of Biological Sciences and Health, Federal University of São Carlos (UFSCar), held in 2012. Part of these reflections were published on: Lopes, R. E.; Malftano, A. P. S. (2017). Social occupational therapy, citizenship, rights and policies: connecting the voices of collectives and individuals. (pp. 245-256). In: Dikaios Sakellariou, Nick Pollard. (Org.). Occupational therapies without borders. 2ed. London: Elsevier.

the Partidão *[the Communist Party], in that order. In the assemblies, there was the vanguard of a part of the youth, united by their contempt for the conservative habits and tactical alliances of the traditional left.*

(Gaspari, 2004, p. 408)

I was part of that crowd.

What mattered was individual and collective liberty, the valuation of people. The late 1970s was characterized by a political boom in which there was space in Brazil for the participation of the population, which was mobilized and discussed a large number of issues, with the basic axes being democratization, the struggle for the rights of citizenship, the contestation of the then-current status quo, and the corresponding debates on alternatives to the economic, social, and political exclusionary order established by the military regime. Civil society was organized into different representations—labor unions, popular movements, religious institutions, and professional associations—and political parties began to resume their space in the Brazilian scene (Lopes, 1999).

The permanent, daily suppression of the rights of "the insane," who were subjected to authoritarian repression in institutions, also became a focus of questioning. The theme of psychiatric reform in Brazil emerged as part of the process of the liberation of the mentally ill. However, beyond that, the struggle against the situation of these people in psychiatric institutions, which was denounced by the media and scandalized public opinion, was part of a more general feeling of rebellion against the suppression by force of the will of "the weaker"—not only of the mentally ill but also of the workers, the unemployed, political prisoners, and excluded people of all kinds (Amarante, 1995). Authors such as Franco Basaglia, Felix Guattari, Robert Castel, Erwing Goffman, and Michel Foucault, representatives of the currents of critical thought in the area of mental health, came to exert great influence among the professionals working in that area with their theoretical elaborations and practical propositions in the most varied forms.

It was thrilling to attend Basaglia's (1979) speech at the Pontifical Catholic University of Sao Paulo (PUC-SP) and to hear him address, based on Gramsci, the pessimism of reason and the optimism of practice. We were particularly optimistic at that time. We were growing professionally. It was the time of the first boom in occupational therapy courses, and through the Association of Occupational Therapists of Brazil (ATOB), we were fighting for the consolidation of quality professional education that was technically and politically competent and for the definition of a new minimum curriculum (Lopes, 1997). Occupational therapy was becoming professionalized and beginning to perceive individuals in society. It was essential for a large part of that generation to understand the general, macro-social

references; to be able to design the desired occupational therapy; to understand the role of the professionals and especially of occupational therapists; and to more autonomously determine their professional paths (Lopes, 2004). It was a matter of seeking an instrument of understanding, a theoretical framework that would assist us with unveiling the contradictions and possibilities of technical action. What did it mean to transform/enable the everyday lives of people at whom occupational therapy was directed and for whom it intended to "care"?

Historical materialism, seized and relocated by Antonio Gramsci (1977, 1987, 2002), helped me delimit the possible spaces for the professionals to consolidate the hegemonic consensus involving the conservation of the interests of the dominant social class or to construct a counterhegemonic dissent that sought to transform the then-current establishment. It was a continuous construction/deconstruction movement. One of the pillars of the old model was worthless: the biopsychosocial individual—the individual on whom interventions should be focused. Under the traditional occupational therapy model, collectives and social groups with their own identities were not a focus of attention (Galheigo, 1997). According to Sandra Galheigo (1997), by questioning the role of social adapters, occupational therapists began to participate in the construction of the collective, the construction of public space, albeit quite timidly in the professional category in general.

Liaison with other fields of knowledge was essential for those who tried to offer paths of understanding and, perhaps, solutions to problems/issues we were faced with.

Professionals who intended to specify their social mission would need to seek a new way of conceiving knowledge, and their technical knowledge should be based on the needs of the group or population to which their actions were directed. In order to reach an understanding of what these needs are, it would be necessary to recognize in the population the true interlocutors, who have a history and knowledge of their own.

(Barros, Ghirardi, & Lopes, 2002, p. 97)

It was believed that provoking collective consciousness and broadening the spaces of freedom would enhance a different type of relationship in which the assisted individuals would be the subjects of personal and social processes and would be recognized as such (Barros, Ghirardi, & Lopes, 2002). In other words: what should we do and how should we do it so that the real people with whom we are in contact in our daily professional life—the mentally ill, the handicapped of all kinds, the personally and socially vulnerable children and adolescents, the poor elderly—could aim to be autonomous, participatory, inserted people? Working based on this premise, it was necessary to struggle to transform the places of exclusion, and hence the studies of many of us, occupational therapists, focusing on the problem and processes of institutionalization/deinstitutionalization, together with the commitment to achieve innovative proposals of intervention. Nevertheless, the possibility of these practices was also due to the incorporation of the populations to which we directed our actions as people we should seek to "care for," from a perspective of health and social assistance as derived from the rights of citizens who are also a part of these groups.

"Citizenship" and "public policies" were included in the lexicon of Brazilian civil society, in its interlocution with the democracy and rights that then existed in Brazil. This was also true for occupational therapists, who were then focusing on the processes involving the creation, invention, and construction of the demanded care, services, and professionals. To this end, the Brazilian health reform and the implementation of the Unified Health System (SUS) were of paramount importance, as well as the incorporation of the Unified Social Assistance System (SUAS) into the field of social security, which occurred with the 1988 Constitution (Brasil, 1988). Health as a right of all—with "all" meaning *all*, not just the majority—entails providing assistance to special population groups. This means understanding social assistance not as charity or philanthropy but as the right of all citizens to a guaranteed social minimum in terms of income, goods, and services. Access to health care and social goods was operationalized through the implementation of social policies and their concrete employment in services and actions, including occupational therapy (Oliver, 1990; Lopes, 1999). In the early 1990s, there was an important incorporation of occupational therapists into social services, with an emphasis on health care and assistance associated with childhood and youth in the Brazilian municipalities that adopted the implementation of constitutional precepts as a guideline (Lopes, 1999).

It can be said that Brazil reached, with a delay of over 40 years, what had been experienced by the most central countries of the world economy during the postwar period. Labor and capital were at the core of struggles for the constitution and access to the public funds of the state. Thus, these concepts, strategies, and processes were submitted to the scrutiny of Brazilian civil society, including occupational therapists.

THE CAPITALIST STATE AND SOCIAL POLICIES

At various moments and spaces, we were and continue to be faced with a certain view of public policies, especially social policies, that immediately leads us to a conception of a "reparative," "access broadening" policy that would interfere with the field of inequalities and social divisions to bring about social change. We propose that this concept be defined based on a theoretical and historical framework, within a materialist conception that parameterizes the general context of the democratic, capitalist state in which the problem of social policies is included.

One of the central and always current issues in the analysis of the contemporary state is the understanding of the genesis of public policies—in our case, with particular focus on social policies—from the existing economic and political-institutional structures. In the capitalist state, based on private valorization of capital and on the sale of labor as commodity, in which these structures are intrinsically classist, some questions are pertinent: What are the functions inherent to those policies? What are the objective limits to which they are subject, within the paradigmatic array of elasticity of the capitalist state, regardless of the actors situated before it? What are the possible actions in this context, and to what extent do they define observable and stable changes? How can the themes of citizenship and social transformations, in the sense of constructing a socially fairer world, be included in this analysis?

Democratic capitalist states can be understood as institutional forms of public power that, in their relation to material production, are basically characterized by three functional determinations: privatization of production, structural dependence on the process of accumulation, and democratic legitimation. This state undergoes a double determination of political power: from the standpoint of content, it is defined by the development and requirements of the process of accumulation; as an institutional form, it is subject to the rules of representative-democratic government through the mechanism of periodic elections. Thus, the *policies of the capitalist state* can be defined as a set of strategies according to which agreement and compatibility between the structural determinations of that state are constantly produced and reproduced. Nevertheless, their general strategy of action is to create conditions under which each citizen is included in the exchange relationships (Offe & Ronge, 1984).

This definition indicates the strategy that should parameterize the creation of those policies, so that determinations of the capitalist state are fulfilled, as a condition for the continuity of its existence. Therefore, the elected officials have to govern within the limits of the self-preservation of the system. To a great extent, however, policies arising from the executive power will have to be articulated and employed within and by the system of political institutions that exist in the state, which in principle presents great temporal stability and is the most internal and effective guardian of the status quo. Consequently, we should seek in its internal structure the elements that, by exerting filtering power and preventing the effective concretization of events that are potentially harmful to the continuity of the accumulation process, can ensure that only strategies that preserve it are executed, while addressing the following three problems: (1) the integration of interests resulting from the valorization process—that is, reconciliation of the internal edges between the various sectors of capital inherent to the very logic of competition, with the establishment of a common global denominator; (2) the protection of capital against anticapitalist interests and conflicts; and (3) the concealment of these two actions, because the votes of individuals of all social classes are needed in the processes of democratic legitimation (Offe, 1984).

In contrast, *social policies* of the capitalist state are defined as a particular case of public policies: they constitute the organized relationships and strategies that aim to create conditions for labor-force owners to be included in the terms of trade. Sociopolitical innovations are needed to expand social policies: changes adopted in the way state managers generate, finance, and distribute social services, reconciling the accepted requirements and already sanctioned human needs (Offe & Lenhardt, 1984). Thus, from the standpoint of domination in the capitalist state, the social classes act on a system of political institutions that outline the range of potentially achievable events. As a result, the actions of these classes delimit, by reflecting the result of the correlation of forces between the various segments of capital and between capital as a whole, labor, and other social actors, in which region—among the structurally permissible—the equilibrium of the system will occur at a given moment and conjuncture.

The social question spells out its genesis in the way people organize themselves to produce in a given society and historical context, and this organization is expressed in the sphere of social reproduction; that is, the social question is determined by the singular and peculiar trait of the capital/labor relationship: exploitation. Without destroying the exploitative devices of the regime, in every struggle against its sociopolitical and human manifestations, the social question is bound to confront symptoms, consequences, and effects (Netto, 2001); however, we do not find it difficult to face them and, in this space, we also seek to move forward. It is important to analyze the social question as a political, economic, social, and ideological matter that refers to a specific correlation of forces between different classes, included in the broader context of social movement of the struggle for hegemony. Certain moments are more favorable to express the demands of work and its inclusion in the political scene of society, demanding their recognition by capital and the state, and requiring other types of intervention apart from charity and repression, and this occurs, within the limits of capitalist society, by means of citizenship and social rights.

CITIZENSHIP

On the Concept of Citizenship

In the last decade of the 20th century, we witnessed a multiplicity of studies on the theme of citizenship worldwide, as part of a great analytical effort to improve the conceptual approach to the notion of citizenship. *Citizenship and Civil Society* (1998) by Thomas Janoski highlights three theoretical strands of thought addressing phenomena related to citizenship: Marshall's theory of citizenship rights, Durkheim's approach to civic culture (previously anticipated by Tocqueville), and the Marxist/Gramscian theory on civil society.

The concept of citizenship as the right to have rights, among several approach perspectives, has as a classic reference the writings by Thomas Marshall of 1949, which proposed the first sociological theory of citizenship in developing the rights and obligations inherent to the condition of citizen. Focusing on the British reality of the time, which majorly addressed the conflict between capitalism and equality, Marshall established a typology of citizenship rights, namely, civil rights, achieved in the 18th century; political rights, achieved in the 19th century; and social rights, achieved in the 20th century (Marshall, 1950). Subsequently, several authors analyzed their national realities using this typology, adding theoretical nuances. Based on the studies by Vieira in her book *The Argonauts of Citizenship* (2001), we present a summary of the theme. Durkheim's theories point out that citizenship is not restricted to that enacted by law, focusing on civic virtue. As a result, space is opened for volunteer, private, nonprofit groups to form civil society in the public sphere. Marxist theories, in turn, emphasize the reconstitution of civil society, an idea previously explored by Hegel, taken up by Marx, and significantly revisited by Gramsci. Gramsci operated a paradigm shift with his threefold view: state, market, and civil society, considering that for Hegel and Marx, civil society encompassed all organizations and activities outside the state, including the economic activities of companies. The current reference to civil society evokes the Gramscian bias of protection against abuses on the part of the state and market. For some authors, this could be understood as an intermediation between the state's approach adopted by Marshall and the focus on civic virtue centered on society based on Durkheim. Looking for other theoretical frameworks to better understand citizenship, it is interesting to point out that citizenship is not a central idea in the social sciences (Vieira, 2001). Addressing the attributes of the term, Janoski (1998) defines the sociological perspective that citizenship is the passive and active belonging of individuals to a nation-state, with certain universal rights and duties at a specific level of equality.

Belonging to a nation-state is understood as the establishment of a personality in a geographical territory. Historically, citizenship was provided to restricted groups of the elite—wealthy men of Athens, English barons of the 18th century—and only later was it extended to a larger portion of a country's residents. Thus, there would be two possibilities of belonging: one that defines how a noncitizen, within the limits of the state, acquires rights and recognition as a citizen (population groups stigmatized by ethnicity, gender, and class), and another that establishes how foreigners obtain entrance and naturalization to become citizens. As for the second element of this definition—the distinction between active and passive rights and duties—it can be said that citizenship consists of both passive rights of existence, legally determined, and active rights that provide the present and future ability to influence the political power. The third aspect of this definition excludes the informal or particularistic character of citizenship rights, which should necessarily be universal rights enacted by law and ensured to all. People and collectives may have their own moral imperatives and specific customs or rights, but these will only become citizenship rights if they are universally applied and guaranteed by the state. The fourth element refers to the idea that citizenship is an affirmation of equality, which balances rights and obligations within certain limits. Equality is formal, and access to courts is ensured. It is not a complete equality, but in general it guarantees increased rights to the subordinates in relation to the dominant elites. The rights and duties of citizenship exist when the state validates citizenship norms and adopts measures to implement them. From this perspective, the processes of citizenship—the struggle for power between groups and classes—are not necessarily citizenship rights but independent variables for their formation; that is, these processes would be constituent parts of the theory but not of the concept that defines citizenship. In this sense, citizenship concerns the relationship between the state and its citizens, especially with regard to rights and duties. Theories on the theme of civil society, concerned with the institutions that mediate citizens and the state, add a varied range of possibilities to the understanding of this relationship (Vieira, 2001). Civil society is constituted mainly in the public sphere, where associations and organizations engage in debates so that most struggles for citizenship occur within it through the interests of social groups, although civil society cannot constitute the locus of citizenship rights because it is not a sphere of the state that ensures official protection through legal sanctions (Vieira, 2001).

It is necessary that political theory and empirical reality be discussed in the search for and understanding of the relationship between civil society and citizenship. *Liberalism*, which is dominant in industrialized Anglo-Saxon countries, with an emphasis on the individual, proposes that most rights involve freedoms inherent to each and every person; despite a few obligations (taxes, military service, etc.), civil liberties and property rights are central issues. Individual rights are vital, whereas social rights or those of groups represent a violation of liberal principles. The relationship between rights and duties is essentially contractual, entailing a heavy burden of reciprocity: each right corresponds, in general, to an obligation.

Communitarianism prioritizes the community, society, and nation, appealing to solidarity and the sense of common destiny as a touchstone of social cohesion. Society exists through the action and support of groups, in a way contrary to liberal individualism. Its main objective is to construct a community based on core values such as common identity, solidarity, participation, and integration. Thus, duties predominate over rights. From this perspective critical of liberalism, the decline of solidarity between citizens and the absence of common destiny would be at the root of the great evils of modernity. Communitarians give citizenship the character of virtue. Under the liberal view, citizenship is an accessory, not a value in itself. In the communitarian view, individuals are members of units that are larger than themselves, such as the political community, which can be understood as a social unit and space for the exercise of the virtue of participation. Citizenship would then be fundamentally an activity, a practice, and not, as advocated by liberals, a "status" of *belonging*.

The theory of *expansive democracy* (Janoski, 1998) is a third strand. It advocates the expansion of individual or collective rights to historically discriminated people—notably based on their class, gender, or ethnicity—claiming increased collective participation in decisions and greater interaction between institutions and citizens. Despite sharing a critique of liberal centralization of the individual, it emphasizes the right to participate, resisting the secondary role assigned to rights, as in the communitarian perspective. A balance between individual rights, group rights, and obligations is claimed, resulting in an identity system built on the notion of individuals as participants in community activities.

As early as 1949, Marshall envisioned citizenship as a true element of social change in the context of industrial reality and the correlated experience of the *welfare state* in the postwar period. The expansion of rights would correspond primarily to the strengthening of previously acquired rights, as well as to the incorporation of new groups into the state. The territorial basis of citizenship has historically been transformed, from the Greek *polis* to the Roman Empire, then to the medieval city, and finally to the modern state. The centralization process from which the state emerged corresponds to the expansion from the local to the institutional form of citizenship. From this point of view, the expansion of rights is part of a democratization process, understood as the popular classes' acquisition of rights that were originally created by and for the elites.

Three generations of citizenship rights can thus be labeled: civil, political, and social, as previously described. First are civil rights, corresponding to rights necessary for the exercise of freedoms; next are political rights, established in the 19th century, which guarantee active and passive participation in the political process; finally, in the 20th century, are the social rights of citizenship, corresponding to the acquisition of a minimum standard of well-being and social security that must prevail in society. However, the recurrent ambiguity of equating welfare state rights with social citizenship should be avoided. The former is based on means and highlights vulnerable individuals who need protection, whereas the latter is universal and acquired as a right by belonging to the community (Vieira, 2001).

Addressing the conflict of cumulative expansion of rights, Marshall (1967) focused his attention on the antagonism between civil rights, which establish protection of the individuals before the state, and social rights, which must ensure the right to real income through benefits guaranteed by the state. Thus, social citizenship collides with the conditions of capitalism, and its exercise creates conflict. Marshall concludes that social citizenship and capitalism are at war, but he argues that citizenship and social class are compatible in democratic, capitalist society insofar as citizenship has become the architect of legitimized social inequality. Such ambiguity echoed loudly in the debate between Marxists and social democrats in later decades.

Empirical studies have demonstrated the multiplicity of relationships between different types of rights in various forms of social organization. In contrast to the linear evolutionary model outlined by Marshall, it can be said that in the United State of America, the traditional struggle for civil rights hindered the growth of social rights of citizenship. Fascism and communism were presented as forms of social achievement at the expense of civil and political rights. The social democratic strand was also criticized for leaving gaps in the critique of the liberal perspective, having restricted its attention to the working class to the detriment of other conflicts, such as those of gender, ethnicity, nationalism, and so forth (Vieira, 2001).

Multiple Citizenship

In this context, contemporary concern is fundamentally directed toward the search for compatibility of the existence of different possibilities and levels of citizenship: life in small communities, reformulation of citizenship in the nation-state or at a global level. Within this collective effort, citizenship can no longer be seen as a set of formal rights, but as a way of incorporating people and groups into the social context. To solve the conflicting relationship

between the multiple traditions of citizenship based on status, participation, and identity, some authors have sought to formulate a complex system, with access to rights guaranteed by local, national, and transnational institutions (Vieira, 2001).

Two main approaches are highlighted. The first, based on Iris Young (Shafir, 1998), addresses the need to institutionalize multiple citizenship, aiming to ensure justice and equity. It is necessary to materialize rights in relation to social groups because, under the auspices of universality, exclusion has always existed and will continue to exist: ironically, formal equality generates substantive inequality. Specifically, the question of oppressed groups in the North American context is raised (Afro-descendants, women, "Chicanos," indigenous people, LGBT people, the elderly, the poor, people with disabilities). Will Kymlicka's (1996) proposal of differentiated citizenship is endorsed, which states that rights should not be guaranteed only to individuals but also to groups. The purpose of the identity criterion, as in the specific case of immigrants, does not consist in a movement of self-exclusion of the social body but rather in ensuring its inclusion while maintaining respect for its culture. An extension of Marshall's linear scheme is proposed: the guarantee of a fourth generation of rights—the cultural rights of citizenship.

In the second approach, based on Michael Walzer (1992), the center of this diversity of citizenship lies precisely in one of its traits: politics. He makes clear his admiration for the Greek tradition, in which political participation assumes the highest form of humanity as a principle of social incorporation and unity. It also explores the concept of civil society as an arena of confrontation: while citizenship is the basis of social unity, civil society, by allowing critical confrontation between several social demands, performs its classic task of generating civility. Respect for diversity and social pluralism should be an integral part of the citizenship discourse.

The Challenges of Citizenship and the Articulation of Rights

There is renewed interest in citizenship at the beginning of the 21st century. The concept of citizenship seems to integrate central notions of political philosophy, such as the claims of justice and political participation. Citizenship, however, is closely associated with the idea of individual rights and belonging to a particular community.

The numerous studies of the 1990s seem to point toward a theory of citizenship. There is no overriding accepted theory of citizenship to date, but important theoretical contributions have already been made regarding the tension between the various elements that compose this concept, clarifying the reasons for its timeliness (Vieira, 2001). Two interpretations are put forward in this context. In the first version, the role of citizens is seen in an individualistic and instrumental way, according to the liberal tradition initiated by Locke. People are considered private individuals, external to the state, and their interests are prepolitical. In the second form, a communitarian conception originating from the tradition of Aristotle's political philosophy prevails, with the proposition of active citizenship. Individuals are integrated in a political community, and their personal identity is a function of common traditions and institutions. There are two models: the first is based on individual rights and equal treatment, whereas the second defines participation in self-government as the essence of liberty, a critical component of citizenship. There would be passive citizenship, from "above," via the state, and active citizenship, from "below." Thus, there would be conservative citizenship (passive and private) and revolutionary citizenship (active and public). It is from this premise that we advocate the context of citizenship and rights, the expansion of equality, and the recognition of differences as presuppositions for social occupational therapy or citizenship and rights as axis (Galheigo, 1997; Lopes, 1999).

OCCUPATIONAL THERAPY IN THE SOCIAL POLICY

As previously stated, in the early 1990s, there was an important incorporation of occupational therapists into social services in Brazilian municipalities adopting the precepts of the Constitution. At that moment, a new generation of occupational therapists was poised to take the lead. They had been educated by the theoretical and practical courses developed by the first generations; they possessed a more general understanding of Brazilian society, of their professional role based on Gramsci's and Basaglia's concepts, and of the role of their interventions in the production of life.

Questions were posited about how occupational therapists acted. How did they practice a type of occupational therapy that was feasible in the 1990s? How could occupational therapists, considering the education they had been receiving, be able to respond to the needs of users of the different public assistance services? That question was an important motivation for my doctoral research. How were the categories of citizenship, rights, and public policies articulated in the case of occupational therapy? Seeking to produce responses, I concretely studied the experience of the city of Sao Paulo between 1989 and 1996 (Lopes, 1999). In my study in particular, at a more general level, the experience in Sao Paulo City Hall revealed, in a very hard and direct way, the magnitude and complexity of the tasks involved in the struggles for citizenship endured by most of the population, of which the implementation and consolidation of policies in the field of mental health and for the disabled constituted a small fragment. The enormous effort required to implement any such projects was evident.

Human resources were an issue of vital importance throughout the process; they have the power to convert (or not convert) the sociopolitical innovations theoretically proposed by managers into practices and real improvements to be made available for the population. With respect to occupational therapists specifically, there was a genuine identification between those professionals and the ongoing projects, and there was a joint and spontaneous effort to implement them to offer the population services and alternatives in which they believed (Lopes, 1999).

SOCIAL OCCUPATIONAL THERAPY: A FIELD OF COMPLEXITY AND BORDERS

In the late 1990s, we were facing a neoliberal avalanche in Brazil—an avalanche that still stifles our hopes. In the world of the minimal, privatizing state focused on selective actions, in a society that trivialized the word "citizenship," where democracy seemed restricted to bourgeois precepts of the cyclical exercise of voting, and, fundamentally, with the intense transformations that have occurred in the world of work, leading to intensification of the exploitation of labor and degradation of the associated protection systems—against this background, the growing vulnerability of groups and people has brought a new configuration of the old "social question" (Castel, 1999; Donzelot, 1984). This transformation process of social rules has contributed to the emergence of people considered "cyclical invalids" (Donzelot, 1986) or "superfluous people" (Castel, 1997), who develop "integration deficits" (in work, housing, education, or culture) and undergo disqualification, social invalidation, the dissolution of ties, and even explicit threats of exclusion with discriminatory treatment. It was in this context that Denise Barros, Sandra Galheigo, and I started the Metuia Project in 1998, which was a part of what we named the resurgence of the social issue for occupational therapy in Brazil (Barros, Lopes, & Galheigo, 2002).

In the article "Social Occupational Therapy," which I wrote in partnership with Denise Barros and Maria Isabel Ghirardi, we identified, from a sociological standpoint, two target groups of the action of disciplinary discourse, both medical (in a broad sense) and legal, which constitute a population to be assisted by social occupational therapy:

I. Individuals who undergo processes of social exclusion that justify their institutionalization aiming at their recovery, education, and/or repression; namely, those who have populated and continue to populate closed and isolated spaces of the community, such as psychiatric hospitals, therapeutic communities, nursing homes and institutions for people with disabilities, and prisons; poor children and youths; the institutionalized elderly deprived of their rights.

II. Groups that, owing to social transformations, are exposed directly to precarious work or relational vulnerability and, therefore, remain on the social margins and experience the disruption of their social networks. For these individuals, the integration deficit is associated with the degradation of the world of work and its consequential impact on quality of life: housing, education, sociability, and culture, leading to processes of disaffiliation (Barros, Ghirardi, & Lopes, 2002).

Constitution of the social field, as one of occupational therapy's subareas, was highlighted at the end of the 1990s by the disconnection of occupational therapy from the area of health and, therefore, from the necessary mediation between health and disease. The processes involving social participation in Brazil created an environment that enabled the identification of serious social problems, and broad sectors of society and professionals were involved in the search for solutions. Occupational therapists were not left out of these processes.

"Occupational therapy mirrors what its professionals think and produce" (Barros, 2004, p. 92) and how they position themselves politically in the face of social demands. "Their methods are conditioned to certain problems perceived and incorporated as pertinent and, for these problem areas, possible solutions are articulated" (Barros, 2004, p. 92). Inequality and poverty are relevant problems and are important factors in the origin of the Brazilian social question, as in many other countries, acquiring configurations that require a revision of the professions and the pertinence of the professional role.

Since the mid-1980s, citizenship has been positioned as the guiding principle for the action of occupational therapists. Initially, [there was] a political struggle through active participation in various social movements. . . . Then citizenship became a parameter of a new way of acting professionally, transforming itself in an axis that articulates the action of occupational therapists. Individual and collective interventions have been, since then, perceived as inserted in their contexts and as part of historical processes of production of meaning and cultural negotiation.

(Barros, Lopes, & Galheigo, 2007, p. 352)

Thus:

Without losing sight of the fact that the struggle against exclusion implies combating the deregulation of labor and the distribution of wealth, without neglecting the fact that actions must be embedded in a conscious political process; we believe that through its history, the accumulation of discussions built on criticism of segregation institutions and, above all, through

knowledge about mediation of the activity, occupational therapy can contribute in intervention fields that have traditionally been outside its area of concern.

(Barros, Ghirardi, & Lopes, 2002, p. 101)

We can consider these arguments to constitute the basis of social occupational therapy, which is reformulated by the challenge to create links between the demands of the social process and the actions of occupational therapists (actions that grow out of the knowledge and experience that the profession has collectively accumulated). This link needs to be established based on the use of the activities as a mediation process (and their concepts and implications) carried out by occupational therapists.

It is also worth mentioning two fundamental elements borrowed from Paulo Freire to design social occupational therapy: awareness and dialogue. Awareness refers to the transition from immersion into reality to distancing from this reality; this process goes beyond the level of awareness through the unveiling of the reasons for being of a given situation followed by a transforming action of this projected reality (Barros, 2004). Paulo Freire (1978, 1979), as well as Basaglia and Ongaro-Basaglia (1977), do not dissociate professional action from political action; or, to put it in terms of a Gramscian formulation, intellectual equals technical plus political (Gramsci, 2002).

Considering these assumptions, since 1999, we have been developing several intervention projects, working in partnership with governmental and nongovernmental organizations that act for the universalization of citizenship rights and for the strengthening and/or creation of social networks to support populations that face processes of disaffiliation. We have also sought to educate occupational therapists to work in the territory, community spaces, and social institutions, working based on the demands of the population, to contribute to meeting their needs and to listen and intervene in the lives of people who have been understood as the "other." But they, the "others," need to be approached professionally, with an understanding of their context and history (Barros, Lopes, & Galheigo, 2002; Lopes et al., 2012; Lopes, Malfitano, Silva, Borba & Hahn, 2012.).

Today there is another generation of occupational therapists developing their professional practices and paths of research and knowledge production, looking at how to work in a complex field of borders—for example, that of children, adolescents, and youths who do not have the means for their realization as individuals and are subjected to violence and that of adults in street situations—and seeing how to take advantage of opportunities (such as several current focal projects/programs) and instrumentalize them in the struggle for rights.

Different demands call for the construction of specific knowledge and methodological procedures. The experience accumulated by the core of the Federal University of São Carlos in Metuia Project (Metuia/UFSCar) has produced social technologies that have been able to foster new possibilities of action, integrating and articulating macro- and micro-social actions. From this perspective, the following social technologies are highlighted: (1) *Articulation of Resources in the Social Field*—understood as an intervention strategy that weaves actions focused on certain people, groups, collectives, and communities with those at the level of civil society, political action, and management; (2) *Dynamization of the Assistance Network*—to certain population groups and/or communities and their interaction with different sectors and levels of intervention; (3) *Workshops on Activities, Dynamics, and Projects*—taking advantage of the formative and transformative potential of the activity, because the sociopolitical and cultural dimension of the different actions pervades every life, favoring the self-valorization of people and enabling production of life with senses, with a view to personal and social emancipation; and (4) *Individual Territorial Follow-Ups*—starting from the attentive listening to the needs of people and population groups, seeking to address essential questions in their lives, often determined by social inequality and lack of access to social services and goods (Lopes, Silva, Borba, & Malfitano, 2011). These experiences are, therefore, aimed at gathering materials that translate into the production of knowledge about this reality and parameters on intervention possibilities. The experiences also aim to educate occupational therapists based on action directed toward the territorial dimension, for the development of living together and the overcoming of the approach based on the clinical/individual dimension, respecting, however, the singularities of people, having as presuppositions the principles concerning the search for the radical exercise of democracy and the rights and duties resulting from citizenship.

In contemporary Brazil, the search for expanded citizenship is a process that cannot be ignored, although many obstacles still have to be overcome. Even after over 30 years of the Citizen Constitution, Brazil has still not been able to account for the social debt it was seeking. On the contrary, the current conservative political ideology threatens to reverse significant gains, particularly with regard to universality and the scope of social rights. Unfortunately, this direction of restriction of rights and, therefore, of citizenship has also manifested in many other countries, underlining the importance and timeliness of this struggle.

Resuming what was exposed in the opening of this presentation, the theme addressed here led me to reflect on how social needs and actions are articulated in social reality; on how, on the one hand, to systematize specific knowledge and, on the other hand, to solve problems of real people and/or population groups; and on how to integrate disciplinary knowledge and, within it, concepts, methodologies, and techniques of occupational therapy, with interventions that occur in a field of complex knowledge production. If the specificity of occupational therapy lies in the quest to enable people and encourage them to have greater autonomy and social insertion and participation, how should we act professionally without advancing from their core of knowledge to an interdisciplinary, intersectoral, interprofessional field? In my opinion, this can be achieved by articulating citizenship, the universalization of rights, social policies, the radicalization of democracy, public power, social movements and participation, labor, education, health, justice, housing, art, culture, and recreation in a technical and political way. In other words, being and acting in the social field. That was how I and the occupational therapy with which I dialogue entered the 21st century.

REFERENCES

Amarante, P. (1995). *Loucos pela vida: trajetória da reforma psiquiátrica no Brasil* [Crazy for life: the trajectory of the psychiatric reform in Brazil]. Rio de Janeiro: SDE/ENSP: Fiocruz.

Barros, D. D. (2004). Terapia ocupacional social: o caminho se faz ao caminhar [Social occupational therapy: the path is open with the walking]. *Revista de Terapia Ocupacional da Universidade de São Paulo, 15*(3), 90–97.

Barros, D. D., Ghirardi, M. I. G., & Lopes, R. E. (2002). Terapia ocupacional social [Social occupational therapy]. *Revista de Terapia Ocupacional da Universidade de São Paulo, 13*(2), 95–103.

Barros, D. D., Lopes, R. E., & Galheigo, S. M. (2002). Projeto Metuia – terapia ocupacional no campo social [The Metuia Project – Occupational therapy in the social field]. *O Mundo da Saúde, 26*(3), 365–369.

Barros, D. D., Lopes, R. E., & Galheigo, S. M. (2007). Terapia ocupacional social: concepções e perspectivas [Social occupational therapy: concepts and perspectives]. In A. Cacalcante & C. Galvão (Eds.), *Terapia ocupacional - fundamentação & prática* [Occupational therapy – Foundations and practice] (pp. 347–353). Rio de Janeiro: Guanabara Koogan.

Basaglia, F. (1979). *Psiquiatria alternativa: contra o pessimismo da razão o otimismo da prática. Conferências no Brasil* [Alternative psychiatry: Against the pessimism of reason, the optimism of practice. Conferences in Brazil]. São Paulo: Brasil Debates.

Basaglia, F., & Ongaro-Basaglia, F. (1977). *Los crimenes de la paz: investigación sobre los intelectuales y los técnicos como servidores de la opresión* [The crimes of peace: Research on intellectuals and technicians as servants of oppression]. Madrid: Siglo XXI.

Brasil. (1988). *Constituição da República Federativa do Brasil* [Constitution of the Federative Republic of Brazil]. Brasília: Centro Gráfico.

Castel, R. (1997). As armadilhas da exclusão [The pitfalls of exclusion]. In M. Belfiore-Wanderley, L. Bógus, & M. C. Yazbek (Eds.), *Desigualdade e a questão social* [Inequality and the social issue] (pp. 15–48). São Paulo: EDUC.

Castel, R. (1999). *As metamorfoses da questão social: uma crônica do salário* [From manual workers to wage laborers: Transformation of the social question] (2nd ed.). Petrópolis: Vozes.

Donzelot, J. (1984). *L'invention du social: essai sul le déclin des passions politiques* [The invention of the social: An essay on the decline of political passions]. Paris: Fayard.

Donzelot, J. (1986). *A polícia das famílias* [The policing of families] (2nd ed.). Rio de Janeiro: Graal.

Freire, P. (1978). *Ação cultural para a liberdade e outros escritos* [Cultural action for freedom and other writings]. Rio de Janeiro: Paz e Terra.

Freire, P. (1979). *Pedagogia do oprimido* [Pedagogy of the oppressed]. Rio de Janeiro: Paz e Terra.

Galheigo, S. M. (1997). Da adaptação psicossocial à construção do coletivo: a cidadania enquanto eixo [From psychosocial adaptation to construction of the collective: citizenship as axis]. *Revista de Ciências Médicas da PUCCAMP, 6*(2/3), 105–108.

Gaspari, E. (2004). *A ditadura encurralada* [The endangered dictatorship]. São Paulo: Companhia das Letras.

Gramsci, A. (1977). *Escritos políticos* [Political writings] (Vols. I–IV). Lisboa: Seara Nova.

Gramsci, A. (1987). *Cartas do cárcere* [Letters from prison] (3rd ed.). Rio de Janeiro: Civilização Brasileira.

Gramsci, A. (2002). Cadernos do cárcere. Os intelectuais. O princípio educativo. In: *Jornalismo* [Prison notebooks. The intellectuals. Educational principle. In: *Journalism*] (Vol. 2). Rio de Janeiro: Civilização Brasileira.

Janoski, T. (1998). *Citizenship and civil society: A framework of rights and obligations in liberal, traditional, and social democratic regimes.* Cambridge: Cambridge University Press.

Kymlicka, W. (1996). *Ciudadanía multicultural: una teoria liberal de los derechos de la minoria* [Multicultural citizenship: A liberal theory of minority rights]. Barcelona: Paidós.

Lopes, R. E. (1997). A direção que construímos: algumas reflexões sobre a formação do terapeuta ocupacional [Ways we build up: reflections on the professional formation of occupational therapists]. *Revista de Terapia Ocupacional da Universidade de São Paulo, 4*(7), 27–35.

Lopes, R. E. (1999). *Cidadania, políticas públicas e terapia ocupacional, no contexto das ações de saúde mental e saúde da pessoa portadora de deficiência, no Município de São Paulo* [Citizenship, public policy, and occupational therapy in the context of health and mental health services for people with disability in Sao Paulo in 1999]. 539f. 2 v. (Doctoral dissertation in Education). Campinas, SP: Faculdade de Educação da Universidade Estadual de Campinas.

Lopes, R. E. (2004). Terapia ocupacional em São Paulo: um percurso singular e geral [Occupational therapy in Sao Paulo: A general and singular way]. *Cadernos de Terapia Ocupacional da UFSCar, 12*(2), 75–88.

Lopes, R. E., Malfitano A. P. S., Silva, C. R., Borba, P. L. O., & Hahn, M. S. (2012). Occupational therapy professional education and research in the social field. *WFOT Bulletin, 66,* 52–57.

Lopes, R. E., Silva, C. R., Borba, P. L. O., & Malfitano, A. P. S. (2011). [0]Tecnologias para a terapia ocupacional no campo social [Technologies for occupational therapy in the social field]. In *IX Congresso Latino-Americano de Terapia Ocupacional e XII Congresso Brasileiro de Terapia Ocupacional,* São Paulo. Cadernos de Terapia Ocupacional da UFSCar - ATOESP - ABRATO e CLATO, 19: 1.

Marshall, T. H. (1950). *Citizenship and social class and other essays.* Cambridge: CUP.

Netto, J. P. (2001). Cinco notas a propósito da "questão social" [Five notes on the "social question"]. In *Temporalis - Revista da Associação Brasileira de Ensino e Pesquisa em Serviço Social (ABEPSS).* Brasília: ABEPSS, 3: 41–49.

Offe, C. (1984). Dominação de classe e sistema político. Sobre a seletividade das instituições políticas [Class domination and political system. On the selectivity of political institutions]. In C. Offe (Ed.), *Problemas estruturais do Estado capitalista* [Structural problems of the capitalist state] (pp. 139–177). Rio de Janeiro: Tempo Brasileiro.

Offe, C., & Lenhardt, G. (1984). Teoria do Estado e política social [Social policy and the theory of the State]. In C. Offe (Ed.), *Problemas estruturais do Estado capitalista* [Structural problems of the capitalist state] (pp. 9–53). Rio de Janeiro: Tempo Brasileiro.

Offe, C., & Ronge, V. (1984). [0]Teses sobre a fundamentação do conceito de Estado capitalista e sobre a pesquisa política de orientação materialista [Theses on the foundation of the concept of capitalist state and on the political research of materialistic orientation]. In C. Offe (Ed.), *Problemas estruturais do Estado capitalista* [Structural problems of the capitalist state]. Rio de Janeiro: Tempo Brasileiro.

Oliver, F. C. (1990). *A atenção à saúde da pessoa portadora de deficiência no sistema de saúde do município de São Paulo: uma questão de cidadania.* [Health care of people with disabilities in the health system of the city of São Paulo: A question of citizenship] (Master's thesis in Public Health). Faculdade de Saúde Pública da Universidade de São Paulo, State of São Paulo, Brazil.

Shafir, G. (Ed.). (1998). *The citizenship debates: A reader.* Minneapolis, MN: University of Minnesota Press.

Vieira, L. (2001). *Os argonautas da cidadania* [The argonauts of citizenship]. Rio de Janeiro: Record.

Walzer, M. (1992). The civil society argument. In C. Mouffe (Ed.), *Dimensions of radical democracy: Pluralism, citizenship, community* (pp. 89–107). London: Verso.

2

Social Occupational Therapy in Brazil: A Historical Synthesis of the Constitution of a Field of Knowledge and Practice

Sandra Maria Galheigo

Achar	To find
A porta que esqueceram de fechar.	The door they forgot to close.
O beco com saída.	The alley with exit.
A porta sem chave.	The keyless door.
A vida.	Life
	(Leminsky, 2013)

INTRODUCTION

The production of knowledge and practices, carried out by a given profession in a given field of knowledge and practice, must, in my view, be understood as a sociohistorical construction. The concept of a field is used here to refer to a broad interdisciplinary area of knowledge and practice, such as health, mental health, collective health, social care, rehabilitation, and education, among others. From this perspective, individual professions develop their practices or areas of practice within different fields. Practitioners may use various perspectives and references to provide consistency in their work, which might follow previous standardized recommendations or engage in a completely new initiative, due to an ethical and political commitment to a cause.

To start, some concepts need to be clarified. In this context, the use of the concept of a field is inspired by the notion of field put forward by Pierre Bourdieu (1989), who argues that the social space is composed by the articulation of diverse autonomous social microcosms, with their various logics, orders, and needs. In addition, naming an occupational therapy area of practice as one developed in the "social field" is a result of an initiative that has been developed in Brazil since the late 1970s, as we will show later. Although this may be a conception mainly referred to by

Brazilian occupational therapy scholars, it is possible to trace parallels with the debate on social field or terrain as developed by British social scientists such as Squires (1990). A discussion on the use of the concepts of *field* in Bourdieu and *social field* in Squires (1990) in relation to occupational therapy in the social field is more thoroughly developed in Galheigo (2011a).

Perspective is used here as the set of theories and methodologies related to certain currents of thought that express a particular vision of human beings and society. In this chapter, positivist/functionalist, humanist, and critical perspectives are addressed. Reference is used here both for the theoretical knowledge produced by authors within certain theoretical-methodological perspectives and for practices developed according to approaches, methods, and techniques applied to certain existential conditions related to life, health, and access to rights, among others.

Having established the concepts used in this chapter, it is important to address what is meant by the creation of new practices and initiatives motivated by an ethical-political commitment. In my view, the inaugural moment in which a new area of practice or a new perspective is born occurs in response to events, contexts, and perceptions about the needs of persons and groups and to a sensitive, comprehensive, and critical reading of collective, institutional, or political demands. It arises, therefore, when professionals feel uncomfortable with their practices and become aware of undetected problems or conditions; thus, professionals are able to deconstruct them in their preconceptions and forms and learn about their complexity. From this moment on, they begin to reflect on possibilities, strategies, and courses of action, as well as seeking to ensure the success of their efforts. The questions posed at such moments could be described as follows: *What contributions can this body of knowledge and practice bring to the human condition before me? To what extent can professional activity, informed by the social, cultural, and political scenario, contribute to changing the conditions of life faced by these people, groups, and collectives?*

Undoubtedly, there is a theoretical and methodological belief underlying these initial reflections. An ethical-political commitment can be perceived behind the intention to change a condition, situation, or cause, and this commitment is established by listening to the needs and demands of people, groups, and collectives. A responsive discourse is constructed through a critical reflection on the "instituted," the "hegemonic," the "normalized," and the "given."

This conception of professional practice, therefore, does not result from the search for evidence or the construction of hypotheses, nor from the implementation of previously defined procedures. It is not committed to achieving pre-established goals. Moreover, it does not propose to comply with an "established" norm, nor to reach a previously established standard of normality as an adequate condition of personal existence.

Summing up, in economic and political terms, a professional practice inspired by an ethical and political commitment does not result from the neoliberal perspective according to which professional practice is seen as offering products to potential consumers and that dictates that a "niche market" should be sought. In addition, it is not guided by a corporate logic that defines professional practice by what is unique to professionals: their roles and merits, resulting from their skills and competencies.

HISTORICAL MILESTONES IN THE CREATION OF OCCUPATIONAL THERAPY IN THE SOCIAL FIELD IN BRAZIL

I've been thinking what I could characterize as Social OT. The ideas that I put forward will not end here, because social occupational therapy will not be defined in one meeting. . . . [W]e still have twenty years to define it.

(Galheigo, 1981, p. 2)

Occupational therapy in the social field emerged in Brazil in the late 1970s based on an ethical and political commitment, as it would be referred to some decades later. It originated out of a concern with the social issues of its particular time and context and the possibilities envisioned by some occupational therapists on developing alternative practices.

The first initiatives in this new area of practice focused on marginalized groups such as the youth who lived institutionalized in the State Foundation for the Well-Being of the Youth (FEBEM), poor children and adolescents attending public day care and community youth centers, adults in prison, and the institutionalized elderly living in precarious nursing homes.

The term "occupational therapy in the social field" first appeared in the Fifth Scientific Meeting of Occupational Therapists in the State of São Paulo, Brazil, in 1979, when Jussara de Mesquita Pinto delivered an oral presentation entitled "Report of an Experience in Occupational Therapy in the Social Field" about her practice with young people institutionalized at FEBEM (Pinto, 1979).

As important historical milestones, it is vital to note that at the end of the 1970s, the occupational therapy programs of two universities—the Federal University of São Carlos and the Pontifical Catholic University of Campinas—introduced into their curricula a discipline called Occupational Therapy Applied to Social Conditions, offered at the two institutions, respectively, by Jussara de Mesquita Pinto and Maria Heloísa Medeiros. In July 1980, the Associação dos Terapeutas Ocupacionais do Brasil (Association of Occupational Therapists of Brazil, ATOB) (1980) submitted to the Ministry of Education and Culture its *Proposal for the Reformulation of the Minimum Curriculum for Occupational Therapy*, conceived by its Education Commission. This proposal presented, for the first time in an official professional document, the request to include the discipline "Occupational Therapy Applied to Social Conditions: Including Situations of Social Marginalization," among other disciplines within the Cycle of Professional Topics (ATOB, 1980, pp. 15–16).

It can be seen, then, that occupational therapy in the social field began to be developed in Brazil by a double initiative: the design of intervention proposals for marginalized populations and the creation of disciplines in undergraduate courses in occupational therapy. In this, it had to overcome some challenges: to develop its own theoretical bases and to design appropriate methodologies of action for people living in marginalized conditions. It also had to deal with the difficulties of proposing emancipatory speeches and practices during the dictatorial civil-military dictatorship, as some scholars pointed out at the time and since:

Given the range of existing problems and the lack of specific occupational therapy resources, occupational therapists have attempted to adapt, at first, the methods and techniques already known to [fit] the aims of this type of practice.

(Pinto 1979, p. 5)

The processes of institutionalization of the populations living in marginalized conditions . . . opened a new reality in the area of social programs: how to characterize this population? How to deal with the marginality, language and culture of these populations?

(Soares, 1991, p. 174)

The definition of so-called occupational therapy in the social field, the formalization of its object and objectives of intervention, and the establishment of its theoretical bases were the initial concerns explored in the first academic events to delve into the subject. The very first one was a panel entitled "Social Occupational Therapy: Philosophy, Definition, and Fields of Action," which was presented in the Second Scientific Occupational Therapy Week, held at the Federal University of São Carlos in 1981, an event at which oral presentations on practices in public childcare centers and prisons were offered. Also, one presentation reflected on the creation of occupational therapy in the social field, an extract of which is presented here:

> What would this theoretical and practice body consist of? . . . Could a public childcare centre always be considered a social area? The prison? The asylum? So, in this sense, is the psychiatric hospital? Community work? . . . [T]o be able to define an area [of knowledge and practice], we will have to discuss the criteria, since our proposal here is to reflect on what Social OT is. . . . Considering that the object, objective and priority of Social OT has to be different from the object, objective and priority of other areas of practice . . ., what would it be? . . . [W]e lack a sociological basis.
>
> (Galheigo, 1981, pp. 3–4)

Therefore, the search for theoretical and methodological bases for occupational therapy in the social field, which was perceived to be needed, started to take place during the 1980s; however, it is noteworthy that it happened under the influence of a singular historical-political context. On one hand, professors and researchers of occupational therapy sought postgraduate training in related areas of knowledge, such as social sciences, philosophy, education, and psychology. On the other hand, the new proposals were largely influenced by the political effervescence for country redemocratization, the emergence of new social movements, the debate on sanitary reform, and the anti-asylum movement.

> The regular participation of the occupational therapist in social programs has become reality in the 1980s. This fact, associated with a vaster debate on the National Mental Health Policy and the process of redemocratization of Brazilian society, has contributed to the discussion about the social and political roles of occupational therapy.
>
> (Galheigo, 1988, p. 79)

In theoretical terms, the ideas of Althusser, Basaglia, Bourdieu, Castel, Donzelot, Foucault, Goffman, Gramsci, Illich, Marx, and Paulo Freire, which constituted the critical framework of the time, were also partially incorporated into the content of the existing disciplines of social occupational therapy. Besides these authors, the bibliographical references of these disciplines also included scholarship from the social sciences on marginalized populations, as well as journalistic texts of social critiques. The experience of the discipline of occupational therapy in the social field, offered by the Pontifical Catholic University of Campinas, revealed that the studied topics and literature varied throughout the following years, according to the historical, political, social, and epistemological trends of the time. Practical settings were predominantly developed by university projects in public childcare centers, community programs, orphanages, and institutions for adolescents in conflict with the law, among others.

Certain strategies were crucial to the development of the occupational therapist role in the social field, namely: (1) listening to people's life stories, which served as a means of learning about social realities, and (2) reflecting critically on daily professional practice, demystifying the professional as the one who holds the knowledge. These strategies enabled occupational therapists to get to know people's unique ways of being, existing, and surviving and to grasp their perspectives, living conditions, needs, and demands (Galheigo, 2011b).

The first reflections of the social field were based on the critical theoretical and methodological frameworks used at the time in Brazil, which were derived from the propositions of the occupational therapy philosophical models developed by Pinto (1990) and Francisco (1988). Their works identified three possible occupational therapy perspectives: positivist/functionalist, humanist, and historical-materialist. Some studies in the area began to explore how a situation within a session could be differently viewed according to these different standpoints, as well as how social occupational therapy practices could either reproduce the status quo or be transformative, as the following session extract and analysis show:

> Youth: Have you ever been arrested, madam?
> OT: No.
> Youth: No? But someone in your family, for sure. There is always a black sheep in the family. I am the black sheep of mine. Everyone there is worthy, except me.
> For Miguel the world was a reproduction of his house. He did not clearly distinguish social classes and their mechanisms. He referred to the Judge of the Juvenile Court as the highest rank in the social hierarchy, who [in his view] was powerful and wealthy—"very rich indeed" [in his words].
>
> (Galheigo, 1988, p. 77)

This master's dissertation first presented how this dialogue could be understood within a more conservative standpoint:

According to the first perspective [positivist], Miguel would be attributed to a disease or "weakness" of personality since his brothers did not opt for delinquency and were raised under the same conditions. Yet the second conception [humanist] would highlight the social background that caused Miguel's delinquency. Both, however, would propose therapeutic strategies that ensured his adaptation to society. Either would no doubt lead to an alienated and alienating understanding.

(Galheigo, 1988, p. 79)

Then the author considered how the dialogue could be understood within a critical perspective:

An occupational therapeutic practice can only be said to be transformative when: it enables Miguel, Claudinéia, João and Maria to understand the historical dimension of their lives; [the practitioner] does not take ownership of knowledge and, instead, shares with them the construction of the therapeutic process/project; [the practitioner] does not impose a direction, but instead, gives them elements for reflection on their position and the choice of their life path; when [the practitioner] perceives, denounces, denies and repositions oneself against the traps of power implicit in social relations; when [the practitioner] carries out a self-critique in relation to the disciplinary mechanisms rooted in professional practice since its creation.

(Galheigo, 1988, p. 79)

This example shows how occupational therapists in Brazil started to address the first guiding questions of the social field: How do we make the practice of occupational therapy not serve as a mechanism of social control? How can we do it to enact social transformation?

Despite these first academic works during the late 1970s and the 1980s, the activities of practice, teaching, and research in occupational therapy in the social field were not sufficient to produce a body of knowledge that clearly affirmed its domain of action and its theoretical-methodological bases. In fact, although not clearly documented, the constitution of social occupational therapy suffered a setback in the early 1990s, when the naming of a field of professional knowledge and practice as "social" came to be seen as a reductionism.

This movement was partly the outcome of the proposition of the philosophical models of occupational therapy (Pinto, 1990; Francisco, 1988) mentioned earlier that sought to establish the epistemological differences between professional practices. At the end of the 1980s, the idea that epistemological perspectives mattered more than specificities of the areas of occupational therapy practice prevailed in some circles for a few years. The fragility of the maintenance of a field of knowledge and practice called social occupational therapy resulted in the elimination of its specific disciplines from the undergraduate courses of the two universities where this area of practice originated. Thus, teaching, research, and academic production in the area ceased to gain institutional status during the early 1990s, a period when, in contrast, the occupational therapy practice in other fields actively sought dialogue with the ongoing social policymaking restructuring. Not even the enactment of the Organic Law of Social Assistance (LOAS) (Brazil, 1993), which could foster the practice in the field, was enough to invite an organized professional response to sustain this area of practice; however, a few teaching, research, and extension projects in the social field, although scarce, continued to take place.

During the 1990s, with the restructuring of social policies in Brazil, the philosophical models proved insufficient to provide theoretical bases for the diversity of fields of practice engaged within the profession (Galheigo, 1999). Even so, it took nearly a decade for social occupational therapy to re-establish itself again in Brazil (Galheigo, 2003). In 1998, however, this situation was reversed with the creation of the Metuia Project, a university-based joint effort to develop theoretical and methodological bases for social occupational therapy.

PROPOSAL OF SOCIAL OCCUPATIONAL THERAPY BY THE METUIA PROJECT: WAYS OF DOING OF THE SOUTH

An epistemology of the South is based on three orientations: to learn that there is the South; learn to go to the South; learn from the South and with the South.

(Santos, 2010, p. 15)

The interinstitutional group of studies, education, and practice for the citizenship of children, adolescents, and adults in the process of the breakdown of their social support networks (Metuia Project) was created via a partnership of professors from three universities in the state of São Paulo: the Pontifical Catholic University of Campinas, the Federal University of São Carlos, and the University of São Paulo. The main motivation of this initiative was to reinsert the social field in the academic agenda by producing what they would call social occupational therapy, as the project's objectives in its inaugural website in 2000 described (see Box 2.1).

BOX 2.1   Objectives of the Metuia Project

1. To develop and disseminate knowledge in the field of social occupational therapy.
2. To create partnerships with governmental and non-governmental organizations, developing initiatives for granting citizenship rights.
3. To study the features and living contexts of the population undergoing a breakdown in social support networks to develop practice methodologies that consider the complexity of their living social conditions.
4. To enable occupational therapy students and professionals to develop studies and practices with children, adolescents, and adults undergoing a breakdown in their social support networks.
5. To enable professionals and students to develop practices where the people's and communities' stories are heard, and the solutions for their own needs are fostered in an action that is jointly built and historically contextualized.

Source: Metuia's former website (now defunct), 2000.

From the start, the development of Metuia's teaching, research, and university practice and learning projects, carried out in partnership with nongovernmental organizations, followed a strategy of promoting the field through theoretical and practical articulation. Thus, through systematic meetings, Metuia's members sought to create a theoretical-methodological alignment between university professors and practitioners working in the services involved to ensure the cohesion and coherence of their proposals. The strategy entailed the periodic holding of seminars, workshops, and discussion groups that presented and debated (1) the theoretical bases produced for the field, (2) ongoing research conducted by the group members, (3) practice projects developed with partner nongovernmental organizations, (4) methodologies of action used in teaching and care, and (5) the very structuring of the Metuia Project through the elaboration of its guidelines for action and the preparation of dissemination materials, such as folders and the website.

In these meetings, some points of debate were important. First, the professional role was problematized to deconstruct traditional practices; the intention was to make students and professionals aware that practices should not produce institutional conformism or the reproduction of the status quo. Second, the discussion moved around the idea that a different social and political commitment should be entailed by social occupational therapists by criticizing practices guided by the functionalist perspective

of "adapting the individual to society" and creating ones where professionals worked as "social mediators" (Galheigo, 1997, 2003). The research and practice projects developed by Metuia's members aimed at urban and rural youth, people living on the streets, and children and adolescents in public schools, in shelters, or in conflict with the law. These studies and practices served as resources for critical reflection on the field, resulting in a constant process of the production and problematizing of theory and practice. Paraphrasing the title of an article by Denise Dias Barros (2004), the path of social occupational therapy was made while walking.

Therefore, social occupational therapy was constituted as a professional knowledge and practice based on a critical reflection on the social place of the occupational therapist, seeking to characterize the population form whom their actions were designed and to develop methodologies of action that aimed at autonomy, citizenship, and access to rights of persons and collectives:

Social occupational therapy is intended for people whose greatest needs are based on their exclusion from access to social goods and whose problems are manifested by the worsening of living conditions to which they are subjected. Such a problem can be acknowledged as poverty or also understood as a situation of vulnerability, of "apartheid," since access to the rights of citizenship, even if constitutionally guaranteed, is unequally distributed, translating itself into an experience of no-citizenship, of not-belonging.

(Galheigo, 2003, pp. 34–35)

The aim [of social occupational therapy] is to develop theoretical and applied studies on activities in occupational therapy as resources for self-valorisation and the production of personal and social meaning that aims at the expansion of opportunities and personal & social emancipation by means of focused (but always contextualized) projects of improvement of quality of life.

(Barros, Lopes, & Galheigo, 2002, pp. 367–368)

Metuia's academic production, using Castel (1994, 2003) as a reference, placed the debate on the social question—and its production of vulnerability and disaffiliation—as the result of the extreme social and economic inequality lived by a large contingent of the Brazilian population (Barros, Ghirardi, & Lopes, 1999, 2002, 2005; Galheigo, 2005, 2011a; Barros, Lopes, & Galheigo, 2007a, 2007b, 2011a; Barros, Lopes, Galheigo, & Galvani, 2005, 2011). This theoretical framework helped social occupational therapy approach the social question by articulating the understanding of the social, cultural, and political contexts lived by the people in the process of breakdown of their social support networks:

> *The occupational therapist devotes him/herself to a reading of everyday life and its contexts, the intermediation between the macro and micro-social structure, the re-signification of doing, the individual and collective intervention, developing strategies that seek to strengthen personal and social support networks, with the objective that these will translate into a greater autonomous sustainability of people in the complex social structure in which they are inserted.*
>
> *(Malfitano, 2005, p. 6)*

Social occupational therapy therefore appears as a proposal that differs completely from the perspectives of Anglo-Saxon occupational therapy, both those perspectives focused on the recovery of functionality and those centered on the person. On the contrary, its knowledge and practices are produced in the South by using epistemologies of the South, viewed by Santos and Menezes (2010) as a metaphor for the epistemic challenges used by the countries of the South to confront capitalism and colonialism.

The dissemination of social occupational therapy on the international level (Barros, Ghirardi, & Lopes, 2005; Barros, Lopes, & Galheigo, 2011; Barros, Lopes, Galheigo, & Galvani Barros, 2005, 2011; Galheigo, 2005, 2011a), which was mainly carried out in the two volumes of the book *Occupational Therapy without Borders* (Kronenberg, Algado, & Pollard, 2005; Kronenberg, Pollard, & Sakellariou, 2011), ended up revealing its similarity with practices that had already been developed in Latin America and South Africa. This perspective shares concerns for economic, social, ethnic, and gender inequalities; the rescue of the knowledge proper to its peoples; the search for community/territorial intervention alternatives; and the education of new professionals with a focus on political literacy (Duncan, Buchanan, & Lorenzo, 2005; Lorenzo, Duncan, Buchanan, & Alsop, 2006; Trujillo, Camacho, et al., 2011; Trujillo, Torres, Méndez, & Carrizosa, 1991; Watson & Swartz, 2004).

The close ties among academics and practitioners in scientific and academic events have also contributed to the development of a sense of the South. In 2010 and 2011, several international events contributed to bringing Brazilian social occupational therapy closer to coming into action in other countries in the South: the 15th Congress of the World Federation of Occupational Therapists, the 12th Brazilian Occupational Therapy Congress/9th Latin American Congress of Occupational Therapy, and the 2nd International Symposium of Social Occupational Therapy. Since then, there has been an expansion of Latin American, Ibero-American, and South African–Brazilian–Indian

cooperation projects that point to the creation of new international exchange networks (Galheigo, 2011b; Galvaan, Galheigo & Saha, 2013).

Exchanges imply intercultural and intersocial actions in which reciprocal recognition and availability for exchange are present. They allow for the articulation of ideas, practices, processes, and contexts, but they require, on the other hand, the clarification of differences, which points to the importance of sustaining academic dialogue (Galheigo, 2011b).

This conceptual, historical, and epistemological dialogue is also necessary at the national level. After all, from the beginning of the 21st century, occupational therapy in the social field in Brazil has expanded and diversified, coming to include teams from sectors such as social assistance as well as expanded academic dissemination in congresses, seminars, and journals.

In this new scenario, the theoretical-methodological issues and tensions of the past seem to persist, as Lopes and collaborators (2012) point out when studying the papers approved for presentation at the 12th Brazilian Congress of Occupational Therapy and 9th Latin American Congress of Occupational Therapy. This study identifies the fragility of the conceptual basis of the references used and "a simultaneous use of different approaches, in a kind of bricolage of conceptual references" (Lopes, Borba, Silva, & Malfitano, 2012, p. 29). The study also pointed to the core of the contemporary problems related to occupational therapy in the social field when it criticized practices in fields where professional action is reduced to the developmentalist approach, decontextualized from the social, political, and existential scenarios of institutional emergency placements:

> *An example of such a situation is related to the reports of interventions in shelters, which represented a significant number of works. In these, approaches to child development and the use of play as a beneficial resource for the child were predominant, elements certainly related to childhood; they lacked, however, what effectively hinders the development and play of our children: poverty, family and/or social abandonment, vulnerability and violence to which they are subjected, that is, the immense inequality with which we must deal in Brazil and in Latin America as a whole.*
>
> *(Lopes et al., 2012, p. 29)*

For an academic dialogue *without borders* in the context of occupational therapy in the social field, it is fundamental to give voice to differences, to go in search of their contexts, and to problematize existing tensions or contradictions. It is a necessary exercise as well as one of the most important contemporary challenges in the area.

INTERVENING IN THE SOCIAL FIELD: ON THE IMPORTANCE OF THE REFRAMING OF THE EPISTEMOLOGICAL DEBATE

To intervene. *1. Take part voluntarily; get in the way, come or put yourself between, on your own initiative; interfere: Intervened in the contest. 2. Interpose your authority, or your good offices, or your diligence. 3. Be present; help. 4. Occur incidentally; to emerge.*

(Ferreira, 1999, p. 961)

Every social experience produces and reproduces knowledge, and in so doing presupposes one or more epistemologies. Epistemology is any notion or idea, reflected or not, on the conditions of what counts as valid knowledge.

(Santos & Meneses, 2010, pp. 15–16)

The professional practice of the occupational therapist is characterized by intervening, whether or not one likes the term and whether or not one prefers to use other concepts that seem more appropriate in their meaning. Based on the Portuguese definition of the term "to intervene" in the dictionary *Novo Aurélio Século XXI* (Ferreira, 1999), it is possible to sustain that, when **intervening,** practitioners voluntarily take part; they interpose their good tasks or diligence in the face of any problematic situation, need, or demand. Therefore, they intervene along with their colleagues from other professions who share practices in health, education, culture, work, and social support services.

The character of the intervention, the principles that define the act, the ideas that give it meaning, and the act that reveals the *habitus* are what bring practitioners and social actors closer or farther apart, reveal their consonances or differences, and lead them to partnerships or dissents. It is important to highlight that differences and dissent may occur not as an outcome related to professional training but instead by the way practitioners understand and relate to social actors who come from different backgrounds and henceforth different *habitus*. This is a central concept, in Bourdieu's theory, that can be defined as

a system of enduring dispositions acquired by the individual during the process of socialization. Dispositions are attitudes, inclinations to perceive, feel, do and think internalized by individuals as a result of their objective conditions of existence, and which function as unconscious principles of action, perception and reflection.

(Bonnewitz, 2003, p. 77)

The social practice of intervention, attention, or care, as one may prefer to call it, generates understanding and, as a

result, new (though not always) practices and knowledge are produced and reproduced:

There is therefore no knowledge without practices and social actors. And since both exist only within social relations, different types of social relations can give rise to different epistemologies.

(Santos & Meneses, 2010, pp. 15–16)

Since the late 1970s, epistemological questions related to occupational therapy in the social field have emerged as essential for the definition of this area of knowledge and practice, among them: *What are the central ideas of this field, beyond which it loses its legitimacy?*

In the early 1990s, Soares (1991) argued that the first experiences in the so-called social field did not differ from those developed by other areas of action; furthermore, they did not address the issue of social marginalization or institutionalization, at least as far as the methodological approaches used are concerned:

He/she [the occupational therapist], working with the child and youth clientele, aimed at correcting development delays and accelerating the integration process. In working with the elderly population, in turn, the therapist focused on organic degenerative processes or support for emotional problems such as loneliness, terminal illness, etc. In relation to both clienteles, the charitable nature of the program and its institutionalizing logic were evident.

(Soares, 1991, p. 174)

Going further, Soares problematized the theoretical-methodological question of occupational therapy in the social field as follows:

The limited adequacy of professional models to this reality raises the following controversy: should we develop a new specific model—social occupational therapy? And does the psychosocial approach, elaborated by North American professionals, respond to these needs? Or do we have to focus on Brazilian occupational therapy and look for alternatives within it?

(Soares, 1991, p. 174)

Of course, today the debate takes place differently from 20 years ago because there is already a scholarship that unequivocally establishes the bases of social occupational therapy. However, differences exist in Brazil, both in terms of the interventions carried out and in the theoretical arguments that support them, which need to be better known. Thus, the debate can be enriched by the ideas of Santos and Meneses (2010), who, when discussing epistemological differences, affirm that

The differences may be minimal but, even [if they were] large, they may not be the subject of discussion, but in any case, they are often the source of the tensions or contradictions present in social experiences, especially when, as it is usually the case, these are constituted by different types of social relationships.

(Santos & Meneses, 2010, pp. 15–16)

To resume the debate on the epistemological differences that underlie social interventions, it is essential to indicate ways of approaching the social field. Three perspectives that, to a certain extent, may be rooted in social practices and influence interventions in the social field are highlighted here: the structural-functionalist, the humanist, and the critical. These perspectives demarcate both great differences of approach to the social question and different understandings about the human being in its relationship with the world. Therefore, these perspectives are not interchangeable, and if they overlap, they reveal an important lack of theoretical-methodological cohesion.

The structural-functionalist perspective of Talcott Parsons had a strong influence on Brazilian health and social services, including those designed to deal with what was conventionally called the "problem of the minor," relating to adolescents and youth (Galheigo, 1996). Parsons (1991) argued that social integration was the result of the process of socialization experienced by individuals, a process that produced in the individual the desire to internalize rules and adapt to social norms. Thus, from his perspective, social order was the result of the sharing of a culture of common values by social actors (Turner, 1991). The deviant or dysfunctional attitude was understood by Parsons as the tendency of some people to oppose the system of values standardized institutionally, which brings imbalance to the process of social interaction. This view, therefore, applied to unrelated conditions, such as disease, poverty, and crime.

In Parsons' view, social control mechanisms must thwart deviant tendencies "by teaching the social actor not to embark on them" (Parsons, 1991, p. 298). Thus, in case of failure of the socialization process, social control mechanisms should be used to impose limits. Parsons (1991) established a relationship between the processes of socialization and social control, where the former would serve as a reference for the latter. Thus, socialization would teach "what to do," while the mechanisms of social control would teach "what not to do" (Parsons, 1991, p. 298). The professional role could thus be equated with that of executor of social control.

Based on this perspective, interventions with the marginalized population should be based on a thorough knowledge of this population. Thus, "case studies" have become widely diffused to peripheral countries (Midgley, 1981), making it one of the main strategies used worldwide

by health professionals and social workers to deal with social issues. This strategy was also highly recommended by the National Policy on the Welfare of Youth (underage), implemented by the civil-military dictatorship in Brazil (Galheigo, 1996). Case studies, incorporating a biomedical perspective, use clinical, psychological, psychiatric, and social references to know and prescribe interventions for people and families considered "deviant," "unstructured," or "dysfunctional." They are based on the idea that it is a professional responsibility to perform a psychosocial diagnosis of the individual and to prescribe interventions.

Critics of this theoretical perspective maintain that these interventions resulted in what came to be seen as the psychologization or medicalization of social problems (Galheigo, 1996). Social care, education, and health in contemporary Brazil are still rooted in this perspective.

The humanist perspective is usually considered to be phenomenological inasmuch as it deals with "subjective individual experience, the personal 'worldview' that each individual develops as a result of his/her unique life, feelings and perceptions" (Hagedorn, 1997, p. 64). Its most influential theorists are Maslow, Frankl, and Rogers.

According to this perspective, each individual's position on one's own life should be valued. Authenticity, honesty, and respect for the other are regarded as important, and the search for meaning for the subject is essential. Thus, self-knowledge and control over one's own life are the conditions that lead to self-realization. The client-centered approaches that underlie psychotherapeutic practices and occupational therapy models in Anglo-Saxon countries have originated from this perspective (Hagedorn, 1997).

The humanist perspective was widely discussed in Brazil in the works of Pinto (1990) and Francisco (1988). For these authors, the humanist perspective began to be used by Brazilian occupational therapists in the 1970s as a way of opposing the positivist perspective. It aimed at replacing "man at the center of the universe . . . through the main argument that there is no opportunity without exercise of subjectivity" (Pinto, 1990, p. 42).

According to Francisco (1988), in the humanistic occupational therapy model, the role of the occupational therapist is to "facilitate learning in new ways, offering a model of relationship in which it is possible to learn, rehearse, make mistakes, teach and accomplish something that could not happen in another place" (Francisco, 1988, pp. 63–64).

Among the critiques of the humanist perspective is the view that "the opportunity for the individual to control, direct and shape his/her own life may be minimal and, whilst choice may be beneficial, some clients are overwhelmed by being presented with too much of it" (Hagedorn, 1997, p. 64). The client-centered approach, therefore, is limited since it starts from a liberal conception that man is naturally free, disregarding the social and political inequalities that lead to the core of the social question. By not recognizing this sociopolitical context, it also disregards the importance of popular social organization and collective action (Galheigo, 2012).

The humanist perspective manifests itself in a pluralistic way, and there are different approaches whose detail does not fit the scope of this discussion. It is a perspective that provides a foundation for social practices that aim at facilitating people's self-knowledge and autonomy but having only individuals in their personal development as the focus of intervention.

Summarizing critical perspectives is a difficult task, given the breadth of theories that would have to be discussed in an examination of their nuances, consensuses, and dissent. Therefore, what can be done in this chapter is to present some key issues that guide critical perspectives. Luckily, the main authors who have contributed to the critical debate within occupational therapy have been presented earlier in this chapter.

Some problematizations are highlighted in the formulation of critical perspectives. In general terms, critical perspectives question (1) scientific knowledge as a statute of truth, produced in a neutral way; (2) knowledge produced by distancing subject and object and by subordinating the object to the subject; and (3) knowledge that understands the social fact as a natural and universal phenomenon.

In contrast, critical perspectives recognize both the production of subjectivity and social relations as sociohistorical processes. Thus, they hold that to address society's problems, it is important to understand historically the macro-processes that influence social relations and the material conditions of existence. Critical studies, as well as emancipatory practices, highlight the importance of local and contextual knowledge and the value of diversity and culture. The question of power also permeates the critical debate, whether in the search for an understanding of the role of the state, an understanding of institutional power, or an understanding of the capillarity and inequality of power relations.

Critical perspectives have been an important marker for the discussion of the technical application of knowledge. In the hegemonic conception, the practitioner ends up being a reproducer of the dominant discourse and the status quo. When "applying knowledge, [he/she] is outside the existential situation to which the application is referred and [he/she] is not affected by it" (Santos, 2012, p. 157). The practitioner does not mediate between the universal and the particular; he or she does not value the subjective and local knowledge and so adopts one-dimensional thinking (Santos, 2012).

In a critical conception, the ethical aspect guides the application of knowledge. From an ethical-political commitment, the professional "takes sides with those who have less power" (Santos, 2012, p. 159) with an inclination toward social transformation. As Santos (2012) states:

> The enriching application [of knowledge] seeks and reinforces the emerging and alternative definitions of reality; for this, it delegitimizes institutional forms and modes of rationality in each of the contexts [domestic, work, citizenship, and world], in the understanding that such forms and modes promote violence instead of argumentation, silence instead of communication, alienation instead of solidarity.
>
> (Santos, 2012, p. 159)

The contemporary social practices developed in Brazil by social and health care workers have been largely influenced by critical—theoretical and methodological—bases. In parallel, in the scope of occupational therapy, the critical perspective is increasingly based on Brazilian and Latin American experience:

> These new theoretical positions, comprehensive in occupational therapy, require a permanent questioning. From a critical position, which is transformative of the social world we are part of, [the world requires] asking ourselves about the assumptions of OT, the obvious, the natural. [This means] [n]ot only thinking about the political, ethical and economic considerations of the problems that affect the community and the implications for OT, but also considering that criticism is the privileged place to produce knowledge. Criticism as knowledge.
>
> (Guajardo, 2012, p. 23)

SOCIAL OCCUPATIONAL THERAPY IN ITS CRITICAL AND COMPLEX PERSPECTIVE: FINAL CONSIDERATIONS

Social occupational therapy, as conceived by the Metuia Project, uses a critical perspective to ground its theoretical-methodological bases. The guiding principles that define what is meant by occupational therapy in the social field are unequivocal, even when some differences in framing projects and theories may appear within the various practices.

The practices of social occupational therapy are supported by an ethical and political commitment that takes place through a sensible listening to the stories of persons and collectives with whom projects are developed and by a critical perspective of their social and political contexts. It is sensible by listening to and holding people's ideas, affections, and experiences, and critical by problematizing macro-processes in which their everyday lives are interwoven. It has an ethical commitment by intervening in life and in movements of resistance and affirmation. It has a political commitment by the continuous clarification of the existing macro- and micro-political forces; by the defense of autonomy, citizenship, and rights; and by the search for new strategies for the construction and/or strengthening of collective action.

REFERENCES

Associação dos Terapeutas Ocupacionais do Brasil (ATOB). (1980). *Proposta de Reformulação do Currículo Mínimo de Terapia Ocupacional* [Proposal of Reformulation of the Minimum Curriculum of Occupational Therapy] [Original archive document]. Rio de Janeiro: Associação dos Terapeutas Ocupacionais do Brasil.

Barros, D. D. (2004). Terapia ocupacional social: o caminho se faz ao caminhar [Notes for a social occupational therapy: The way is done by the way we go]. *Revista de Terapia Ocupacional da USP, 15*(3), 90–97.

Barros, D. D., Ghirardi, M. I. G., & Lopes, R. E. (1999). Terapia ocupacional e sociedade [Occupational therapy and society]. *Revista de Terapia Ocupacional da USP, 10*(2/3), 71–76.

Barros, D. D., Ghirardi, M. I. G., & Lopes, R. E. (2002). Terapia ocupacional social [Social occupational therapy]. *Revista de Terapia Ocupacional da USP, 13*(3), 95–103.

Barros, D. D., Ghirardi, M. I. G., & Lopes, R. E. (2005). Chapter 30: Social occupational therapy: A social-historical perspective. In F. Kronenberg, S. S. Algado, & N. Pollard (Eds.), *Occupational therapy without borders – Learning from the spirit of survivors* (pp. 140–151). London: Elsevier Churchill Livingstone.

Barros, D. D., Lopes, R. E., & Galheigo, S. M. (2002). Projeto Metuia – Terapia Ocupacional no Campo Social [The Metuia Project – Occupation therapy in the social sphere]. *O Mundo da Saúde, 26*(3), 365–370.

Barros, D. D., Lopes, R. E., & Galheigo, S. M. (2007a). Chapter 38: Novos espaços, novos sujeitos: a terapia ocupacional no trabalho territorial e comunitário [Chapter 38: New spaces, new subjects: Occupational therapy in territorial and community work]. In A. Cavalcanti & C. Galvão (Eds.), *Terapia Ocupacional - fundamentação & prática* [Occupational therapy: Foundation & practice] (pp. 354–363). Rio de Janeiro: Guanabara Koogan S.A.

Barros, D. D., Lopes, R. E., & Galheigo, S. M. (2007b). Chapter 37: Terapia Ocupacional Social: Concepções e Perspectivas [Chapter 37: Social occupational therapy: Conceptions and perspectives]. In A. Cavalcanti & C. Galvão (Eds.), *Terapia Ocupacional - fundamentação & prática* [Occupational therapy: Foundation & practice] (pp. 347–353). Rio de Janeiro: Guanabara Koogan S.A.

Barros, D. D., Lopes, R. E., & Galheigo, S. M. (2011). Chapter 22: Brazilian experiences in social occupational therapy. In F. Kronemberg, N. Pollard, & D. Sakellariou (Eds.), *Occupational therapies without borders* (Vol. II): *Towards and ecology of occupation-based practices* (pp. 209–216). Edinburgh: Churchill Livingstone/Elsevier.

Barros, D. D., Lopes, R. E., Galheigo, S. M., & Galvani, D. (2005). Chapter 30: The Metuia Project in Brazil: Ideas and actions which bind us together. In F. Kronenberg, S. S. Algado, & N. Pollard (Eds.), *Occupational therapy without borders - Learning from the spirit of survivors* (pp. 402–413). London: Elsevier Churchill Livingstone.

Barros, D. D., Lopes, R. E., Galheigo, S. M. & Galvani, D. (2011). Chapter 34: Research, community-based projects and teaching as a sharing construction: The Metuia Project in Brazil. In F. Kronemberg, N. Pollard, & D. Sakellariou (Eds.), *Occupational therapies without borders* (Vol. II): *Towards and ecology of occupation-based practices* (pp. 321–332). Edinburgh: Churchill Livingstone/Elsevier.

Bonnewitz, P. (2003). *Primeiras lições sobre a sociologia de Pierre Bourdieu* [First lessons on the sociology of Pierre Bourdieu]. Rio de Janeiro: Vozes.

Bourdieu, P. (1989). Social space and symbolic power. *Sociological Theory, 7*(1), 14–25.

Brazil. (de 7 de dezembro de 1993). Law nº 8.742. Retrieved January 15, 2019, from www2.camara.leg.br/legin/fed/lei/1993/lei-8742-7-dezembro-1993-363163-publicacaooriginal-1-pl.html

Castel, R. (1994). Da indigência à exclusão, à desfiliação. Cap. 4: Precariedade do trabalho e vulnerabilidade relacional [Chapter 4: From indigence to exclusion, to disaffiliation. Precarious work and relational vulnerability]. In A. Lancetti (Ed.), *SaúdeLoucura* [HealthMadness] (pp. 21–48). São Paulo: Hucitec.

Castel, R. (2003). *From manual workers to wage laborers: Transformation of the social question.* New York, NY: Routledge.

Duncan, M., Buchanan, H., & Lorenzo, T. (2005). Chapter 29: Politics in occupational therapy education. In F. Kronenberg, S. S. Algado, & N. Pollard (Eds.), *Occupational therapy without borders – Learning from the spirit of survivors* (pp. 390–401). London: Elsevier Churchill Livingstone.

Ferreira, A. B. H. (1999). *Novo Aurélio Século XXI: o dicionário da língua portuguesa* [New aurelio XXI century: The dictionary of Portuguese language]. Rio de Janeiro: Editora Nova Fronteira.

Francisco, B. (1988). *Terapia Ocupacional* [Occupational therapy]. Campinas: Papirus.

Galheigo, S. M. (1981). Terapia Ocupacional Social [Social occupational therapy]. In UFsCar. Terapia Ocupacional Social: *filosofia, definição e campos de atuação* [Social occupational therapy: Philosophy, definition and fields of action] [Original archive document]. Second Scientific Occupational Therapy Week. São Carlos: UFSCar.

Galheigo, S. M. (1988). *Terapia Ocupacional: a Produção do Conhecimento e o Cotidiano da Prática sob o Poder Disciplinar- em Busca de um Depoimento Coletivo* [Occupational therapy: Knowledge production and the practice everyday life: In search of a collective testimony] (Master's dissertation). Campinas, SP, Brazil: Faculty of Education, State University of Campinas.

Galheigo, S. M. (1996). *Juvenile policy-making, social control and the state in Brazil: A study of laws and policies from 1964 to*

1990 (PhD thesis). Falmer, UK: School of Social Sciences, University of Sussex.

Galheigo, S. M. (1997). Da Adaptação Psicosocial à Construção do Coletivo: a Cidadania enquanto Eixo [From psychosocial adaptation to construction of a collective society citizenship as basis]. *Revista de Ciências Médicas Puccamp, 6*(2/3), 105–108.

Galheigo, S. M. (1999). A transdisciplinaridade enquanto princípio e realidade das ações de saúde [Transdisciplinarity as a principle and reality of health practices]. *Revista de Terapia Ocupacional da USP, 10*(2/3), 49–54.

Galheigo, S. M. (2003). Cap. 2: O social: idas e vindas de um campo de ação em terapia ocupacional [Chapter 2: The social: Comings and goings of a field of action in occupational therapy]. In E. M. Pádua & L. Magalhães (Eds.), *Terapia ocupacional, teoria e prática* [Occupational therapy, theory and practice] (pp. 29–48). Campinas: Papirus.

Galheigo, S. M. (2005). Chapter 7: Occupational therapy and the social field: Clarifying concepts and ideas. In F. Kronenberg, S. S. Algado, & N. Pollard (Eds.), *Occupational therapy without borders – Learning from the spirit of survivors* (pp. 87–98). London: Elsevier Churchill Livingstone.

Galheigo, S. M. (2011a). Chapter 6: Concepts and critical considerations for occupational therapy in the social field. In F. Kronemberg, N. Pollard, & D. Sakellariou (Eds.), *Occupational therapies without borders* (Vol. II): *Towards and ecology of occupation-based practices* (pp. 47–56). Edinburgh: Churchill Livingstone/Elsevier.

Galheigo, S. M. (2011b). What needs to be done? Occupational therapy responsibilities and challenges regarding human rights. *Australian Occupational Therapy Journal, 58*, 60–66. doi:10.1111/j.1440-1630.2011.00922.x

Galheigo, S. M. (2012). Perspectiva crítica y compleja de terapia ocupacional: actividad, cotidiano, diversidad, justicia social y compromiso ético-político [Towards a critical and complex perspective for occupational therapy: Activity, daily life, diversity, social justice and ethical-political commitment]. *TOG (A Coruña), 5*, 176–187.

Galvaan, R., Galheigo, S. M., & Saha, S. (2013). *Educating for change: Occupational therapy experiences across three countries* [Research project]. Cape Town: University of Cape Town.

Guajardo, A. (2012). Enfoque e práxis en terapia ocupacional. Reflexiones desde una perspectiva de la terapia ocupacional crítica [Approach and praxis in occupational therapy. Thoughts from a critical perspective of occupational therapy]. *TOG (A Coruña), 5*, 176–187.

Hagedorn, R. (1997). *Foundations for practice in occupational therapy.* New York, NY: Churchil Livingstone.

Kronenberg, F., Algado, S., & Pollard, N. (Eds.). (2005). *Occupational therapy without borders – Learning from the spirit of survivors.* London: Elsevier Churchill Livingstone.

Kronenberg, F., Pollard, N., & Sakellariou, D. (Eds.). (2011). *Occupational therapies without borders* (Vol. II): *Towards and*

ecology of occupation-based practices. Edinburgh: Churchill Livingstone/Elsevier.

Leminsky, P. (2013). *Toda Poesia/Paulo Leminsky* [All poetry/Paulo Leminsky]. São Paulo: Companhia das Letras.

Lopes, R. E, Borba, P. L. O., Silva, C. R., & Malfitano, A. P. S. (2012). Terapia Ocupacional no campo social no Brasil e na América Latina: panorama, tensões e reflexões a partir de práticas profissionais [The social field of occupational therapy in Brazil and Latin America: Overview, tensions and reflections from professional]. *Cadernos de Terapia Ocupacional da UFSCar, 20*(1), 21–32.

Lorenzo, M., Duncan, M., Buchanan, H., & Alsop, A. (Eds.). (2006). *Practice and service learning in occupational therapy.* Hoboken: John Wiley & Sons.

Malfitano, A. P. S. (2005). Campos e núcleos de intervenção na terapia ocupacional social [Intervention fields and cores in social occupational therapy]. *Revista de Terapia Ocupacional da USP, 16*(1), 1–8.

Midgley, J. (1981). *Professional imperialism: Social work in the third world.* London: Heinemann.

Parsons, T. (1991). *The social system.* London: Routledge.

Pinto, J. (1979). Relato de uma experiência de Terapia Ocupacional no campo social [Report of an occupational therapy experience in the social field]. In *V Encontro Científico Paulista de Terapeutas Ocupacionais* [Fifth São Paulo Scientific Meeting of Occupational Therapists]. São Paulo, Brazil.

Pinto, J. (1990). *As Correntes Metodológicas em Terapia Ocupacional no Estado de São Paulo (1970–1985)* [The methodological currents in occupational therapy in the state of São Paulo (1970–1985)] (Master's dissertation). Faculty of Education, Federal University of São Carlos. São Paulo, Brazil.

Santos, B. S. (2012). *Introdução a uma ciência pós-moderna* [Introduction to postmodern Science]. Rio de Janeiro: Graal.

Santos, B. S., & Meneses, M. P. (2010). *Epistemologias do Sul* [Epistemologies of the South]. São Paulo: Cortez Editora.

Soares, L. B. T. (1991). *Terapia Ocupacional: lógica do capital ou do trabalho?* [Occupational therapy: Logic of capital or labor?]. São Paulo: Editora Hucitec.

Squires, P. (1990). *Anti-social policy: Welfare, ideology and the disciplinary state.* London: Harvester Wheatsheaf.

Trujillo, A. R., Camacho, L. S., Ferrer, L. C., Esquivel, E. P., Vizcaya, S. R., Sarmiento, J. U., et al. (2011). *Ocupación: sentido, realización y libertad* [Occupation, meaning, realization and freedom]. Bogotá: Universidad Nacional de Colombia.

Trujillo, A. R., Torres, M. C., Méndez, J. M., & Carrizosa, L. F. (2011). *Terapia Ocupacional: conocimiento y compromiso social* [Occupational therapy: Knowledge and social commitment]. Bogotá: Universidad Nacional de Colombia.

Turner, B. (1991). Preface to new edition. In T. Parsons (Ed.), *The social system* (pp. xviii–xlv). London: Routledge.

Watson, R., & Swartz, L. (2004). *Transformation through occupation.* London: Whurr Publishers.

3

Occupational Therapy and Socioeconomic Processes

Maria Izabel Garcez Ghirardi, Ana Paula Serrata Malfitano,
Roseli Esquerdo Lopes

INTRODUCTION

When it comes to consolidating courses of social participation in scenarios that make up the landscape of the working world, socioeconomic processes articulate the encounter between occupational therapy and daily life activities. This chapter intends to discuss some forms of these encounters, based on the premise that the world of work and the world of assistance materialize in different places, at their own times, unyielding between themselves. However, with reference to occupational therapy, there are possible synergies that establish different ties of sociability among the assistance recipients.

The Social Question and Occupational Therapy

One of the purposes of occupational therapy is to intensify conditions of social integration and democratic participation. This requires professional care that comprises a set of professional, political, and ethical actions that translate into complex social interventions, such as interventions directed at resolving suffering and daily seclusion, which result in the deterioration of social ties and individuals' marginalization.

Often social ties weaken due to the restricted access to employment resulting from processes of economic globalization, which, since the second half of the 20th century, defined new concepts with reference to the old *social question* (Castel, 2003). Historically, the concept of the *social question* has been dependent on the popular reaction of denouncing the exploitation of the labor force in the industrialization process and the liberal capitalism that emerged in 19th-century Europe (Ferreira, 2008). In Brazil, the *social question* deepened with salaried employment and the exploitation of the labor force that was required for the capitalist reproduction of the coffee industry, and the

demand for rehabilitation services formed the basis of the need to restore and maintain the workforce available to that market (Soares, 1991).

Occupational therapy was a component of those rehabilitation services and began to be used to reduce the damage caused by the capitalist mode of production. However, dealing with the social question from a clinical perspective of health overlooks the causal relationship between damage to workers' health and the social question.

Thus, the issues of the world of work were integrated into the field of rehabilitation and, more specifically, into occupational therapy by the health – disease matrix and by an intersubjective therapeutic relationship. This reduced the social question to a binary conformation in the exclusion-inclusion syntax. With reference to its current globalized form, this social question keeps alive the dispute on the liberal contradiction that intends to individualize social problems and thus destroy bonds of trust that create social cohesion (de Leonardis, 1998).

It is important to emphasize that the transposition of the health care model to the field of social care resulted in a paradox in the practice of occupational therapy, since this practice tended to imprison the minds of social participation in an individualized and culturally decontextualized relationship, insofar as it isolated the complexity of insertion in daily life, leaving it out of the clinical environment (Barros, Ghirardi, & Lopes, 2005). In a certain way, this movement of the transposition of the clinical model to address social phenomena produced a *disconnect* in professional practice, a specialization of knowledge in rehabilitation that contributed to the *capture of individual experience* of those for whom this practice was intended. This specialization of knowledge that produces the *capture of individual experience* when dealing with social phenomena operates a typical specialist disjunction of modernity and allows rehabilitation actions to be circumscribed to the health universe, limiting the conditions of the understanding of social determinants of participation in social life (Giddens, 1990).

In Brazil, at the beginning of the 1980s, a movement of critical formulation of the profession sought to analyze social phenomena in the context of occupational therapy and resize the ethical and political aspects of the profession. This point had been overshadowed by discussions around instruments, techniques, and clinical procedures of the biomedical model (Barros et al., 2005). However, despite every effort to defuse this contradiction, there is still a tension between paradigms in occupational therapy. Particularly, with regard to the world of work, there is a simultaneity of practices, incompatible among themselves, that operate, sustained by the discourse of citizenship and social inclusion. Hence, interventions in *workshops, cooperatives,* and *job support,* among other designations of technical-social instruments, are operated in the field of rehabilitation and occupational therapy, sustained by the discourse of social inclusion and the proposals of varied clinical settings, which do not provide an account of the complexity of the phenomena that make up what is recognized as a *social question.*

Reflecting the *social question* and, more than that, proposing practices in occupational therapy that address this question depend on unique conditions of intervention, which demand different methodological procedures and courses of action, conditioned by the capacity to analyze and to interfere in social phenomena whose nature is irreducible to the isolated individual fact. These conditions have been pursued in the field of social occupational therapy based on the proposal of interventions guided by humanities and social sciences, which are outlined by means of solid field analyses (Cefaï, 2006). We intend, therefore, to compose collective actions aimed at creating conditions for democratic intensification and social integration as a response to the ailments exposed by the fraying social fabric, which also derives from the processes of economic globalization.

Economic-Social Processes and Occupational Therapy

The proposal in this chapter is to highlight the socioeconomic processes that interfere in the panorama of occupational therapy actions aimed at creating conditions to overcome, at least in part, the *capture of experience* to which some practices of rehabilitation contribute. These practices tend to insulate the intrinsic sociological complexity in the world of work by reducing it to a type of panacea for the social problems, which would be overcome in rehabilitation

processes oriented toward productive action with an inclusive profile. The unveiling of the reductionism covered by rehabilitation actions in the field of health care, directed by the proposal of inclusion in the world of work, is a condition for discussing the possible technical deeds in the context of economic and social complexity under which any form of work falls.

By wishing to contribute to the intensification of democratic participation in the world of work, occupational therapy should consider the complexity of collective and social dimensions that such participation involves. To plan action strategies that contribute to tackling the social question (i.e., to reverse situations of isolation, vulnerability, and the weakening of social bonds), social occupational therapy seeks to create social intervention methodologies that strengthen the conditions necessary for participatory paths guided by creative capability and collective self-organization. In other words, occupational therapy undertakes the social object of action, proposing strategies for the facilitation of participatory paths, which, if successful, should create the conditions for an individual to overcome the status of a recipient of assistance services and proceed toward the status of a producer of social goods and services.

Thus, when the authors of this chapter intend to understand the complexity of a social phenomenon, the care context is necessarily a hybrid place in which one produces social value from the creation of bonds of trust and there is a decrease of uncertainty and mistrust in oneself and in others. It is a place in which one avoids negative discrimination based on physical, psychological, or social exceptions and which moves from the universe of the exception of individual conditions to the universe of communities of collective doing, organized in projects that allow an opening up to the perception and valuing of the exchange of knowledge that potentiates a community of doing. Therefore, the development of tools that forge common places in the midst of exceptional situations is a prerequisite to any practice of occupational therapy that aims to engage in social care.

The economic theory developed by Amartya Sen (1992) is a theoretical framework that allows one to observe and activate organizational resources that can be used effectively in favor of a social valorization. This economic theory proposes to operate from the granting of credit and recognition of individual capabilities to create the necessary conditions for those capabilities to operate in the production of values of use and social exchange (Mozzana, 2008). Put another way, it opens up the possibility of moving from one place to another or from a fixed place of exception and of guardianship to transitional, common places, in multiple shared production networks, based on the power of collective capabilities and possibilities

(Sen, 2006). This interpretative key can assist the occupational therapy field when it comes to dealing with economic issues linked to the production of social value and to participation in the world of work, taking into consideration the complexity of social phenomena that anchor the whole mode of material production.

Economic production presupposes confidence in oneself and in others. Trust is therefore a valuable social value that is not always available among the situations occupational therapy deals with. Addressing work with reference to occupational therapy in economic and social processes presupposes that work is central in what is known as the social question and acknowledges that it is important to consider ways to connect the world of assistance to the world of production, thus avoiding welfarism and the fetishization of income. Thus, the rationale that one should follow economic-social processes in occupational therapy in economic-social processes is this analytical displacement in which collective and common dimensions are prioritized, which is in detriment to the individual clinical relationship and the particularist dimension of action or doing. This idea is supported by the horizontality of care, with places in which the common doing gains power. In contrast, it is avoiding the maintenance of interventions sustained by the verticality of places of care in which the exceptionality of individual situations is addressed by health in a clinical perspective (de Leonardis, 2008).

Work is a collective right, not a special need. Thus, the interventions of occupational therapy in socioeconomic processes propose the observation of the collective place of work, understanding its dimensions and relations of knowledge and power, the contradictions and social determinations that are established in the process of the organization of work, and the everyday context of collective production. Exercising the right to work is therefore a collective challenge, especially when the indices of disengagement and flexibility, added to the globalized forms of work organization, transform this right into a privilege; it is necessary to invest in collective actions that allow the redrawing of the valuing pathways of the capabilities of the many people excluded from the productive market. When addressing socioeconomic processes, occupational therapy considers that a collective of production is not a place where people meet to discuss their individual problems and seek support to face them; it is the opposite and refers to the ability to, for example, generate income and overcome economic misery. A collective of production is a place in which common reflexivity may be enabled and a social condition can be criticized and eventually overcome in the encounter of collective solutions that escape the liberal and individualistic logic of economic production.

When addressing the economic-social aspects of *doing* within the context of a less personalist and more systemic vision, it is possible to find similarities in *doing* that overcome any differences in the modes of *being*, especially considering that poverty does not designate an individual condition but is instead a collective and complex position of specific sections of the population. The approach of occupational therapy cannot maintain a posture alien to the social question, remaining in a universe of actions bounded by groups of individuals recognized by their particularities of paths, as if the lack of economic resources was due to an individual failing of any order, and likely to be treated in the universe of the rehabilitation actions that understand work as a factor of social inclusion.

Occupational therapy, proposed with a focus on socioeconomic processes, considers collective positivity instead of individual negativity, observes affinities of capabilities in place of exclusivity of limitations, and operates considering the systematics of doing and of social organization around doing that are needed for the collective economy. This approach emphasizes the public and common sphere, the collective dimension of everyday social life that occurs in the encounter between differences in various orders—gender, class, and culture, among many others—and that determine variations in the way of being and of creating worlds. Occupational therapy is interested at this time in the multiplicities and the singular conditions that lead to the creation of places of encounter and exchanges, sustained by the diversity of doings and forms of production. It is possible, then, to establish another syntax to expand the professional image to discuss the collective occupations in public places, in a pragmatic shift that brings into play what is common in social phenomena.

Social issues are irreducible to forms of therapeutic or clinical relations (with specific groups or individuals); therefore, the challenge is to enable the encounter of radical differences in the process of the production of goods and of social values, without wishing to adapt either of them to pre-established conditions. It is not, therefore, the learning of techniques or relations of production that ensures the inclusion of people who do not have this right assured in the labor market; rather, it is proposing alternatives to the production of added social value to material production. However, it is not compromised by the pacifying logic and conformist relations of guardianship.

It is important to remember that participation in the world of work, in whatever form, does not refer to health contexts, rehabilitation processes, or equipment, since work is not an inclusive therapy, but a collective social right shared between actors of equal social conditions. The social place of work cannot be reduced to a space shared by subjects in the processes of recovery from individual ills.

The workplace, conquered through the struggle of many workers, is a place inhabited by people with limitations and possibilities that complement one another in everyday action, which unfolds through flashes of being with others. The workplace is therefore a common and temporary place in the cultural universe of exchanges of symbolic values in which people come and go, searching, with diverse stories that weave new social bonds daily. Experimentation, on the border between provision of care and economic production, shows the feasibility of promoting social participation from real contexts of work by means of strategic pathways that result in a scenario of improving conditions of social justice (Vitale, 2005).

As Hammel and Iwama (2012, p. 386) affirm, "occupational therapy is clearly concerned with the conditions that enable or constrain actions, and particularly with doing," and consequently we should be focused on rights and social conditions, but "much of the occupational therapy theoretical literature focuses predominantly on individual issues" (p. 388).

Therefore, it would be naive to think that occupational therapy can contribute to *the generation of income* in economically marginal populations. Generating income is not the same as the allocation of technical care actions, nor is it a sufficient condition for the transformation of social relations. An occupational therapy intervention can, at most, contribute to the generation of social value to the extent that it manages to establish collective dynamics conducive to common reflexivity, from redemption of confidence in oneself and in others to the appreciation of the collective know-how. The *reconnect* that stems from this reflexive activation enables the subversion, through shared doing, of the alienating inertia that intends to define income as a value in itself.

Assuming income as a value in itself is the basis of the various social welfare programs that operate the logic of *should be* to *can do*; that is, the possibility of access to work and income depends on the acceptance of a place of assistance and, with that, of institutional guardianship by the institution that shapes the forms of sociability through the fetishization of income (de Leonardis, 2004). Thus, it is important that occupational therapy finds courses of action that, guided by collective doing, recognize the rights and voices of the recipients of professional actions and promote the visibility of their participation in the activation of individual capabilities in the context of collective production. The course of actions involves creating places that facilitate interactions and confidence. It requires places that overcome practices that understand work as a form of rehabilitation and that desire productive meetings, which, by means of public action that is guided by the logic of negotiation rather than hierarchical logic, render the

displacement of the status of a recipient of assistance actions to the status of a producer of social goods and services (Mozzana, 2008).

The Italian paradigm of social enterprise is another theoretical framework that can provide tools for the systematization of a methodological approach of socioeconomic issues in occupational therapy. This focuses on the communicative action, on individual and collective skills producing their own solutions to everyday problems. It is guided by the organization of services that they use to produce goods, adding social value by investing in the productive capabilities of human capital, and valuing the collective path of economic production as a way to overcome individual limitations of social participation. In spite of the cultural differences between the European and South American contexts, it is believed that this paradigm is an innovation in the field of assistance because it proposes courses of participation that seek to move from the dependent condition of assistance servicing to a position of a producer of social goods and services (de Leonardis, Mauri, & Rotelli, 1994). Thus, the epistemological assumptions that consider the economic-social dimensions of interventions in occupational therapy unveil elements in a field of reflection and research. These assumptions are concerned with investment in the capacity of collective self-organization and in individual creativity to define participatory work pathways that establish conditions of displacement from the position of simple recipients of actions of assistance. Additionally, this would help us proceed toward the position of the producer of social goods and social values.

A Possible Encounter Between Occupational Therapy and Economic-Social Processes

As an example of what has been outlined previously, the following presents a brief report of a case that articulated the field of occupational therapy in an encounter with economic-social processes. This case followed the everyday lives of people in a care project that aimed to generate income for the homeless population. A goal was to create conditions for sociocultural transformation and the intensification of democratic participation on the margins of the socioeconomic welfare system, considering the contradictions concerning care limits when it comes to investing in the social participation of economically marginal populations (Malfitano, Lopes, Magalhães, & Townsend, 2014). This section entails examples from a report based on past studies.

A nongovernmental organization (NGO) oriented toward providing assistance to the homeless population in Brazil produces a street magazine that has the dual purpose of being a vehicle of social communication and, at the same time, constituting an alternative project of generating income for the homeless population. To achieve this goal, the NGO proposes that the sale of copies of the magazine will be carried out exclusively by homeless persons, resulting in a joint venture in the context of urban movements with global bindings that characterize a new global political economy (Appadurai, 2002). Therefore, the magazine would be an instrumental aspect of an occupational course par excellence, aimed at strengthening social ties and creating the conditions for the homeless to migrate from a place of dependence, tied to care services, to a place of autonomy in the management of their own life. The magazine may be classified as a socioeconomic strategy since it intends to contribute to the rehabilitation of an economically and socially stigmatized, marginalized population.

Undertaking an economic activity and offering a cultural product in the information and communication market requires investment in human resources and in conditions of cooperation between all those involved in the joint venture (Sennett, 2012). In this case, a larger part of these resources is composed of homeless persons, whose workforce and *labor* are socially and technically not adequately qualified. Consequently, they are also recipients of care services. Notwithstanding the proposal, it was observed that the adherence of the homeless population to the magazine sales project was not accomplished. This led to the implementation of occupational therapy in an intervention project, based on the assumption that the search to understand the resources and the difficulties surrounding occupations of daily life is an integral part of the occupational therapy practice, an approach that avoids diagnosing and instead intends to consider the various occupations that shape individuals (Piergrossi, 2006).

The methodological approach that guided this intervention was based on the Italian methodology of social enterprising (de Leonardis et al., 1994) and the economic theory of capabilities approach (Sen, 1992). The aim was to delineate a course of intervention that permitted the displacement of deeds to migrate from occupational rehabilitation with a focus on subjectivity to a perspective of community of deeds with a focus on public and collective action. The matrix of research-action enabled the approach of institutional cognitive organization and the conditions of expression of the target population in a hybrid context, whose operation was unveiled by means of dense observation and description in a form of pragmatic ethnography (Cefaï, 2006). From the point of view of occupational therapy intervention, we sought to encourage the creation of bonds of trust and the decrease of uncertainty and mistrust in oneself and in others through a common doing mediated by economic production. It also sought to enable organizational resources so that their effective use favored the projects of the target population.

The intervention started from the approach of an occupational social phenomenon (i.e., the low adherence to the magazine sales project) through the observation of care actions that were involved in this project, as a way of avoiding approximation with an individual focus and relational character inappropriate to studies in the social field. The intervention also aimed to experiment to create an approach that would avoid the perspective of individual action and, at the same time, bring elements of complexity to the observation of the collective *doing*, based on the theoretical framework of the social, economic, and work field. This approach facilitated the outline of an initial picture of the socioeconomic context of the population with potential for adherence to the sales project, as well as the organization of care actions. Thus, the magazine—its organization and operation, its production, and its divulgation policy—featured the observation of the common doing and of creating collective action in its production and sales, in detriment to listening to the unique demands of each person, in order to value the sales organization and the sociability of the active and potential sellers.

The intervention was based on the shared doing and its analysis, taking into account the conditions peculiar to that population facing the production process. The intervention was intended to create a reflexive environment through an initial observation directed toward daily sociability, which grew around the assistance proposed based on an economic deed and avoided the interpretation guided by individual signals or *symptoms*. A delicate approach was pursued by means of observation and description of the field through incursions to the various places where the production and the dissemination of the magazine occurred and concurrently with an analysis of the workplace responsible for the reception of sellers and the mapping of the assistance facilities of the central region of the municipality. The publicization actions of the magazine sales project and awareness of potential sellers were followed, and the actions that organized the sales taskforce of the magazine at public events were monitored. The observation and analysis of these various field elements enabled the identification of relevant aspects of the cognitive organization of NGOs through the analysis of vocabulary, institutional grammar, and organizational practice.

The process of occupational therapy intervention that stemmed from preliminary observations was guided by the organizational capabilities imposed and the conditions of expression (voice capacity) of the target population in the decision-making process regarding magazine design and sales strategy development. The contact with active sellers put into motion a form of activation and visibility of the *place of sales*, contrary to what was proposed, which until then was the visibility of the *seller* and his or her access to care. This displacement wished to forsake the personalist logic of the assistance of care and establish, starting with weekly meetings, a scenario in which it was possible to get closer to the sales project of the magazine.

As such, these meetings, which came to be known as the sales meetings, created a valuation environment of the participants' occupational backgrounds and the recognition that their experiences could enable recovery pathways from a place of productive social insertion from their own occupational skills and not just the institutional expectations. Thus, these weekly sales meetings, which lasted 2 hours each week, were formulated and led to strategies of activation of collective ability, focusing on the complexity of the sales exercise, as well as the necessary conditions to occupy the place of the seller of a cultural product.

The sales meetings focused on collective ability and collaborative action to encourage the strategies of approximation with the occupation of magazine sales. They were, in practice, stages of conversations whose emerging themes included conditions of collective production, of production and sales strategies, of difficulties, and of institutional obstacles that hindered adherence to the magazine sales project. The consolidation of the sales meetings was not always able to count on the mobilization of active sellers, who complained of excessive debates proposed by the institution and, until then, of their own suggestions having limited repercussions for the institutional dynamics. This was an interesting strategy to leverage the voice and participation of the homeless population in the magazine project and to create conditions of collective reflexivity in relation to the care project. This point was important for the intermediate conflicts that occurred during the sales meetings, since some arose out of a conception that the occupation of the seller was eminently of an individual and competitive character, which meant that the *point of sale*[1] became, in a sense, the owner of its seller, evidencing a logic sustained by the design of a liberal market. The logic of possession was contrasted by the logic of the shared use of points of sale, suggesting that a point of sale does not result from the isolated capacity of a seller, nor is it restricted to a defined geographical area, but rather is the sum of variables such as geographical location, frequency of the seller's presence, and nearby cultural events, among other factors. The discussion was guided toward natural elements that constitute the *place* of sales and the conditions for building a shared place that is recognized by the consumer as a *place of sales*. That is, we sought to

transition from a position in which the individual conferred value to a *point of sale* that became a kind of individual and fixed property, a kind of showcase for the seller constituted a priori, to discuss the *place of sale* as a transient condition settled in common agreement, a collective configuration built by the know-how of various sellers. This strategy was proposed to create the activation of collective reflexivity in the displacement of occupational therapy action so as to migrate from an approach of the meritocratic doings of an individual and the rehabilitative perspective to an approach of collective action in the organizational qualification of a community of doings.

During the year in which the sales meetings were conducted, various suggestions emerged on the management of the NGOs' assistance projects. The participants suggested, for example, that in events oriented toward the dissemination of magazine sales, the expression "sales representative" be used instead of "seller." According to the opinion of the participants, being identified as representatives of the magazine confers value on the sales activity, whereas being identified as a seller deferred them to a place of dependence of care, as the magazine is recognized for its purpose of generating income. It was possible, on the other hand, to understand that the existence of the magazine depended on adherence to the sales project, without which the institution of assistance has no visibility, and not just conversely, as propagated by the care team, making us believe that salespeople are the sole beneficiaries of the magazine sales. It was identified that the magazine also depends on the sales performed by the homeless, which it depends on to define its identity as an organization. The aim was to outline an occupational therapy pathway that activated the collective reflexivity when considering the power of the capacities of choice and collective action and to observe the modalities of organizational logic and practices that can make dependence on the system chronic.

On the other hand, examining the demands of the population that arrives at the organization's port of entry allowed for identifying strategies for institutional opening for those interested in knowing and trying the magazine sales project. In general, the requests that appeared at the institutional reception evidenced the dependence on assistance services of those who presented there. Whoever arrives seeks recognition of their own needs and immediate solutions for them in an attempt to *capitalize* on the assisted condition.

The approach of capabilities sought to establish a transition from the condition of being assisted to that of being a producer, constituting a middle layer in the process of approximation of the *place* of sales—the seller in

---

[1]Point of sale is how we denominate defined locations and times determined in the streets of the city in which a seller offers copies of the magazine.

training—which tended to minimize the fear of not being able to perform sales. Finally, it is important to consider that the freedom to participate in economic exchange has a fundamental role in collective life (Sen, 1992) and that occupational therapy can offer various forms of benefits when it comes to dealing with economic-social issues.

What has been reported here is one of these possible ways of conferring positivity onto collective production to intensify social participation and to enable confidence in oneself and others by means of constructing a place of collective belonging that values the individual's know-how regarding economically relevant production in the market of cultural goods and services.

REFERENCES

Appadurai, A. (2002). Deep democracy: Urban governmentality and the horizon of politics. *Public Culture, 14*(1), 21–47. doi:10.1215/08992363-14-1-21

Barros, D. D., Ghirardi, M. I. G., & Lopes, R. E. (2005). Social occupational therapy: A socio-historical perspective. In F. Kronenberg, S. S Algado, & N. Pollard (Eds.), *Occupational therapy without borders: Learning from the spirit of survivors* (pp. 140–151). London: Elsevier Science Ltd – Churchill Livingstone.

Castel, R. (2003). *From manual workers to wage laborers: Transformation of the social question* (R. Boyed, Ed. & Trans.). New York, NY: Routledge.

Cefaï, D. (2006). Due o tre cosette sulle associazioni . . . Fare ricerca su contesti ibridi e ambigui [Two or three little things about associations . . . Doing research on hybrid and ambiguous contexts]. *Rivista delle Politiche Sociali, 3*, 201–217.

de Leonardis, O. (1998). *In un Diverso Welfare. Sogni e Incubi* [In a different welfare. Dreams and nightmares]. Milano: Feltrinelli.

de Leonardis, O. (2004). *Le Istituzioni. Come e Perché Parlarne* [The institutions. How and why talk about it] (2nd ed.). Roma: Carocci.

de Leonardis, O. (2008). Da luoghi di cura allacura dei luoghi [From places of care to the safety of places]. *Animazione Sociale, 226*, 3–11.

de Leonardis, O., Mauri, D., & Rotelli, F. (1994). *L'impresa Sociale* [The social enterprise]. Milano: Ed. Anabasi.

Ferreira, S. (2008). A questão social e as alternativas da sociedade civil no contexto das novas formas de governação [The social question and civil society alternatives in the context of new governance forms]. *Ciências Sociais Unisinos, 44*, 28–38.

Giddens, A. (1990). *The consequences of modernity*. Palo Alto, CA: Stanford University Press.

Hammell, K. R., & Iwama, M. K. (2011). Well-being and occupational rights: An imperative for critical occupational therapy. *Scandinavian Journal of Occupational Therapy, 19*(5), 385–394. doi:10.3109/11038128.2011.611821

Malfitano, A. P. S., Lopes, R. E., Magalhães, L., & Townsend, E. A. (2014). Social occupational therapy. *Canadian Journal of Occupational Therapy, 81*(5), 298–307. doi:10.1177/0008417414536712

Mozzana, C. (2008). I servizi a servizio delle capacità delle persone. Capacità personali e capacità istituzionali nei percorsi verso l'autonomia [Services at the service of people's abilities. Personal skills and institutional capacities in the paths towards autonomy]. *Animazione Sociale, 37*, 14–22.

Piergrossi, J. C. (2006). *Essere Nel Fare. Introduzione Alla Terapia Occupazionale* [Being in doing. Introduction to occupational therapy]. Milano: Franco Angeli.

Sen, A. (1992). *Inequality reexamined*. Oxford: Clarendon Press.

Sen, A. (2006). *Identity and violence: The illusion of destiny*. New York, NY: Norton & Company.

Sennett, R. (2012). *Together: The rituals, pleasures and politics of co-operation*. New Haven, CT: Yale University Press.

Soares, L. B. T. (1991). *Terapia Ocupacional: Lógica do Capital ou do Trabalho? Retrospectiva Histórica da Profissão no Estado Brasileiro de 1950 a 1980* [Occupational therapy: Logic of capital or work? Historical retrospective of the profession in Brazil from 1950 to 1980]. São Paulo, Brazil: Hucitec.

Vitale, T. (2005). *Contradiction and reflexivity in social innovation. A case study from the deinstitutionalisation movement*. European Urban and Regional Studies. Social Innovation, Governance and Community Building. Oxford: Oxford University Press.

4

Occupational Therapy: Social, Cultural? Diverse and Multiple![1]

Denise Dias Barros and Debora Galvani

MULTIPLE PERSPECTIVES ON THE INTERPRETATION OF REALITY: CHALLENGES

In this chapter, we address the need to construct methodologies of action for social occupational therapy. Social occupational therapy practice calls for constant questioning about the space occupied by practitioners and the nature of their action. It demands reflexive action in the midst of interpretations that are in dialogue; thus, social occupational therapy assumes a hermeneutic that is also characteristic of interpretative anthropology (Geertz, 1989), which is a highly narrative form of description in which cultural realities are inscribed by the researcher in texts that attempt to capture the layered meanings and nuances of lived experience. Because of their rich or "thick" descriptiveness, these texts then require careful interpretative engagement by readers and become understandable through multiple readings and intertextual perspectives. Interpretation must be present in ethnographic work. Potential conflicts and alignments of interpretation are always present in ethnographic work, since the researcher has a position in relation to social groups, communities, and the personal trajectories of specific individuals described through the research. Therefore, multiple perspectives occur and need to be assessed both during fieldwork and in the analysis process. This same plurality of perspectives also needs to be analyzed during the construction of social actions and technologies in social occupational therapy.

Since 1998, the Metuia Project (Barros, Lopes, Galheigo, & Galvani, 2011), conducted by a group of university academics in occupational therapy who have been developing actions, research, and teaching, has been engaged in a collective effort to construct experiences in social occupational therapy in dialogue with the problems of populations that, for social, cultural, and historical reasons, find themselves disconnected from social and affective support networks. The Metuia Project therefore provides an opportunity to reflect on the profession's role relating to the social and cultural dynamics of situations and spaces in which people experience inequality and disqualification of identities (Barros, Ghirardi, & Lopes, 1999). The Metuia Project further aims to develop approaches for action by social occupational therapists that can meet the theoretical, technological, and methodological challenges in such situations or spaces. Thus, social occupational therapists working in this manner have had to make theoretical and practical choices for each new project, drawing on a dense archive of experiences and reflections relating to social and cultural matters in a range of settings and situations: urban, rural, and peripheral, with various sectors of society in Brazil and in Africa.

With the reflections in this chapter, we intend to revisit the aspects of this work associated with the practices of university research and activities of teaching and extension work (i.e., partnerships between the university and communities). We will do so by selecting emblematic situations for description and analysis in terms of social occupational therapy's key concepts and methods (Barros, 2004; Barros et al., 1999; Barros, Lopes, & Ghirardi, 2002; Barros, Almeida, & Vecchia, 2007). Emphasis is placed on the experiences and strengths that ethnography brings to our work and its processes.

The term "ethnography," an anthropological method based on prolonged immersion in a culture and rich narrative description, can be translated as "writing about a culture" (Atkinson, 1992). Understanding that there are multiple ways of seeing culture informs the attention that professionals need to take when they are working in the social field, where the actions they take as practitioners

---

[1] We are grateful to all the people mentioned in this study, with whom we have shared discussions, ideas, experiences, and productions and have learned together.

must be carefully designed to fit specific situations and contexts. Since the beginning of the 21st century, we have developed this approach by engaging in dialogue with those for—and with whom—we anticipate that our actions and activities can help to expand or even guarantee possibilities of social and educational life, support aesthetic and cultural expression, and strengthen social development and rights among socially and culturally diverse groups. We initially began this undertaking while working with children and adolescents, later expanding to work with adult street people. These practice-related encounters included discussions about housing, quality of life, and community action in both urban and rural environments.

This chapter, then, concerns our university research and the extension of social occupational therapy in projects we developed in the states of Sao Paulo and Minas Gerais, Brazil, as well as in the Dogon Country of Mali, West Africa. It is important to keep in mind that the projects

in Brazil and Mali were developed also to provide opportunities for undergraduate and graduate students in the Metuia Project of the University of São Paulo (USP). Thus, in the selected ethnographic descriptions from our work in social occupational therapy in Sao Paulo, we highlight the theoretical, political, social, cultural, practical, and educational dimensions of life on the streets and in activities associated with the Casa das Áfricas community center. Finally, we touch on public policies related to social assistance, culture, human rights, and migration.

The Streets Open to Our Inquiries about Occupational Therapy

Our first contacts with social groups—including the so-called street people in the city of Sao Paulo—were rooted in the need to cross borders and break down mutual misunderstandings. The narrative in Box 4.1 reconstructs one of our initial visits to the group's spaces of everyday living, such as

---

BOX 4.1   Preliminary Approaches[3]

It was a scene of devastation, as in a science fiction movie based on pessimistic global predictions about there being no more water for everyone, machines controlling the world, or monkeys dominating humans. In this case, the mice reign. As a man living under the viaduct said: "Rats are more organized than men!" One sleepless night, he could observe their routine of leaving and bringing food to their shelter!

The Minha Rua, Minha Casa Association (AMRMC) is located under this viaduct. On top of it: traffic, speed, passage. Under it: the street and the home of few people, undoubtedly a borderline place. AMRMC appropriates a public space (the area under the viaduct) and gives it a private sense, with organization, established routines, and space limits. The tables arranged on the association's patio give a family atmosphere to the place. We met Eduardo in this protected space. It was curious to observe how he daily brought materials here: pieces of rope, wool, umbrellas, magazines, etc. At that time, Eduardo lived on the streets and, over the course of the 2 months that we knew him, he explained and demonstrated his "strategies," as he used to say. Without denying that we were in a situation of rights violation in which there was a lack of access to housing, work, health, safety, and culture, we wanted to look *closely at it and into it*. What were Eduardo's "strategies"? What could we learn from them? Eduardo was our guide during two strolls around the neighborhood; he showed us the first police station in the city and told us that one of the "strategies" he uses to have lunch is to be arrested and taken to this police station. He reported that he hangs around the police

station "provoking," aiming to be arrested for a while. But before doing this, he finds out which police chiefs are on duty, because some of them are tough guys.

Across from the police station, on a street from which it is possible to observe the frantic movement of cars, Eduardo showed us the tree where he sometimes sleeps. According to him, sleeping on top of the tree is safer, because the thieves come out at night: ". . . during the day, street people are all good people, inoffensive . . . at night, they are all thieves."

Besides the tree, other places to spend the night include under a cart, a shack built from wood or cardboard, under a viaduct, on a square bench, and some unusual spaces, such as inside the structure of a viaduct. According to Eduardo, the preferred spot is right in the middle of this structure, because the floor is not flat on the sides: ". . . in these spaces, people put sofas, beds, rugs, and even stoves." But how do they come in? Only after Eduardo showed us was it possible to understand. When viaducts are being restored, small holes are made at their base, big enough for a person to pass through, and that becomes an entrance. Eduardo reported that he had even met a person who had made a rope ladder that could be rolled up and down, which was very practical to climb up to his makeshift home.

We learned from our experience with Eduardo that street people make many efforts to guarantee a living space: it requires that different situations and resources need to be articulated and there are established relationships that ensure the protection of people and space. There is also the availability of resources in the region and

---

BOX 4.1   Preliminary Approaches—cont'd

what it can offer. In the vicinity of 25 de Março St., a busy commercial region in Sao Paulo, Eduardo invited us to search through the garbage and showed us one of his sources of materials. When we returned to the area under the viaduct, at dusk, Eduardo pointed at Laurinda, whom we had previously met at AMRMC. As we approached her, she said gently: "Please, don't mind the mess; come in!" That scene of devastation became familiar, intelligible. We could identify the rug, the door, the sofa, the kitchen, the bedroom; we had some coffee and chatted, and one of the most important themes is the fear of the *rapa*.[1] And we could understand many things, including the most important: the *rapa* takes away much more than just the belongings of street people.[2]

---

[1]An expression used to refer to city hall's actions to remove the objects and belongings of homeless people; sometimes even documents are taken.

[2]Claudia Turra Magni (1994) explored the cultural dynamics established by urban nomadism relating to space, body, and things in the experience of homeless people in Porto Alegre, state of Rio Grande do Sul, Brazil.

[3]This text is part of the research field diary Circuits and religious practices in the lives of adults living on the streets in the city of São Paulo, developed by Debora Galvani. (Galvani, 2014, p. 28)

---

the Minha Rua, Minha Casa Association (AMRMC)[2] (Galvani, Sato, Reis, & Almeida, 2006), a reference center for the homeless, where we met one of its users, Eduardo.

We started at the AMRMC social center because of its mission to meet the needs of the street people as a social group. Once there, we adopted strategies of proximity and territorial mapping, inviting users of AMRMC's services such as Eduardo to construct narratives about the city from their own perspective. Such strategies were needed to initiate us and allow us to understand the social dynamics among users and be able to break though spatial frontiers in the city that we would not typically be able to cross given the differences between our and their everyday experiences.

We were also motivated to use this mapping strategy because of the presence of our students in social occupational therapy. Given the perspective of most of the street people whom we were accompanying, it would not be possible for occupational therapy practitioners and student interns to do research and work with this social group "from within an office." We came to understand the mapping strategy as a way to construct shared knowledge. Barros et al. (1999) articulated:

It is based on knowledge about the reality, necessities, and way of understanding the world of these people that we should direct our investigations and search for answers. (p. 70)

We also realized that while social welfare services were important in the everyday organization of this social group, social services are by no means the only thing that is important for this social group. This was demonstrated in an undergraduate term paper on the survival strategies adopted by street people living in the central region of Sao Paulo by Ushidomari (2005), who argued that existing social services offered to this population were insufficient to satisfy the varied everyday needs of each individual.

As the Metuia/USP Project continued to develop, students and professionals discussed the central ideas on urban anthropology developed in Sao Paulo by José Guilherme Cantor Magnani (1996, 2002, 2003), whose work focuses on networks of belonging (social membership) among urban social groups. Bringing together urban studies and ethnography, Magnani proposes to "look closely at and into" the experiences of the social actors, versus "looking distantly and from the outside." This involves seeing street people

not as isolated, dispersed elements subjected to inevitable massification, but which, through vernacular use of the city (of space, devices, institutions) in spheres of work, religiosity, leisure, culture, survival strategies, are responsible for their everyday dynamics.

(Magnani, 2002, p. 18)

Concerned with the dynamics of sociability, Magnani understands that social practices provide meaning or resignify the conventional meanings of urban spaces. Based on the work of identifying and analyzing different forms of use and appropriation of such spaces, Magnani proposes key concepts to interpret the dynamics of the city that have helped us in the Metuia/USP Project to gain a deeper understanding of the social groups with which we develop university research, teaching, and extension activities.

Thus, the concept of a "part" seeks to explain a particular type of social relations established in a space that becomes a reference point for belonging to a specific network of relationships, regardless of territorial limits. As described by Magnani, the part interests its *habitués* and the

---

[2]Community center for homeless adults located in the central region of the city of Sao Paulo, under the Glicério viaduct. More information and images are available at http://www.usp.br/jorusp/arquivo/2003/jusp666/pag03.htm.

relationships established between its members through the handling of symbols and common codes, which are the determinants. The notions of "part," "itineraries" (moving about in the city), and circuits (network of spaces, parts, and devices referring to certain practices or service offers) would serve as a foundation to understand the dynamics of the city associated with specific social groups: adult street people, people in permanent interaction with the streets, street artists, and immigrants.

Julia Nascimento (2012, p. 3), an intern linked to the Metuia/USP Project, described one day of circuit in downtown Sao Paulo guided by two street people, Pilar and Salvador. The theme Pilar chose to show the students was the experience of "Pilar who has fun selling *Ocas*[3] magazines and her poetry books. It strengthens and creates new relationship networks."

During the visit to the center region, I joined the group guided by Pilar. First, we visited the Lâmina[4] Studio to get to know the work and the points of view of artists about the city center. The works exhibited in the gallery are very interesting and inspiring, they show each artist's perspective on the city center in unique ways, and it was interesting to hear from the artists themselves about what they meant with their works. I believe that the comments made by Salvador enriched the discussion and brought many elements of reflection for all, as well as the comments of Pilar and Paulo (Salvador's friend). The work of the cart touched everyone in different ways. Salvador, for instance, was disturbed by the work. A cart, a working tool used by some street people, turned into a work of art in an exhibition, in his view, appealed to the use of an image that represents this social group. It was possible to realize how important it is that each person understands that there are several points of view, and that there is not only one reality.

After our visit to the gallery, we gathered to decide what to do next, and many students left because it was past the finishing time for the activity. Those who stayed decided after a brief meeting to go to Vale do Anhangabaú, where there was a celebration in honor of the 100th birthday of the musician Luiz Gonzaga. Pilar took advantage of the movement to show us how

she sold the Ocas magazines and had fun at the same time. We could observe Pilar's work, the way she involves people as she joyfully tells her history with pride and presents her literary productions, sometimes with a few declamations. It was interesting to note that even when she realized that a person would not buy the magazine, she still showed the same friendliness. We also noticed that, quite often, Pilar met someone she knew, and who admired her. From these encounters, invitations to conduct poetry soirees and proposals of new places to sell the Ocas magazine and her poetry books were made, and we could clearly observe the possibilities of strengthening and enlarging affective ties and of work. Those who stayed until the end of the day could understand how Pilar works, has fun, and is always producing art and culture.

Finally, Salvador showed his interaction with a sculpture located in the region. In his opinion, it was a way of occupying the city and expressing himself. The circuit and the reflections of our guides have led us to perceive different ways of defining art and culture.

In partnership with our interlocutors, we developed an understanding of different perspectives of Sao Paulo city. From singular histories, we participated in parts, circuits, and itineraries that are invisible to the "look distantly and from the outside of it" approach, which configures possibilities of social belonging in movements opposed to social disaffiliation (Castel, 2005) and disqualification (Paugam, 1999), seeking to uncover singularities in the process of constructing identities capable of redimensioning and conferring historicity to the experience of street situation (Galvani, 2008).

Some students affiliated with the Metuia/USP Project shared with us the perception that the guided circuits around the city by our interlocutors, in addition to providing critical reflection, were situations of intense learning. Camila Exner (2012, p. 2), dialoguing with the concepts of Magnani, discussed this in her internship report:

The circuit aroused an essential perception for the construction of my career in occupational therapy. Walking through places that are part of the everyday life of another person has transported me to a new place, full of things to discover, learn, and rethink. It is remarkable how people who are exposed to situations of vulnerability/disaffiliation are grouped in a homogeneous mass, characterized by absence and necessities, and thus seen as having nothing to offer. However, what I noticed were people with many ideas, experiences, desires, and enriching stories to share, who are actively searching for spaces and resources through

---

[3]The Civil Organization of Social Action (OCAS), affiliated with the International Network of Street Paper (INSP), is the publisher of *Ocas* magazine, which is purchased by the seller for R$3,00 or U$1.08 and sold for R$7,00 or U$1.89 exclusively on the streets of Sao Paulo and Rio de Janeiro (reference values of 2018).
[4]http://spcultura.prefeitura.sp.gov.br/espaco/635/.

income-generating programs, political organizations, and religious and artistic circuits.

Lack of housing was one of the main issues we faced, whether in the experience with street people or with organized groups struggling for urban housing (Barros, Lopes, Malfitano, & Galvani, 2001; Lopes, Barros, Malfitano, Galvani, & Galluzzi, 2001; Lopes, Barros, Malfitano, & Galvani 2002; Lopes, Barros, Malfitano, Galvani, & Barros. 2002). In the case of street people, plenty of money[5] and energy[6] are spent on solving the lack of access to what would be a constitutional right. The shelters have been the main public policy alternative offered to this social group. Alternatives such as provisional dwellings[7] seem to offer, during the period in which a person may stay in them, a welcoming space that provides the homeless with greater freedom and possibilities of everyday life management than the shelters. Amanda Campana (2005, p. 7), in her undergraduate final term paper for the occupational therapy course at USP, sought to understand the operation dynamics of the Dormitory Assistance Service and its meaning for users based on her experience in the streets. She understood that the project

> *offers a better quality of life for people during their stay in the provisional dwelling, providing better conditions to meet their basic needs (bath, rest, feeding, etc.), as well as fostering a sense of living together with the people in the dwelling and allowing greater autonomy for the residents, who begin to manage their everyday life activities.*

However, she also found that most people remain dependent on the homeless support network after being assisted by the Dormitory Assistance Service. We understand that the Dormitory Assistance Service has brought important demands to social occupational therapy. The project

A Casa Acolhe a Rua,[8] a pioneer in the construction of housing alternatives for this social group, was one of the spaces of action for occupational therapy practitioners and students linked to the Metuia/USP Project. We shared concerns with the residents and the project staff: How can the coexistence of such different people in a single space be improved? How can the new demands of everyday housing be met, considering that most residents had previously experienced situations of living in the streets and staying in shelters? What can be done when the maximum term of stay in the project (6 to 24 months) expires?

We then proposed to remain in the community space, seeking to establish relationships with the residents. In addition to the five dwellings that housed approximately 10 residents each, the project had a community center for the collective use of residents and community members. That was where we met a group interested in cinema. The group began to gather around the film collection of Gilvan, one of the community center's residents. After having slept in the streets and in shelters for a long time, he proudly explained that he had managed to keep them in his luggage. Many of his belongings had been lost, but not these! In a negotiated manner, a common project named Cultural Tuesday was born among residents and team members of the Metuia/USP Project. Occupying the community center with cultural activities pertinent to its residents, in addition to participating in other cultural spaces of the city, guided the construction of the activities. We reflected together on the importance of culture, especially because social policies aimed at this social group were not directed at addressing this aspect of life at that time. We were immersed in a field of contradictions where the dominant discourse emphasized the need for work and housing. In this sense, the thoughts that Armand—one of the residents interested in cinema—expressed in an interview led us to reflect on the importance of culture:

> *When you have access to culture, you have the possibility of formulating ideas, and in formulating ideas, you have the possibility of getting out of the situation you're in. You can think better about these things, can't you? Because the ideas are fantastic! You can also see another world, that there is much beyond. Yesterday, I was watching a program on backyards. Some people said: What is your yard? Some people believe that the backyard is just that, it's a small thing. Then they interviewed a man in the Northeast, and he thought his yard was his simple life. A famous writer was saying*

---

[5]In downtown Sao Paulo, the rent of a tenement can reach R$50,00/m^2 (reference value of 2015). The tenements serve people with no access to the formal labor market and no guarantor or permanent job to facilitate renting a house/apartment, but who need to live in the central part of the city to be near work possibilities and infrastructure. See Kohara, Comaru, & Ferro (2015).

[6]It is not so simple to find a place in a shelter for the homeless, and on many occasions it is necessary to wait hours until a vacancy is available, especially in winter. The vacancy may be in a shelter far from the region where the person performs his or her activities and concentrates his or her relation networks, hindering the person's already precarious everyday life organization.

[7]With the National Typification of Social Welfare Services (Brasil, 2014), the provisional dwellings were named Dormitory Assistance Services, configured as a high-complexity special protection service within the Brazil Social Welfare System (SUAS).

[8]An OAF that temporarily responds to the demand for housing for the homeless who already have some alternative income. This project's name translates as "The House Welcomes the Street."

BOX 4.2 **Excerpt From the News Report Rebellion at Provisional Dwellings in Sao Paulo**

"We've had enough of alms; we want a future!" This is how the letter written by Sebastião Nicomedes, a user of the Dormitory Assistance Service who lives in a provisional dwelling located at 518 Mercúrio Ave., downtown Sao Paulo, begins. Somehow his letter ended up circulating in the 11 provisional dwellings scattered in the city and had the adherence of many residents who intend to demand the continuity of this program of the Municipal Department of Social Assistance and Development (SMADS).

The Dormitory Assistance Service began in 2003 and functions as follows: people living on the streets or staying in shelters are interviewed at the SMADS, and if they can prove conditions to generate some income, they are allowed to live in a provisional dwelling, a house rented by city hall, with a 6-month contract renewable for a further 6 months, paying a condominium fee that ranges from R$25 to R$35. Before becoming a modality of city hall, over 10 years ago, the nongovernmental organization (NGO) Fraternal Assistance Organization Program (OAF) rented houses and invited the homeless population to inhabit them, but these houses were called "dormitories"

or "community dwellings." Today, the OAF, in partnership with the SMADS, maintains five houses, each with room for 10 people and a communal kitchen equipped with a stove, refrigerator, shelves, and tables. Close to these houses there is a community center that serves as an area of sociability and leisure for the residents.

Now, many contracts are coming to an end, and the users of different provisional dwellings are disgusted at the possibility of having to return to shelters or the streets. In the shelters, they do not have the freedom to come and go whenever they want, take a shower whenever they want, or stay during the day (they can only stay overnight). There was a claim to extend the 6- to 12-month contract to an 18-month contract, but "the real problem does not lie in the length of the contract, but in the issue of provisional dwelling." The issue is that there is no continuity. The residents claim "Bolsa Aluguel," social housing. "Instead of being managed by the Secretary of Social Assistance, the Dormitory Assistance Service should be managed by the Secretary of Housing," explains Regina Maria Manoel, general coordinator of the OAF.[1]

[1]Available at http://www.midiaindependente.org/pt/blue/2006/04/350461.shtml.

---

that her yard was the world, everything. And for an astronaut, it would be the universe! What is your backyard? What do you allow yourself to do? Today I can say that my backyard—I can't say that my backyard is the world or the universe, but I can say that it is ample, because I know it has other possibilities.

(Interview available in Galvani, 2008, p. 131)

Cultural Tuesday also included more individualized projects and situations involving larger collectives. An interesting, though tense, moment was the mobilization of residents of several provisional dwelling projects in the city around the discussion of access to housing. Box 4.2 shows an excerpt from the news report by Graziela Kunsch (2006) on this issue.

Cultural Tuesday, a day on which there was already a certain mobilization of residents for collective activities, was chosen by the National Movement of Street People (MNPR) to hold an assembly to discuss such mobilization. Members of the Metuia/USP Project supported and participated in this historic moment. In the assemblies, the need to discuss housing as a right was clear, and the voices against the mobilization drew attention, and in this sense, one of the most forceful and paradoxical opinions was the assumption that "homeless people need to work before complaining about housing." What was evident was, on the one hand, the

strength of the people in this social group that does not accept alms and, on the other hand, the need to discuss and reflect on the construction of necessity hierarchies.

In the experience with the adult street people in the city of Sao Paulo, relationships with different public policies (health, social assistance, culture, housing, human rights) and other resource networks were widely used. In the territorial activities, for instance, we were given information about people, projects, and services that could be used, including in emergency situations, as in the case of finding a night shelter, which we observed to be a frequent occurrence.

As posited by Magnani, there are circuits and parts in the city that are invisible to those who "look distantly and from the outside of them." Through close contact with street people and nongovernmental organizations (NGOs), we were able to map a circuit of political participation involving forums, assemblies, social movements, public demonstrations, parties, special dates (e.g., the Street People's Day of Struggle[9]), and historically established rituals (e.g.,

---

[9]Every year since 2005, the MNPR has organized demonstrations on August 19 against the lack of public policies and violations of the rights of street people in several Brazilian cities. This date was chosen because on August 19, 2004, homeless people were murdered at Sé Square, downtown Sao Paulo, in one of the most violent actions against the street population in Brazil.

the March of the Excluded). This circuit of political participation gathers people and groups into a joint struggling for the guarantee of rights and public policies for this social group (Costa, 2007). The circuit provides possibilities for exchanges that often transcend the typical hierarchical relationships between researchers/researched, therapists/population, and coordinators/subordinates. We recommend that mapping, knowing, and participating in such activities—which have become part of the practices of social occupational therapy—should be seen as an important part of what occupational therapists do. Such activities provided privileged spaces for discussing and understanding problems associated with the social group. They also helped to establish contacts and expand the possibilities for exchange, and, as was observed in a few situations, participation in the circuit strengthened networks of belonging in a wider movement against social disqualification. The narrative of Francisco, a proactive participant in the Forum of Debates on Street People[10] and one of the early leaders of the MNPR, invites us to reflect on the importance of political participation and of the discussion and controversies that occur in such spaces:

In the last general strike during the Figueiredo government, I was beaten. I remember it as if it were today, I dream about it sometimes, those truncheons. We were taken onto the buses that took people away. In the afternoon nobody worked, there was no commerce. It was a victory, really, a lot of fighting, the union was really united, people that fought, as if they were at war . . . so this is very important, feeling useful, not doing it for yourself, looking at your bellybutton! . . . It is necessary to know that others have the same rights as you and have to have the same possibilities as you do. I've never accepted that, since I was young, I've never accepted it! We have to look at people the way they really are, as human beings, nothing else, forget the rest, as human beings that have the same right that you have, the same amount, they are in a poor condition, without money, maybe without a home, they're just like you, there's no other difference other than that, social difference is nothing, so it is very important that crowds come and fill the Forum of Debates, it is necessary to bring these people closer to us, so that we can change this situation. We are putting into the minds of those people that it is worth politicizing, fighting for something better. . . . So when I went to the Forum of Debates, right in the beginning,

another participant told me to be careful 'cause there were several college students participating, and he believed that I would diverge too much. I told him that that was exactly what I wanted! This is the reason, because if everyone is going to say the same thing, I don't need to go, they already know what I'm going to say and I already know what I'm going to hear! If we want to reach a consensus, the ideas have to diverge, otherwise we will only see one side of the question! So I went there, and that's important! The other day, I said that the Forum is a family, every 15 days I had to go there, and I would go there with the greatest affection, but sometimes I would miss it, when things were too rough! There will always be a split of ideas, and this is very important, it's no use imposing one thing; for me, taking a position is something else, I've always fought for it and I'll fight the rest of my life, there's no point in imposing something on me, sure you won't get anything!

(Galvani, 2008, p. 240)

Castells (2002, p. 20) conceptualizes social movements as "collective actions with a specific purpose whose result, both in case of success and failure, transforms the values and institutions of society." These are processes that, according to Castells, are the basis for building collective identities. For this analysis, it is also interesting to resume Castells' discussion on territorial identities. He concludes based on his observations and studies of urban social movements in various regions of the world during the 1970s and 1980s that people resist the process of individualization and atomization, tending to group into community organizations that, over time, generate a sense of belonging and, in many cases, a communal identity. Regarding urban social movements, Castells understands that, regardless of the more evident achievements, their existence in themselves produces meaning for social actors and the community—both at the time that they take place and as part of the community's collective memory.

It seems appropriate to include the description of the Solidarity Christmas of 2007 (Galvani, 2008), one of the activities of the MNPR in Sao Paulo, in which students and occupational therapists participated actively for some years (Box 4.3).

Culture as Articulating Axis: Diversity and Cohabitation of Difference

On the one hand, we understand, in agreement with our interlocutors, culture as a right and, on the other hand, culture as mediation and the possibility of strengthening the person, collective identities, and networks of interdependence. The relationships that occurred in the experience of Cultural Tuesday, in the Forum of Debates on

---

[10]The Forum of Debates on Street People was held in biweekly meetings with predetermined themes. Researchers, professionals, students, welfare service users, and leaders of social movements participated in these meetings.

BOX 4.3　Solidarity Christmas, December 2006

The year-end celebrations are a very delicate time for the street people, a moment when the absence of family is felt more intensely by some of them; the city stops; loneliness reigns. Aiming to "confront" this season with a dose of solidarity, the National Movement of Street People (MNPR) has been organizing the Solidarity Christmas since 2004. If in 2004 its realization seemed like a daydream, in 2005 and 2006 there was anticipation surrounding the event. Anderson, a leader of the MNPR, talked about the meaning of the Solidarity Christmas:

Let's do it at Sé Square again, not because of the massacre or anything, but because it is there that the street population is more concentrated. It's no use taking the Solidarity Christmas to Paulista Ave.; how are they going to get there? The bite to eat[1] is in the central area; those who donate food are downtown. ... And also, we want to go in search of the places where the food is, but for the sake of the culture, not the food. On that day, you eat a lot and forget the person, and we don't want that. We want to show culture, joy, dignity, respect, credibility, and tell who the homeless people are, what they really want, and why they are living on the streets. ... This year, Christmas will be Solidarity Christmas, a "Happy City" for everyone, this is our theme this year. A "Happy City" for the rich, the poor, the black, the white, for whoever uses the city. ... May the city embrace these citizens, make them even more united. This is Solidarity Christmas.

The 2006 Solidarity Christmas was indeed a great party that featured several cultural events (music, dance, graffiti, workshops), adequate stage and sound infrastructure, and the collaboration of many people. Occupational therapists and students affiliated with the Metuia/University of São Paulo (USP) Project participated in the party as collaborators and were assigned to help at a table where people had access to materials to produce their Christmas cards. This intervention in the city center roused the curiosity of passersby, who stopped to appreciate it and wanted to understand what was happening. Many of them asked whether they should pay to have access to the cards; others simply cried. The newspaper *O Trecheiro* published a report on the event that, in our view, conveys the "spirit of the moment":

There was everything: many singers; musical groups of various tones and sounds: rap, Brazilian country music, pop; puppet theater with audience interaction; Christmas trees decorated in real time with recycled material and cards made by passersby; many people,

some just watching, perhaps surprised by the novelty, others happy, who freely danced spontaneously or chatted with friends, and many others working to make everything work out right. And it did! A day of encounter, despite being, as they say, the saddest day of the year for those who live on the streets and in shelters.

The Solidarity Christmas, in addition to marking the existence of the MNPR as an organization and expressing the capacity of the movement, subverts the usual order of things by showing that those who are considered dependent and in need of charity can offer a party to the city. It seems that the various expressions of this movement contribute to the construction of collective identities insofar as even those who are not directly involved with the movement feel themselves responding to its actions. Regardless of its most evident achievements and its constant tensions, the movement seems to contribute to the construction of a feeling of belonging. As noted by Castells (2002, p. 24), actors in social movements construct "identities capable of redefining their position in society and, in so doing, of seeking the transformation of every social structure." In some sense, the MNPR offers participants the opportunity to redefine themselves through an identity of resistance.

Another emblematic event for our discussion is the Street People's Day of Struggle in 2012, which had moments of protest marching and camping, as well as the organization of a meeting with the candidates running for mayor of Sao Paulo. This remarkable act of citizenship involving various social actors (MNPR, clergy, nongovernmental organizations, and the university) gathered three of the candidates running for city hall at the time: Fernando Haddad, Carlos Gianazzi, and Soninha. One of the highlights of the event was the presentation of guidelines and commitments prepared by the MNPR regarding assistance policies to street people, finalized by the signing of a memorandum of understanding with these candidates. Two of these guidelines are:

- active participation of society (movements, organizations, clergy) in the construction of effective public policies for the city, considering that social issues should not be treated as a case of public safety and violence, and
- support and improvement of policies to assist the homeless to leave the streets, such as income-generating projects, social leasing with the possibility of permanent housing, vocational courses and service incubators,

---

BOX 4.3	**Solidarity Christmas, December 2006—cont'd**

cultural projects, opportunities to return to studies, and so forth.

In its first claim, the MNPR draws attention again to the violence of the state by stating that "social issues should not be treated as a case of public safety and violence."

This matter will be mentioned in several situations in this text when addressing the everyday life of street people. In the second claim, it demands that street withdrawal policies involve a series of intersectoral actions, highlighting the idea of cultural projects.

[1]Local expression to say a place with free food.

Street People, and in the actions of the MNPR led us to propose the concept of Point of Encounter and Culture (PEC) as a space of articulation and encounter between diverse forms of knowledge and languages for cultural expression. Freire (2012) showed us that we are authors and actors of our culture, and as we write it, we also experience it. The PEC was constructed by professionals of the Metuia/USP Project, leaders of the MNPR, artists, students of the occupational therapy course at USP, street vendors, volunteers of the OCAS, and other people in the community. PEC meetings were held at Casa do Brás, initially the main office of the *Ocas* magazine and the Landless Rural Workers Movement (MST), and, later, the MNPR.

The PEC experience has been described and analyzed in greater detail in other publications (see Barros, Galvani, Almeida, & Soares, 2013). We excerpt Valdir Pierotti Silva's (2009, p. 2) perception of the PEC from his internship report. After delimiting the concept of culture, Silva sought to discuss its effectiveness as a right, understanding that culture is a fundamental aspect of social occupational therapy practice:

Quite often, the concept of human culture is reduced to a meaning that refers to the field of arts and performances. However, culture does not concern a single area or department; it is, in fact, the result of individual and collective creations, ranging from works of art, thought, values, and even of behaviors and the imaginary. . . . Aware of these issues, the Point of Encounter and Culture seeks to promote, perhaps in a much more instinctive than systematic way, several forms of cultural manifestations. In the soirees held there, for example, there is space for everyone, for everyone's culture and knowledge. The diversity of ideas and actions is celebrated. The poems written with difficulty, there, at the time, are valued; declamations lacking rhythm and with misspellings are valued; any mode of expression is valued and given legitimacy. People sing, recite, and present their performances. People listen to rap, Brazilian country and popular music. Reading ranges from the poems of Castro Alves to ergonomics manuals, from Paulo Freire to Tula Pilar, the house poet. There is

invention and improvisation. There, what counts is the power of plurality: the greater the diversity, the better. And the members of the project also enjoy the city: they go to cinemas, theaters, exhibitions, debates, and everything else they want or suggest. Many among them saw a film projected on a big screen for the first time through the actions of the PEC. Others, likewise, have discovered through the PEC that they can attend cultural events for free on any day of the week—they can go to various SESCs [social and cultural services], cultural centers, movie clubs, etc. We learn that the city is also ours, that it is a place of culture that should be enjoyed, discussed, and ceaselessly constituted in collectivity.

The constant presence of occupational therapy students in university extension activities has fueled the need for context-rich research over the years. One such study was motivated by the arrival of new students at the PEC that coincided with a period of repression of street artists in the city. Our intention was to understand the movement of street performers and performers living on the streets. Among them we found artists who understood the public space as a privileged place to disseminate their art and those who, due to a series of disruptions, were merely existing in the streets.

The study was conducted by a team of occupational therapy undergraduate students, occupational therapists, a street artist who worked in Sao Paulo, and two street people who enjoyed the cultural activities available in the city center. Two meetings were held to define our itinerary, the use of resources, and our purposes. The research began at a historical moment, when city hall had started to restrain the presence of artists and at times seize their musical instruments. Guided by João da Viola, a poet and musician who identifies with *sertanejo de raiz* (original Brazilian backcountry music), we followed the itinerary of his performances, engaging in about 10 significant encounters in these spaces: Sé Square, 15 de Novembro St., São Bento Square, Ramos Square, República Square, and Luz Park.

On 15 de Novembro St., for example, we met Marcos Rasta. Born in the interior of the state of Ceara, he has circulated in several cities in Brazil and Latin America and exemplifies a type of itinerant artist who performs in public spaces and feels that this artistic work is somehow sacred. His criticism of the criminalization of street artists was overwhelming:

> *I am an African-Brazilian and I play African-Brazilian music, but when I'm broke I play Amado Batista, Brazilian country music, whatever the audience asks for! But I think the 50-year-old generation is still supporting the street culture manifesto actively. To perform in the streets, we look for ways, if you stay it is because you are a street artist, you have the courage I do . . . . It's a spiritual wave, I think, it's mystical, it's a guiding force, because it's hard to play and sing in the streets. I make a living through music, singing in the streets, and I've been on the road for about 15 years. It would be great if the street culture manifesto grew in Sao Paulo, and people valued it, especially the authorities who need to learn to distinguish an artist from a bandit! . . . I've seen an officer in a uniform kicking the face of a guy who was sleeping on the street, is that right? And how will people get to know that? That's also why I perform music, this complaint is in my lyrics. (October 2009)*

This particular study resulted in a series of audio (songs, interviews, spontaneous statements) and image (photos and videos) recordings that served as a basis for producing a collective text entitled "On the Streets, Where the People Are," later published by the *Ocas* magazine.[11] It also resulted in the production of a manifesto in support of street artists, prepared by the research group and distributed to the artists and their audience along this same itinerary of downtown Sao Paulo. One of the main demands the artists put to our research group was the possibility of expanding their collection of images, a commitment that the group assumed by ensuring the return of the images produced. In addition, other projects unfolded from this contact. For example, the research group became engaged in the project to record a live album with João da Viola and Nogueira, his partner at the time. Although satisfactory audio quality could not be achieved due to the limitations of our equipment, the event was a great opportunity for the musicians to disseminate their work. In addition, João and Nogueira felt that a live recording attests to the quality of the musicians, and thus it would have better chances to be marketed. Moreover, it is worth noting that the project sealed the partnership between the two musicians. We observed, then, that networks of belonging are constructed

on dimensions complementary to politics, religiosity, education, culture, and work. Such dimensions allow participants to leverage their experiences to bring about new life perspectives (Galvani, 2008; Barros et al., 2013).

Concern with the relationship between researcher and researched group is inherent to the ethnographic method; however, predefined ethical parameters can generate discomfort. In an academic publication, for example, preserving the identity of the interlocutors is not always the expectation. From the ethnographic perspective, ethical care should be taken mainly in a negotiation relationship to produce dialogues between the cultural differences of researchers and interlocutors. Social occupational therapy is enriched by this perspective. However, researchers and occupational therapists are inserted into a historical process that values technical/scientific knowledge excessively, often considering it as the only true form of knowledge; that is a reason the contributions of Paulo Freire are very valuable for reflecting on the dialogical relationship between educators and students. Here we will provide an excerpt from the report by Olívia Ishiki Resende (2009) on her internship experience, because it illustrates something we have observed many times, the surprising discovery by students of almost unimaginable proximities with marginalized people who seemed so distant:

> *The (re)construction of the look begins at the very first PEC, where I meet João and Jesus and can hear their ideas and listen to their life histories. What had been crystallized is somehow dissolved when I am welcomed by João, a person in a situation of social vulnerability who, in describing the PEC, creates an image of it as "a place of welcoming, friendship, understanding, love, and sharing." Furthermore, his ideas impress me by their proximity to Paulo Freire's words: ". . .no one educates anyone, no one educates himself alone, people educate each other, mediated by the world" (Freire, 2012). I begin to notice that those meetings have much to offer me, and so the crystal that was thought to have much to teach these people begins to dissolve, and opens to intent listening, realizing how enriching the dialogue is.*

There are innumerable situations in which we were surprised at these encounters. When the frontiers between social class, generation, gender, and ethnicity become more permeable, we are faced with new challenges. One of them is to think: What are the boundaries between people of this encounter in territorial and community works? When does this work start? In the subway, for instance, when we would meet people who were going to the project and walk together with them? There is a need, therefore, for constant

---

[11]Issue 70, March/April 2010.

reflection on the construction of this praxis, as Resende concluded in her report:

> This shift in learning did not occur with brief contact, in an encounter; but through supervisions and reflective writings (reports), where shared impressions in supervision were instigated to be reflected and elaborated, or discussed and/or clarified.
>
> The experience with people under processes of disruption of support networks impressed me by the richness of exchanges and learning. During this process, many certainties dissolved and became questions. For instance, I imagined that I could offer a lot to the participants through the theories read during my studies, but with practice, I noticed that relating with them taught me many lessons, which may not be a part of any theory. Thus, it can be noted that wisdom is not in only one place (in academia, for example), it is in the contact, in the relationship with what is different, in the questioning, in the multiplicity of sources (practice, theory, the other, poetry, dialogue).
>
> (Resende, 2009)

It becomes evident that the places between those who teach and those who learn, those who observe and those who are observed, are part of a game of "musical chairs," whose rhythm is established according to the context and possibilities and limits of the real.

Concern with the encounter with the other has been a constant theme of our reflections. In the experiences of university research and extension quoted in this chapter, it is a matter of thinking ethnographically within an urban environment, and thus, as suggested by Magnani (2003) and Oliven (1995), of accepting the challenge to the researchers and, in our context, to the occupational therapists to interpret their own culture. According to Magnani, in this type of work, there is a need to try and overcome the feeling of closeness, creating a certain distancing to transform something familiar into something necessarily strange. Magnani emphasized that approaches that isolate social groups should be avoided, reinforcing the need to consider the network of relationships maintained between social groups and the surrounding society.

Diversity and Culture: Territories Covered in the Partnerships With the Casa Das Áfricas

The theme of Africa and African migration in Brazil, and its related challenges and issues for social occupational therapy, has been an important aspect of our work (Barros, 2004; Barros, Bahi, & Morgado (2011); Sato, 2004; Savadogo, 2014; Pastore, 2015). It remains currently significant

in the theory and practice of the Metuia/USP Project, notably in partnering with the Casa das Áfricas.[12]

In 2003–2004, the presence of people from the African continent living in shelters in the city of Sao Paulo was one of the concerns addressed by student Miki Sato (2004) in her final term paper, which was later revised and published (Sato, Barros, & Santos, 2007). At that time, it was possible to observe the increased presence of recent immigrants from the African continent living in shelters; this situation was verified in a survey carried out at Casa do Migrante, a shelter located in downtown Sao Paulo that specializes in welcoming immigrants. Although there was no public policy for the reception and assistance of such immigrants at that time, Casa do Migrante was one of the NGOs associated with the Catholic Church that offered shelter and legal counseling and coordinated action aimed at guaranteeing the rights of these individuals.

In 2011, Metuia/USP resumed working with the theme of human mobility through a program to value the presence and contributions of Africans living in Brazil, as well as to assist and follow up with African students. Partnering with Casa das Áfricas, the program promotes activities to expand the training of occupational therapists in diversity, focusing on racial, gender, generational, religious, and rationality issues. These are concerns endorsed by the World Federation of Occupational Therapy (WFOT, 2006, 2010, 2012). More recently, a proposal has been developed to address African migration more broadly in the Brazilian context, particularly as it relates to student mobility and the circulation of intellectual and cultural products. These preoccupations have been consolidated in projects addressing specific aesthetic and cultural universes, such as contemporary African children and youth literature, cinema, and arts. The concern is to train teachers and cultural agents, as well as occupational therapists, in the understanding of otherness through knowledge about Africa and its aesthetic and linguistic expressions.

With this view, we became a part, in the context of the Casa das Áfricas, of discussion groups that addressed the matter of migration and, in 2013, of the recently created "interinstitutional network in favor of immigrants," a network that unites a series of initiatives and social actors involved with migratory issues in the city of Sao Paulo. One of the main topics on the agenda was the legal framework for immigrants and, consequently, efforts to change law no. 6815 of August 19, 1980, which defined the legal situation of foreigners in Brazil and created the National Immigration Council (Brasil, 1981). Discussions focused on the urgent need to change the paradigm, hitherto supported

---

[12]Institute of culture, training, and studies on African societies.

based on the philosophy of national security, to the paradigm of human rights and full citizenship. In 2017, new immigration legislation (law no. 13.445, May 24, 2017) came into force and, despite failing to meet some of the demands of immigrants and human rights organizations, such as the right to vote, the new law has brought significant advances and no longer views immigrants from the perspective of a national threat (Brasil, 2017).

Within the complexity of social occupational therapy, we have focused our practical and reflexive investments on the possibilities of action in contexts marked by differentiated, multiethnic cultural practices in spaces coinhabited by social groups that are religiously and multiracially diverse. The notion of culture as a collective human right and the theoretical and practical repercussions generated by its application are not new (UNESCO, 2002). But this notion is not yet common among occupational therapists. Nevertheless, applications of the notion of culture as a right in the Brazilian context have helped transform serious situations of disqualification and discrimination affecting African immigrants. For example, activism around the notion of culture as a right and the political recognition of collective identities has resulted in important initiatives at the national level: federal laws no. 10.639/03 and no. 11645/08 now make the teaching of African-Brazilian, African, and Indian history and cultures compulsory in all school curricula in arts education, history, Portuguese, and literature, as well as the roles of academic staff (university extension activities and education) and professionals (professional/political action) in the dissemination of cultural rights as rights to participate in a collective identity.

One of the objectives of this partnership is to develop methodologies (and activities) to work on issues that converge on the theme of recent African migration in Brazil, including issues of gender, religiosity, and artistic expressiveness in contexts marked by racial, socioeconomic, and/or cultural inequality. In general, Brazilian society's perceptions about Africa have been ignorant. We have lived, historically, with the construction of stereotypes surrounding the African continent: misery, wars, backwardness, and naivety. As observed by Sato, Barros, and Santos, (2007, p. 13):

> In Brazil, African immigrants are perceived only as people from a continent known for misery and wars. In addition, they are inserted into Brazilian society through referral services for the homeless, which contributes even more to increasing the stigma and prejudice towards the African population.

Added to these observations, there is need for questioning in two directions, in relation to the ideology of Brazilian racial democracy and the myth of Brazil as a welcoming country with welcoming people. Recalling the words of Chauí (1998, p. 80), "we are the good savages, by nature and divine providence, for we are heirs to the innocence of the natives from Paradise (though we have decimated them in a systematic genocide)."

Senegalese sociologist Alain Kaly treats the idea of the "terrestrial paradise" in his article on "The African Black Being in the Brazilian 'Terrestrial Paradise,'" reflecting on and analyzing racism in his trajectory as a researcher in Brazil and, above all, the experiences of African students in Brazilian universities. Kaly (2001, p. 112) opposes the idea that racial discrimination in Brazil is associated with the social condition of African-Brazilians:

> The so-called African students who came to Brazil left their respective families, neighborhoods, and cities, e.g., Mancagne, Peul, Serere, Diola, Ibo, Banto, Soninké, Bambara, Dioula, Ewe, Touare, Dinka, took the plane as Senegalese, Guinean, Cameroonian, Gabonese, Ivorian, Algerian, Egyptian, Cape Verdean, Angolan, Mozambican, Sao Tomean, and arrived here as "Africans." In the country that welcomed them, cultural, linguistic and ethnic diversities are eliminated, and they find themselves reduced to a single group. While European, Asian, and American foreigners are treated according to their own nationalities, those from Africa are not. We are "Africans," with all the negative burden associated with it.

It is in this context that the project "Africa Circles: Conversation Circles about the Intellectual Production of African Students and Researchers in Brazil" emerged, one of the outstanding projects we have conducted with the Casa das Áfricas. Box 4.4 is based on the report by Ana Carolina de Medeiros Laki (2012), an undergraduate student in occupational therapy, and refers to one of the meetings held in 2012.

We believe that to achieve a society more open to diversity and difference, it is necessary to increasingly favor spaces for debate on the meanings of diversity and on inclusion and participation policies. It is about creating spaces for differences to coexist and sharing the dynamics of the social process. In Brazil, as elsewhere, this must also translate into actions against racism and xenophobia.

Several occupational therapists have been attentive to issues regarding Africa, whether through study or action works, to broaden the worldview and the contribution of occupational therapy. Talita Vechia worked on the project "The Threads That Bind Us," run by Casa das Áfricas and the Songho Dere wo Dere Association (SDDA) together with Denise Dias Barros, between 2003 and 2005. We have worked in support of projects creating means to value the weaver culture of the locality of Songho, Mali; a literacy

---

BOX 4.4   Africa Circle

On September 17, we went to the Africa Circle, where Robert Koofi Badou talked about the troubled presidential elections of 2010 in Ivory Coast. Prior to the meeting, we had learned about the historical political facts in Ivory Coast preceding this fateful election. The talk was mediated by Hadi Savadogo, Burkinabe anthropologist, member of the Casa das Áfricas and monitor in the course of practices in social occupational therapy. I could clearly see very contradictory contents between the seminar presented by Badou and the conversation we had with Hadi; that is, for a "pure" Ivorian who saw his country being populated by immigrants, mainly Burkinabe, the interest was in the perpetuation of the ruling government, something of a dictatorship, which preserved power in the hands of a legitimate Ivorian, whereas for the non-Ivorian people, it was preferable that a new president take office in order to promote participation space for those who were not necessarily Ivorian. This contradiction sparked a heated discussion in the Africa Circle, demonstrating the fragility of relations between African nations and the constant pursuit of a policy directed at self-interest, thus confirming the turbulent relationship between foreigners and nationalists. A converging situation between these two interests lies in the disapproval of the interference of European countries and the United Nations Organization (UNO) with the political decisions taken by Africans in African countries. This fact demonstrates the strong interest of the powers in continuing to prioritize the exploitation of the wealth of Africa by foreign companies. Future prospects of this conflict are bleak, as expectations to establish a democracy in Ivory Coast have been diluted by radicalism that is transformed into violence and persecution, culminating in a process that totally opposes democracy: to silence the voices of those who oppose their ideal.

---

project in the local language, especially for adults; and the training of youth in audiovisual resources, women in handcraft, and schoolchildren. After agriculture, production of artisanal textiles is the main economic activity for the population of Songho. The women, adolescents, and girls are engaged in spinning, dyeing (indigo and brown), and marketing, whereas the men perform weaving and trading in the capital or selling to tourists in the community shelter. In 2005, this partnership was reconfigured with the foundation of the SDDA, an entity created by a group of people from the village of Songho. It unfolds, in part, from the work performed in the 1990s with people and their families with psychological problems and lacking social networks. From the discussions, a proposal arose to make supporting these people one of the association's objectives. Four main objectives were defined: supporting people without social welfare assistance (people with chronic diseases, the elderly, the blind, people with physical and mental disabilities, etc.), supporting literacy (in the local language and French), supporting cultural and sports activities, and supporting youth organizations and local handcraft activities (spinning and weaving, dyeing and painting of fabrics).

The support provided by the Casa das Áfricas program, in collaboration with the Metuia/USP Project, aimed at providing logistical, financial, and technical assistance to the SDDA to favor the achievement of its objectives (Box 4.5).

Audiovisual resources were used as a resource of mediation and a method of comprehending reality and approaching identity. The audiovisual resources also imply a political attitude in which there is dialogue and a search for exchange relationships (in seeking something from others, they also seek to obtain something from us). Based on this formulation, the program developed ways of transferring communication and information technology focused on photography and video work. This intervention strategy enabled youths to work both with the technical question—how to use the equipment—and with the possibilities of communication that this new instrument would allow (Box 4.6).

Pingréwaoga Béma Abdoul Hadi Savadogo (2014), an anthropologist who developed a master's thesis in occupational therapy at the Federal University of Sao Carlos (UFSCar), aimed to understand the strategies of social, religious, and economic reintegration of young Burkinabe Muslims after their return from a study period in Arabic-speaking countries. Marina Di Napoli Pastore (2015) developed a master's thesis in occupational therapy (UFSCar) with a focus on the economics of trade and the concept of child responsibility in the context of city peripheries in Mozambique: she discussed differentiated perceptions of occupational therapy from an ethnic, political, and cultural perspective. She published some of her thoughts on the blog "Moça de bique" (Box 4.7).

These occupational therapists are not isolated voices; they raise concerns that Brazilian occupational therapy—which establishes its basis in human doings in diverse historical, cultural, political, economic, and existential senses—understands as a translocal and transnational vocation integrated in international mobility. Here we accept the challenge of self-criticism and the reformulation of notions and concepts developed within paradigms without connection between techniques and cultures, between

BOX 4.5 Valuing the Local Language

The project Valuing the Local Language was developed to address the demand for literacy, in large part, of the youths. In the region of Songho, the public school was just over 5 years old. The lack of minimum schooling has generated difficulties for the local youths, especially when they go to cities or seek employment outside their hometown. Within this project, forms of support for the teaching-learning of writing of the local language and French were developed. Among the strategies, the preparation of a primer in the local language, Mombo, transmitted only orally, was proposed. During the work period in 2005, an effort was made to create this primer so that it could be used in the literacy of the speakers of that language. This work was performed by the Songho Dere wo Dere Association (SDDA) members who can speak and write languages such as French and Donno So and who also speak the language of Songho, Mombo.

The primer, produced collectively, was organized and transformed into a booklet, which was taken to Songho in 2006–2007 for review, approval, and commencement of use. Since then, it has been used in different situations. In addition to the use of the primer in the activities developed in partnership with the SDDA, contact was made with the Molibemo Association, which is responsible for the production of a Donno So primer, the training of teachers, and the organization of literacy classes. The purpose of this contact was to disseminate this work in Songho and request that this material be analyzed in order to continue the training in Mombo. Two classes with children aged 11 to 13 years (one of girls and one of boys) participated in the experience of the training group in 2007, in which didactic material was used for the first time.

BOX 4.6 Sensitizing the Gaze

The 11 youths in the group (including two girls) participated in six meetings in which they did different types of activities related to photography, from experimentation with the equipment to accomplishment of exercises of photography and recording events in the village. What did they want to say about that? How did they want to convey what they saw? How do you go from the desire to make the image in a certain way to being able to represent it through the audiovisual resources? Those were the motivating questions. Four cameras were made available for the photography workshop.

An effort was made to allow the viewing of photographs and books and present the basic elements of photography. In addition to topics of free choice of the participating young people, this activity allowed the registration of images on topics of interest for the studies that were being conducted, such as everyday life, migration, and tourism. In its initial module, the video workshop—conducted by Gianni Puzzo with support from the occupational therapists of the Metuia Project—had the participation of two youths from Songho: one of them used a camcorder to record the March 2007 circumcision ceremony and the other used a camera.

BOX 4.7 Who Teaches Whom? Who Knows What?

Girl who plays, girl who studies, girl who cries, girl who laughs. Girl who brawls, girl who cares, girl who carries, girl who listens. Boy who plays, boy who runs, boy who sells, who climbs a bucket. Boy who sees, boy who jumps, boy who takes a ride, and boy who returns, boy who is responsible for the house. How many children fit these descriptions? I've been in Mozambique for a month, and today a conversation made me think about things in a different way. When I asked Anabella if Saquena needed a notebook, she replied, "Everyone needs a notebook, but I won't tell who you have to give it to or not. You choose if you want to give it to her." I thought and wondered how we are the ones who define who needs what, who needs more than whom, and what I say for the other. More than that, what is needed when you're an outsider? What can another person, who is not the familiar other, want that is within my reach, but which, just by looking,

I can't see? I come to the school every day and work with 822 children who have a daily life that repeats itself: from home to school, from school to home, and from home to some housework or to aid in the sales of vegetables in front of their homes. I see them working, but I don't often see them playing, except during class breaks. Since most people in the community sell the same things (tomatoes, potatoes, and cabbages, or charcoal, for a change), how does money circulate there? Could I, from the outside and with an outside Western perspective, say that there is trivialization of practices, of economics, or marginalization of childhood, encouragement of child labor? How do I work with a culture concept that is not my culture? How can I be willing to do this, and more than this, how can I act from a Western view, but that has to be "de-Westernized"? How can I be willing to work with the other, in another culture, with other social rules?

technical action and political action, in complexity and diversity. For us, it is also about developing *South-South dialogues* and, above all, relearning our knowledge with complex political parameters linked to the great multiplicity of languages, aesthetic and ethical expressions, and forms of cultural exchange.

SOCIAL OCCUPATIONAL THERAPY AS ORCHESTRATION OF POLYPHONIC EXCHANGES

When we speak of relations of exchange, we speak of dialogicity (Freire, 1987, 2012) and interlocution, in which we seek to mediate the search for possibilities to strengthen the individual dimension of the person while simultaneously strengthening the collective dimension of the sense of belonging. To this end, constant exercise is needed to avoid separating between person and group, individual and collective, but to instead enhance the very notion of historical identity and collective belonging. Thus, occupational therapists become interlocutors—for the understanding and transformation of social and cultural situations of oppression or disqualification—moving away, in this specific context of action, from their social positioning. According to Oliveira (2000), the interlocutors have a voice and reflect on their history and on reality, think about their problems, and find solutions for them. They "think with" and "be with" to achieve disalienation through the recognition of people's capacity to reflect on their realities; design their own everyday lives, culture, economy, languages, and forms of expression; and develop projects and elect their existential priorities.

This reflexive path places us at the forefront of occupational therapy practice, especially in social contexts, when it is faced with communities or social groups that experience situations of personal, social, or cultural disqualification, such as the street people, and cope with racism among other forms of discrimination and violations of rights. What are the needs of the people in these social groups? Is there a hierarchy of needs to be respected? Can this response be produced a priori? In the way that we have construed social occupational therapy, possibilities of action that respect and have dialogue with the social context in question are only found in the relationships and negotiation processes that involve multiple rationalities.

We can still ask ourselves: In our society, is it possible to conceive of street people as artists? Or as leaders of social movements? Is investing in the production of a musical album while homeless less preferable than saving money to rent a tenement? When working with street people, is it our goal to withdraw them from this condition? How do we cope with situations of racial discrimination or xenophobia? Is it really pertinent to continue separating technical action from political and cultural action in the face of social or cultural discrimination, either when it falls upon a person individually or when it disqualifies an entire culture and its history (in the cases of Amerindian societies and those of African descent)?

After all, what needs are we talking about? Of control? Of adaptation? Of the pursuit of guarantee of rights? It is worth remembering, according to Barros (2004), supported by the formulations of Freire (2012) and Basaglia and Basaglia (1979), that the praxis of occupational therapists is part of a historical process and it presents a technical dimension and a political dimension, which are inseparable. It is in this context that Basaglia and Basaglia (1979) invites us to reflect on the dangers of technical practices as actions of colonization and domination:

> *This new type of maladaptation control that recovers most of the social conflicts in psychology, medicine, and social assistance, without having to resort to hospitalization, except in extreme cases, is a new model ready for export, which in fact has already begun in developed countries. Its practical application in regions where this type of control is not yet needed to ensure public order and industrial development leads to the creation of artificial problems and necessities for which the new system has a ready response. But this response occurs to the extent that they are artificial problems and necessities, produced by the control itself, precisely because they are foreign to the concrete reality where they began to occur, and they are used to divert attention from the real problems and necessities. The distance between real necessity and artificial necessity is used as an instrument of domination, because the imposition of domination and colonization, as demonstrated by the missionaries who brought faith and their moral values to new lands, is nothing but preparation of the ground for the arrival of the conquering army.*

It is essential to revise and reflect on the meanings of the concept of activity. Human activities are a privileged instrument in the practice of occupational therapists and constitute the centralizing and guiding element in the complex and contextualized construction of the occupational-therapeutic process (USP, 1997).[13]

---

[13]We believe it is important to differentiate the concept of therapeutic process, based on the health paradigms, from the concepts of occupational-therapeutic processes, based on the paradigm of social occupational therapy.

According to the reflections of Barros et al. (1999, p. 102) on social occupational therapy practice:

> It is situated and significant in the imbrication of a kaleidoscope of interpretations: it is perceived, lived, and interpreted by each one of its actors (the person, the occupational therapist, the mediating group, the culture, and the values sought), and is modified in an attempt to transform the objectives of the program to which it belongs. That is the reason why the concept of social occupational therapy practice is a construct, a mediation of multiple relationships, but situated in cultural time and space; it is an unfinished concept that incorporates this incompleteness in itself, being composed of the movement and the process of communication in language (verbal, gestural and sonic, that is, iconic, indicial and symbolic). It is a concept realized in the experience and the situation lived. The activities show irreducible matter that is lent to signification, but which imposes a condition for its action and defines limits for interpretation. Such activities are objects constructed in communication, experience, and situation lived according to the history, social practices, and cultural values that each person or social group realizes in a particular way.

Therefore, there is a plurality of modes of knowledge that need to be perceived and valued. It is in this sense that the reflections of Boaventura de Souza Santos on the role played by the university and the place of scientific knowledge in Western societies warn us about the importance of breaking with the hegemony of scientific knowledge in relation to other knowledge, such as common sense and popular wisdom. In Santos' opinion, it has become vital to create interpretive communities in which people can construct understandings of the world from the interpretation of the social reality that concerns them (Santos, 2003; Barros et al., 2011). In this way, we understand that

> the work of interpreting the real from multiple perspectives creatively values the forms of rationalities, the singular experiences and their preparation, and the perception that, jointly, we can learn from each other.
>
> (Barros et al., 2013, p. 593)

If social practices give meaning or resignify urban spaces, as suggested by Magnani, it is in the bosom of these practices that we must seek the necessary dialogue for the construction of activities in social occupational therapy, with the notions of citizenship and rights as its core.

Theoretical-methodological reflection has become a requirement in the context of the effort to produce bases for social occupational therapy practice. Over the past 15 years, some experiences and research have been opening up the epistemological path. The dialogue with historical research and anthropology has brought the yarn necessary to weave our studies and rethink the meaning of occupational therapy in the core of cultural and social work.

PATHS THAT GAIN RECOGNITION AND OFFICIALITY

The dimension of cultural work and cultural diversity in occupational therapy (and of human rights as well) has gained momentum in recent years, receiving prominence and recognition within the profession, both nationally and internationally. This is expressed in the WFOT position statements (on Human Rights, 2006; on Diversity and Culture, 2010; on Human Displacement, 2012) and in the Federal Board of Physiotherapy and Occupational Therapy (COFFITO) resolutions (366/2009; 383/2010; 406/2011), which define occupational therapy in the fields of social welfare assistance, education, diversity and culture, and human rights and human displacement, questioning the hegemony of health and broadening the professional horizons and possibilities of the contribution of occupational therapy to society.

The publication of COFFITO resolution 418 (2012)—which establishes occupational therapeutic assistance parameters in the various modalities practiced by occupational therapists, including in social contexts—provides an interesting starting point for the discussion and systematization of programs, services, and projects associated with the national social welfare assistance policy, as well as cultural, education, and environmental policies. Article 5 of this resolution establishes the occupational therapeutic assistance parameters in social contexts in the scope of community, territory, household, or other forms of housing:

I. social assistance services, programs, and projects for basic social protection;
II. social assistance services, programs, and projects for special social protection of medium complexity;
III. social assistance services, programs, and projects for special social protection of high complexity;
IV. cultural services, programs, and projects;
V. formal and nonformal educational services, programs, and projects;
VI. social-environmental, economic services, programs, and projects in various associative modalities and with traditional communities.

Article 6 of this resolution establishes occupational therapeutic assistance parameters in the areas of regular and special education.

Nevertheless, it is worth mentioning that the perspective adopted in the present discussion is based on the guidelines of Brazilian social occupational therapy (Barros et al., 2002, p. 366), historically composed of

- resuming the social and cultural movements and the processes of deinstitutionalization that favored the development of the extra clinical assistance in occupational therapy, through a privileged dialogue with human sciences;
- problematizing the concept of activity from a perspective that inscribes it in a social cultural context, which attributes particular and specific senses to activities through an approach toward occupational therapy as an instrument of personal and social emancipation; and
- analyzing public policies aimed at the target population of occupational therapy, as well as the organization of this population for the defense and guarantee of their rights.

Occupational therapy needs to construct its space in the field of culture to expand and enable expression of the diversity of groups, communities, and people. Thus, we inscribe the initiatives aimed at culture practice as a form of expression, participation, and working on social conflicts and issues associated with the problems that arise in the cohabitation of diversity (cultural, gender, religious, ethnic, and racial). Since the Federal Constitution of 1988, a number of federal, state, and municipal laws and regulations have required changes in training. To educate for inclusion is to promote the exercise of understanding the diversity of logic, values, and needs. This demands that the university conduct a thorough revision of its undergraduate curriculum.

It is our responsibility to subsidize debates and activities to provide bases for the territorial and community action of occupational therapists and the preparation of projects in contexts marked by differentiated, multiethnic, and multiracial cultural practices. In many societies, the coexistence of several cultures can lead to difficult coexistence, conflicts, and even wars. Minority groups often face greater difficulties in exercising their established rights. This challenge is the engine of the projects we have been developing, in which there remains the need to develop approach methodologies/activities and cultural, educational, and social development plans to be applied in contexts marked by racial, socioeconomic, and/or cultural inequality, as in the cases of the projects and studies we described previously.

In the opinion of the authors of this chapter, this is the moment for occupational therapists to focus on teaching-learning processes and action-reflection in contexts marked by cultural diversity. In our case, we do so with emphasis on African and African-Brazilian matters, on the study of migration as a fundamental human right, and on cultural citizenship with freedom (to create), equality (of access), identity (respecting diversity), and exchange (national and international).

REFERENCES

Atkinson, P. (1992). *Understanding ethnographic texts*. London: Sage Publications.

Barros, D. D. (2004). *Itinerários da Loucura no território de Dogon* [Itineraries of madness in Dogon territory]. Rio de Janeiro: FIOCRUZ.

Barros, D. D., Almeida, M. C., & Vecchia, T. C. (2007). Terapia Ocupacional Social, diversidade, cultura e conhecimento [Social occupational therapy: Diversity, culture and knowledge]. *Revista de Terapia Ocupacional da Universidade de São Paulo*, *18*(3), 128–134. doi:10.11606/issn.2238-6149.v18i3p128-134

Barros, D. D., Galvani, D., Almeida, M. C., & Soares, C. R. S. (2013). Cultura, economia, política e saber como espaços de significação na Terapia Ocupacional Social: Reflexões sobre a experiência do Ponto de Encontro e Cultura [Culture, economics, politics and knowledge as meaning-spaces in social occupational therapy: Reflections on the experience of "Culture and Meeting Point"]. *Cadernos de Terapia Ocupacional da UFSCar*, *21*(3), 583–594. doi:10.4322/cto.2013.060

Barros, D. D., Ghirardi, M. I. G., & Lopes, R. E. (1999). Terapia Ocupacional e Sociedade [Occupational therapy and society]. *Revista de Terapia Ocupacional da Universidade de São Paulo*, *10*(2/3), 69–74.

Barros, D. D., Lopes, R. E., Galheigo, S. M., & Galvani, D. (2011). Research, community-based projects, and teaching as a sharing construction: The Metuia Project in Brazil. In F. Kronenberg, N. Pollard, & D. Sakellariou (Eds.), *Occupational therapies without borders* (Vol. 2): *Towards an ecology of occupation-based practices* (pp. 321–327). London: Churchill Livingstone – Elsevier.

Barros, D. D., Lopes, R. E., & Ghirardi, M. I. G. (2002). Terapia ocupacional social [Social occupational therapy]. *Revista de Terapia Ocupacional da USP*, *13*(3), 95–103. doi:10.11606/issn.2238-6149.v13i3p95-103

Barros, D. D., Lopes, R. E., Malfitano, A. P. S., & Galvani, D. (2001). O Espaço do brincante na experiência do Projeto Casarão [Space to play in "Projeto Casarão" experience]. *Revista de Terapia Ocupacional da Universidade de São Paulo*, *12*(1/3), 48–51.

Barros, D. D., Bahi, A. A. & Morgado, P. (2011). » Dogonité » et Internet : une lecture critique de l'essentialisation des identités. Anthropologie et Sociétés, 35 (1-2), 69–86. https://doi.org/10.7202/1006369ar *Anais do 32º Encontro Anual da ANPOCS*, Caxambu (MG).

Basaglia, F., & Basaglia, F. O. (1979). *O homem no pelourinho* [The man in the pillory]. São Paulo: Tradução IPSO - Instituto de Psiquiatria Social.

Brasil (1981). Lei *nº* 6.815, de 19 de agosto de 1980. Define a situação jurídica do estrangeiro no Brasil, cria o Conselho Nacional de Imigração. Diário Oficial da República Federativa do Brasil [Law 6.815, August 19th 1980. Defines foreign juridical situation and creates Imigration National Council]. Brasília, DF, v. 7.

Brasil. (de 24 de maio de 2017). *Lei nº 13.445*. Institui a Lei de migração [Establishes the law of migration] (p. 1). Diário Oficial da República Federativa do Brasil, Brasília. Retrieved March 2019, from http://www.planalto.gov.br/ccivil_03/_ato2015-2018/2017/lei/L13445.htm

Campana, A. B. (2005). Projeto de moradias provisórias: dinâmicas, limites e possibilidades [Provisional housing project: Dynamics, limits and possibilities]. 73f. In *Trabalho de Conclusão de Curso* (Graduação em Terapia Ocupacional). São Paulo: Faculdade de Medicina, Universidade de São Paulo.

Castel, R. (2005). *Metamorfoses da questão social: uma crônica do salário* [Metamorphoses of social question: A chronicle of the salary] (5th ed.). Petrópolis: Vozes.

Castells, M. (2002). *O Poder da identidade* [The power of identity] (3rd ed.). Tradução de Klauss Brandini Gerhardt. São Paulo: Paz e Terra.

Chauí, M. (1998). Cultura Política e política cultural [Political culture and cultural policy]. *Estudos Avançados, 23*(9), 71–84. doi:10.1590/S0103-40141995000100006

Conselho Federal de Fisioterapia e Terapia Ocupacional – COFFITO. (June 16, 2009). Resolução nº 366, de 20 de maio de 2009. Dispõe sobre o reconhecimento de Especialidades e de Áreas de Atuação do profissional Terapeuta Ocupacional e dá outras providências (Alterada pela Resolução nº 371/2009) [It deals with the recognition of specialties and areas of practice of the professional occupational therapist and gives other arrangements]. Brasília, DF: Diário Oficial da República Federativa do Brasil. Retrieved March 2019, from https://www.coffito.gov.br/nsite/?p=3134

Conselho Federal de Fisioterapia e Terapia Ocupacional – COFFITO. (December 25, 2010). Resolução nº 383, de 22 de dezembro de 2010. Define as competências do Terapeuta Ocupacional nos Contextos Sociais e dá outras providencias [It defines the competences of the occupational therapist in the social contexts and gives others arrangements]. Brasília, DF: Diário Oficial da República Federativa do Brasil. Retrieved March 2019, from https://www.coffito.gov.br/nsite/?p=3146

Conselho Federal de Fisioterapia e Terapia Ocupacional – COFFITO. (November 7, 2011). Resolução nº 406 de 07 de novembro de 2011. Disciplina a Especialidade Profissional Terapia Ocupacional nos Contextos Sociais e dá outras providências [Disciplines occupational specialty occupational therapy in social contexts and makes other arrangements]. Brasília, DF: Diário Oficial da República Federativa do Brasil. Retrieved May 29, 2013, from https://www.coffito.gov.br/nsite/?p=3169

Conselho Federal de Fisioterapia e Terapia Ocupacional – COFFITO. (June 6, 2012). Resolução nº 418 de 4 de junho de 2012. Fixa e estabelece os Parâmetros Assistenciais Terapêuticos Ocupacionais nas diversas modalidades prestadas pelo Terapeuta Ocupacional e dá outras providências [It establishes the occupational therapeutic care parameters in the various modalities provided by the occupational therapist and provides other measures]. Brasília, DF: Diário Oficial da República Federativa do Brasil. Retrieved May 29, 2013, from https://www.coffito.gov.br/nsite/?p=3181

Costa, D. L. R. (2007). A rua em movimento – experiências urbanas e jogos sociais em torno da população em situação de rua. [The street in movement – urban experiences and social configurations among the homeless population]. 241 f. *Dissertação (Mestrado)*. São Paulo: Faculdade de Filosofia, Letras e Ciências Humanas – Universidade de São Paulo. Retrieved March 2019, from www.teses.usp.br/teses/.../8/...20122007.../TESE_DANIEL_LUCCA_REIS_COSTA.pdf

Exner, C. (2012). *Terapia Ocupacional no Campo Social: Práticas Supervisionadas III* [Occupational therapy in the social field: Supervised practices III]. Diário de campo. Mimeo.

Freire, P. (1987). *Pedagogia da Autonomia: saberes necessátios a uma prática educative* [Pedagogy of autonomy: Knowledge necessary for educational practice] (3rd ed.). São Paulo: Paz e Terra.

Freire, P. (2012). *Pedagogy of the oppressed* (30th Anniversary ed.) (3rd ed.). New York, NY: Bloomsbury Academic.

Galvani, D. (2008). População em situação de rua em São Paulo: itinerários e estratégias na construção de redes sociais e identidades [Homeless people in the city of São Paulo: routes and strategies in the construction of social nets and identities]. 2008. 261 f. *Dissertação (Mestrado em Ciências da Reabilitação)* – Faculdade de Medicina, Universidade de São Paulo, São Paulo, 2008. Retrieved March 2019, from livros01.livrosgratis.com.br/cp064259.pdf

Galvani, D. (2015) *Circuitos e práticas religiosas nas trajetórias de vida de adultos em situação de rua na cidade de São Paulo. [Circuits and religious practices in the lives of adults living on the streets in the city of São Paulo]* Tese (Doutorado em Ciências) – [Doctoral Thesis]. Instituto de Psicologia, Universidade de São Paulo, Retrieved August 2020, from https://www.teses.usp.br/teses/disponiveis/47/47131/tde-07072015-100223/publico/galvani_corrigida.pdf

Galvani, D., Sato, M. T., Reis, T. A. M., & Almeida, M. C. (2006). Perfil dos usuários da Associção Minha Rua Minha Casa entre 2002 e 2003 [Profile of users of the center of services Associação Minha Rua Minha Casa between 2002 and 2003]. *Revista de Terapia Ocupacional da Universidade de São Paulo, 17*(2), 48–56. doi:10.11606/issn.2238-6149.v17i2p48-56

Geertz, C. A. (1989). *A interpretação das culturas* [The interpretation of cultures]. Rio de Janeiro: Zahar.

Kaly, A. P. O. (2001). Ser Preto africano no « paraíso terrestre » brasileiro: Um sociólogo senegalês no Brasil [The African Black being in the Brazilian "terrestrial paradise." A Senegalese sociologist in Brazil] (pp. 105–121). *Lusotopie*, Bordeaux-França. Retrieved March 2019, from http://www.lusotopie.sciencespobordeaux.fr/kaly.pdf

Kohara, L., Comaru, F., & Ferro, C. (2015). *For the resumption of social rental programs*. ObservaSP. Retrieved December 20, 2018, from https://observasp.wordpress.com/2015/04/22/pela-retomada-dos-programas-de-locacao-social/

Kunsch, G. (2006). Rebellion in provisional dwellings in São Paulo. Centro de Mídia Independente, Brasil, 2006. In Fórum Centro Vivo, *Violações dos direitos humanos no centro de São Paulo: propostas e reivindicações para políticas públicas* [Human rights violations in the center of São Paulo: Proposals and demands for public policies]. Retrieved February 15, 2019, from http://www.polis.org.br/uploads/977/977.pdf

Laki, A. C. M. (2012). *Terapia Ocupacional no Campo Social: Práticas Supervisionadas III* [Occupational therapy in the social field: Supervised practices III]. Diário de campo. Mimeo.

Lopes, R. E., Barros, D. D., Malfitano, A. P. S., & Galvani, D. (2002). Histórias de Vida: Histórias de vida: a ampliação de redes sociais de suporte de crianças em uma experiência de trabalho comunitário [Life stories – Increasing the social support networks for children through the experience of community work]. *O Mundo da Saúde, 26*(3), 426–434.

Lopes, R. E., Barros, D. D., Malfitano, A. P. S., Galvani, D., & Barros, G. (2002). Relato de experiência: video como um elemento comunicativo no trabalho comunitário [Video as an element in communication for the community work]. *Cadernos de Terapia Ocupacional da UFSCar, 10*(1), 61–67. Retrieved from March 2019, from http://www.cadernosdeterapiaocupacional.ufscar.br/index.php/cadernos/article/view/224/178

Lopes, R. E., Barros, D. D., Malfitano, A. P. S., Galvani, D., & Galluzzi, A. M. (2001). Terapia ocupacional no território: as crianças e os adolescentes da Unidade do Brás – movimento de luta por moradia urbana [Occupational therapy in the territory: children and teenagers from "Unidade do Brás" social movement for urban dwelling]. *Cadernos de Terapia Ocupacional da UFSCar, 9*(1), 30–49. Retrieved March 2019, from http://www.cadernosdeterapiaocupacional.ufscar.br/index.php/cadernos/article/view/233

Magnani, J. G. C. (1996). Quando o campo é a cidade: fazendo antropologia na metrópole [When the countryside is the city: Doing anthropology in the metropolis]. In J. G. C. Magnani & L. L. Torres (Eds.), *Na metrópole: textos de antropologia urbana* [In the city: Texts of urban anthropology] (pp. 15–53). São Paulo: Edusp/Fapesp. Retrieved March 2019, from https://edisciplinas.usp.br/pluginfile.php/4246690/mod_resource/content/1/qnd_o_campo_cidade.pdf

Magnani, J. G. C. (2002). De perto e de dentro: notas para uma etnografia urbana [Insider and a close-up view: Notes on urban ethnography]. *Revista Brasileira de Ciências Sociais, 17*(49), 11–29. doi:10.1590/S0102-69092002000200002

Magnani, J. G. C. (2003). Rua, símbolo e suporte da experiência urbana [Street, symbol and support of urban experience]. In *NAU - Núcleo de Antropologia Urbana da USP.* Retrieved March 17, 2019, from http://www.n-a-u.org/ruasimboloesuporte.html

Magni, C. T. (1994). *Nomadismo urbano: uma etnografia sobre os moradores de rua em Porto Alegre* [Urban nomadism: An ethnography of homelles in Porto Alegre]. 198f. (Dissertação de Mestrado em Antropologia Social). Programa de Pós-Graduação em Antropologia Social, Universidade Federal do Rio Grande do Sul, Porto Alegre.

Nascimento, J. (2012). *Terapia Ocupacional no Campo Social: Práticas Supervisionadas III* [Occupational therapy in the social field: Supervised practices III]. Diário de campo. Mimeo.

Oliveira, R. C. (2000). O trabalho do antropólogo: olhar, ouvir, escrever [The work of the anthropologist: To look, to listen, to write]. In R. C. O. Oliveira (Ed.), *Trabalho do antropólogo* [The work of the anthropologist] (2nd ed., pp. 17–35). São Paulo: Edunesp. Retrieved March 2019, from https://www.revistas.usp.br/ra/article/viewFile/111579/109656

Oliven, G. R. (1995). *Antrologia de grupos urbanos* [Anthropology of urban groups] (5th ed.). Petrópolis: Vozes.

Pastore, M. N. (2015). *Sim! Sou Criança eu! Dinâmicas de socialização e universos infantis em uma comunidade moçambicana* [Yes! I'm a child! Dynamics of socialization and children's universes in a Mozambican community] (Dissertação Mestrado em Terapia Ocupacional). São Carlos: Programa de Pós-Graduação em Terapia Ocupacional da Universidade Federal de São Carlos.

Paugam, S. (1999). O debate em torno de um conceito [The debate around a concept]. In M. P. B. Verás (Ed.), *Por uma sociologia da exclusão social: o debate com Serge Paugam* [For a social exclusion sociology: The debate with Serge Paugam] (pp. 115–142). São Paulo: Educ.

Resende, O. I. (2009). *Terapia Ocupacional no Campo Social: Práticas Supervisionadas III* [Occupational therapy in the social field: Supervised practices III]. Diário de campo. Mimeo.

Santos, B. S. (org.) (2003). Democratizar a democracia: os caminhos da democracia participativa [Democratizing democracy: the paths of participatory democracy]. Porto: Afrontamento.

Sato, M. (2004). *Africanos refugiados sobreviventes na Casa do Migrante* [Survey of African refugees at Casa do Migrante]. 64f. Trabalho de Conclusão de Curso. São Paulo: Graduação em Terapia Ocupacional – Faculdade de Medicina, Universidade de São Paulo.

Sato, M., Barros, D. D., & Santos, A. S. A. (2007). *Da África para abrigos públicos: africanos na Casa do Migrante em São Paulo* [From Africa to public shelters: Africans at Casa do Migrante in São Paulo] (pp. 29–62). Rio de Janeiro: Estudos Afro-Asiáticos.

Savadogo, P. B. A. H. (2014). *Desafios de jovens muçulmanos em Burquina Faso no retorno de estudo em países de língua árabe: entre vulnerabilidades e a reconstrução da cidadania* [Challenges of young Muslims in Burkina Faso on return from study in Arab-speaking countries: Between vulnerability and the reconstruction of citizenship] (Dissertação Mestrado em Terapia Ocupacional). São Paulo: Programa de Pós-Graduação em Terapia Ocupacional da Universidade Federal de São Carlos, São Carlos; Casa das Áfricas. Retrieved March 2019, from https://repositorio.ufscar.br/handle/ufscar/6892

Silva, V. P. (2009). *Terapia Ocupacional no Campo Social: Práticas Supervisionadas III* [Occupational therapy in the social field: Supervised practices III]. Diário de campo. Mimeo.

UNESCO. (2002). *Universal declaration on cultural diversity.* Retrieved March 2019, from http://portal.unesco.org/en/ev.php-URL_ID=13179&URL_DO=DO_TOPIC&URL_SECTION=201.html

Ushidomari, I. Y. (2005). *Vida nas ruas: busca por alternativas* [Life on the streets: looking for alternatives]. 108f. Trabalho de Conclusão de Curso. São Paulo: Graduação em Terapia Ocupacional – Faculdade de Medicina, Universidade de São Paulo.

USP. (1997). *Centro de Docência e Pesquisa em Terapia Ocupacional do Departamento de Fisioterapia, Fonoaudiologia e Terapia Ocupacional da FMUSP.* São Paulo: Universidade de São Paulo. Folder do Curso de Terapia Ocupacional da FMUSP.

World Federation of Occupational Therapists. (2006). World Federation of Occupational Therapists position statement on human rights. *Journal World Federation of Occupational Therapists Bulletin, 59*(1), 5. doi:10.1179/otb.2009.59.1.002

World Federation of Occupational Therapists. (2010). *World Federation of Occupational Therapists position statement on diversity and culture.* Victoria Australia: Author. Retrieved from https://www.wfot.org/resources/diversity-and-culture

World Federation of Occupational Therapists. (2012). *World Federation of Occupational Therapists position statement on human displacement.* Victoria Australia: Author. Retrieved from https://www.wfot.org/resources/human-displacement

5

Social Context and Social Action: Generalizations and Specificities in Occupational Therapy

Ana Paula Serrata Malfitano

INTRODUCTION

The motivation for writing this chapter is rooted in debates involving social occupational therapy and discussions on whether this is a distinct field in occupational therapy or part of *every* occupational therapy practice. Is there reason to talk specifically about one area of social action—that is, social occupational therapy?

Two different approaches are proposed. The first addresses social context as an element that should be present in every action in the field of occupational therapy. Regardless of the population group and, consequently, of the subarea being addressed, this approach views the social context of people's lives as an element inherent in all occupational therapy practice. The second approach highlights the specificities of social occupational therapy, what is unique about it, presenting it as a specific field of occupational therapy. In this approach, social occupational therapy is characterized by its theoretical and methodological approach, which is based on working with specific people, groups, and collectives. Finally, the last section of this chapter contributes to the argument for why social occupational therapy should be advocated, highlighting the *dangers* of approaching eminently social issues through the health sector, and discussing the increasingly predominant trend toward the medicalization of life.

THE SOCIAL CONTEXT: A STARTING POINT

A key epistemological concern of occupational therapy is its own social function, which is examined by considering the objectives of developed practices and interventions, the populations assisted, and the results yielded by professional interventions. Why are occupational therapists needed in society? What types of social demands/problems do occupational therapists respond to? What knowledge does social occupational therapy offer to contemporary society? Since the 1980s, several Brazilian authors have addressed these questions by pointing out the inseparability of the technical, political, and ethical dimensions in the practice of occupational therapy (Barros, Ghirardi, & Lopes, 1999; Lopes, 2013). Influenced by theorists such as Antônio Gramsci and their formulations of the role of organic intellectuals (Gramsci, 1971), as well as by real-world experiences based on these theories, such as those developed in the field of mental health by Basaglia and Ongario-Basaglia (1977), Brazilian occupational therapists have discussed the contributions of occupational therapy to contemporary society.

Academics from the University of Sao Paulo (USP) view the function of occupational therapists in society as encompassing interventions in the areas of "health, education and in the social sphere, gathering technologies aimed at the emancipation and autonomy of people who, for reasons associated with specific problems, physical, sensorial, mental, psychological and/or social, temporarily or definitively experience difficulty in social inclusion and participation" (USP, 1997). It is therefore essential to discuss the contexts in which people live, including their historical and collective dimensions. Context refers to the place where occupational-therapeutic practice should occur and where strategies for social inclusion and participation are sought, without disregarding the structural limitations that are always present, so that social inclusion can be achieved. Addressing the social context in which professional action occurs is absolutely essential to any discussion of occupational therapy practice. This means that in addition to applying specific techniques in different subareas (such as physical disability/rehabilitation, mental health, worker health, communities, etc.), regardless of the problems that affect the different groups, which require targeted and focused interventions, occupational therapists should be primarily dedicated to the development of actions that enable/facilitate/create forms of social inclusion and participation.

Occupational therapy's greatest epistemological contribution is that actions can address the social dimensions of people's lives. This assertion is based on a view of occupational therapy that understands its objective to be the emancipation and autonomy of people, a view that is advocated by a critical strand of occupational therapy both in Brazil (Galheigo, 1997; Barros, 2004; Ghirardi, 2012; Lopes, 2013) and elsewhere (Townsend, 1993; Whiteford & Townsend, 2011; Whiteford & Pererira, 2012; Gerlach, Teachman, Laliberte-Rudman, Aldrich, & Huot, 2018). This view is in line with the principles of the World Federation of Occupational Therapists (WFOT), which includes the participation of people and communities in its definition of the profession (WFOT, 2012).

The social field can be defined as an intersectoral *locus* of life operationalization, that is, the real context where life occurs according to the possibilities and limits imposed by socioeconomic factors (Malfitano, 2005). The social field involves the social dynamics, its interrelationships and conformations (Heller, 1984), and, at its root, the relations of power that integrate and define it (Bourdieu, 1993), in which discussions of justice and human rights are indispensable (Wilcock & Townsend, 2000). In this dialogue, it is fundamental to turn to the human and social sciences and rely on theorists who can assist with understanding the social context of our historical moment.

Authors have argued that social dynamics has a materialist-historical basis, influenced by the structure of capitalist society, its implications for the world of work, and the different possibilities of the social inclusion of people (Offe, 1974; Lenhardt & Offe, 1984; Castel, 2003). From a materialist-historical perspective, the sociohistorical view explores the connections between the economic, social, political, and cultural aspects. Such a view delimits social inclusion in an imbalanced economic structure guided by people's relation with the capital.

In this configuration, the action of the state in social dynamics occurs predominantly by means of public policies (Lenhardt & Offe, 1984; Gramsci, 1971), based on the understanding that the contemporary social question requires the modern state to respond to the problems presented by lived reality. Recognizing the presence of social demands and the need for state intervention is a prerequisite for discussing social policies, which are one kind of public policy (Lenhardt & Offe, 1984). Public policies are sometimes regarded as sources of concrete (empirical)

information about a capitalist state, since they can be understood as the state in action, shedding light on its intentions, interests, and priorities (Leca, 2004). Public policies aim to maintain the capitalist exchange relations that are key to the state, facilitating the reproduction of all the values of a capitalist society, while social policies aim to create conditions that allow each citizen to be included in these relations of exchange (Lenhardt & Offe, 1984).

Social policies represent the incorporation of *human needs* according to the *interests* of the system. In many instances, tension is generated to increase the recognition of these needs, which will translate into the implementation of sociopolitical innovations (Lenhardt & Offe, 1984). Social policies can affect directly the outcomes of the tensions arising from the relations of power between civil society, political society, and the market. Amid these tensions, civil society agents engage in social pressure and mobilization actions, ultimately forming social movements. Civil society agents intervene in the cultural and political sphere as actors struggling for the expansion and accessibility of social rights, forming collective actions that assist with determining an expanded view of democracy (Dagnino, 2000). To incorporate new needs, the state takes responsibility, with greater or lesser degrees of involvement, according to recognized and legitimized rights-based democratic and social parameters. According to Lenhardt and Offe (1984), sociopolitical innovations in the field of social policies are implemented to the extent that there are changes in the way the state's agents generate, finance, and distribute social services. These elements determine the scope of social policies, characterized according to the nature of their intervention as promoters of universal or focused actions. Focused policies are, in most cases, directed at the poor, in contrast to the universalization of actions of the state.

But what should the object of social policies be? Which human needs should be prioritized? The debate over which needs should be met by social policies should occur in public spheres; this enables decisions and innovations to be understood as necessary by everyone and to be regarded as a collective responsibility of society. Gramsci (1971) advocates the existence of the political arena so that different projects can operate and coexist in dispute, in the constitution of public spaces and the construction of hegemony. Based on the Gramscian framework, Telles (1990) adds that the existence of the public space will enable discussion to distinguish collective questions from private questions in the current historical-social moment, allowing the creation of an agenda that addresses themes of social interest.

Considering that occupational therapists are professionals who work in this society, seeking means to facilitate the social inclusion of people, participation in public spaces to determine those needs is required. Facing up to social inequality is imperative because it is mainly through public policies that occupational therapists can act in the everyday lives of people to foster social participation and inclusion. Thus, they should have knowledge about public policies, particularly social policies, including the actions and priorities of governments. Therefore, occupational-therapeutic action requires direct participation in social policies and in public discussions on collective projects and needs. Such participation is valuable for occupational therapy practice because it foregrounds the profession's focus on the real lives of people, in their occupations and/or everyday lives. It should be emphasized that occupational therapists work mostly with groups that experience social inclusion difficulties.

It is thus argued that occupational therapists cannot carry out *only* individualized assistance, restricted to the application of particularized techniques or approaches, aimed at individuals or groups. Actions focused on the individual are not sufficient for achieving social inclusion and participation, that is, the purpose of occupational therapy (Gerlach et al., 2018). To achieve this goal, it is essential to include a collective dimension that bridges the association between the micro- and macro-social dimensions, the technical and political analysis of the space, and the target population group, community, and people. From this perspective, this action requires that individual, collective, and institutional needs be reconciled and connected.

With this in mind, the theoretical contribution of Robert Castel (2003) on supportive social networks is of great importance, as it provides a sociological analysis of the conjunction between aspects of individual dimension and macrostructure, the latter determining the conditions and possibilities of life. Castel proposes an interpretation of the processes of social inclusion in two axes: labor relation (from stable employment to the complete absence of work) and relational inclusion (from inclusion in solid networks of sociability to social isolation). He defines three *zones* for the understanding of social dynamics: the *integration zone*, which implies access to permanent work together with solid relational supports; the *disaffiliation zone*, which combines absence of work and social isolation, characterizing social disruption and uprooting; and the *vulnerability zone*, which includes precarious and/or unstable work and relational fragility.[1] However, we are living in a time of crisis with growing unemployment rates and,

more than that, income instability (Castel, 2003). As a consequence, social inclusion processes are fragile, vulnerable, or disaffiliated in most cases. In addition, association with individualistic Western culture has created difficulties for the establishment of social bonds and solidary relationships (Castel & Duvoux, 2013).

Based on these concepts, the work of occupational therapists demands discussion of the context and technical and political actions required for their practice, which means discussing collective recognition of the social needs of different population groups. However, the current configuration of the social fabric is characterized by a predominantly uneven structure, with increased vulnerability and decreased solidarity, hindering the work of occupational therapists. In other words, the contemporary challenge is to develop theoretical and methodological elements that facilitate the development of strategies for the social inclusion of people through the strengthening of their individual and social support networks, beyond the specific problems (physical, mental, social, etc.) that affect them. Therefore, addressing the social context from this perspective should be central to any occupational therapy practice. For instance, considering the most traditional target populations of occupational therapy interventions, such as people with disabilities and those with mental illness, the social context and the search for strategies for social inclusion of these people, groups, and collectives are fundamental. In the subarea of physical disability, although emphasizing the relevance of biomedical interventions to improve physical movement and adaptations that allow greater autonomy requires a focus on individuals, it is also important to plan interventions that also result in increased mobility in public spaces and participation in the spheres of life considered necessary by people—that is, actions that are valuable in their contexts. In the subarea of mental health, it is necessary to move beyond the specific treatments for mental illnesses and their symptoms; the possibility of circulation, the struggle against social stigmas, the spaces of belonging, and the networks of people should be integrated into the work of occupational therapists.

In other areas of practice, called *emerging* in some countries, such as primary health care, professional discussions have concentrated on the contexts and living conditions of people, with a special focus on poor communities (Oliver, Pimentel, Uchoa-Figueiredo, & Nicolau, 2012). Through some experiences in nongovernmental organizations, occupational therapists have been working to integrate people's service networks through informal education (Borba & Lopes, 2010). The social assistance sector is another example that necessitates work in the community, with its local characteristics and culture, and has slowly

---

[1]Robert Castel also describes a fourth zone, the *social assistance zone,* which associates absence of work, due to incapacity to engage in it, and social inclusion, resulting from the assistance provided by the state and other institutions, characterizing a state of dependence strongly influenced by the historical factors of social assistance development.

absorbed an increasing number of occupational therapists in Brazil, establishing a role for occupational therapy (Almeida, Soares, Barros, & Galvani, 2012). The ramifications of cultural accessibility for all (Dorneles & Lopes, 2016; Barros, Galvani, Almeida, & Soares, 2013) touch upon different population groups, demanding actions directed at access to services and cultural goods and their influence on people's everyday and social lives. In the legal sector, occupational therapists have worked with young offenders in community services or secure institutions (i.e., prisons), seeking articulations in the everyday life of these youths (Morais & Malfitano, 2014; Kappel, Gontijo, & Alves, 2014).

Examining these different areas of action exemplifies that, regardless of the population group at which action is directed, emphasis should be placed on the social context as an arena for occupational therapy practice, articulated with social policies (Malfitano, 2005). Thus, regardless of the area or population group involved, working within the social context demands acknowledging the intersectoral and intersectional demands present in people's lives. In conclusion, the social context is a general starting (and finishing) point for the work of occupational therapists. This point involves different practice subareas and population groups, arranged horizontally, requiring questioning and previous knowledge of the action space so that people can be effectively assisted. Only from within the social context can the social inclusion and participation of different people, groups, and collectives be addressed.

SOCIAL OCCUPATIONAL THERAPY: SPECIFICITIES OF A FIELD

Building on what has been previously advocated about the social context's importance to *every* occupational therapy practice, we shall now discuss the specificities and distinct characteristics of social occupational therapy. Social occupational therapy is directed at the development of actions through the search for emancipation and autonomy of people who are faced with socioeconomic impediments and/or difficulties in accessing their social rights. It is a question of focusing on people, groups, and collectives whose social positions and life conditions are marked by the socioeconomic question. The question is whether it is possible for occupational therapists to intervene in the everyday lives of people to create joint strategies for the widening of opportunities in contexts marked by social inequality.

However, the following should be emphasized: it is not a matter of predefining the "correct" form of social inclusion or advocating marginalized integration without discussing the reasons for people's exclusion and even the resistance to reinclusion of some groups (Galheigo, 1997); nor is it about establishing standardized and moral models of participation in social life (Fassin & Lézé, 2013) to define what is correct. It is a matter of recognizing the multiple forms of inclusion and/or integration, including the marginal and illegal ones, and mediating the almost always conflicting process of access to some social goods and the possibilities of autonomous participation in social life. It is worth remembering that it is not the role of occupational therapists to judge people's *choices*.

Social occupational therapy directs its actions to groups for whom the social question is a central impediment to their participation in social life (Barros, Ghirardi, & Lopes, 2005). This is a situation that characterizes the following population groups: populations living on the street, young offenders, prisoners, poor children and youth, poor and institutionalized elderly, people with alternative forms of income generation, poor people living in urban peripheries, migrants and immigrants, and so forth.

Of course, this is not a *new* field. Social occupational therapy has been developing professional practices in Brazil since the 1970s and 1980s (Barros, Lopes, & Galheigo, 2007). The presence of professionals working with populations whose centrality of action was not within the demands associated with health and disease but with socioeconomic factors is well established in Brazil. Based on projects developed in the social field, Denise Dias Barros, Maria Isabel Ghirardi, Roseli Esquerdo Lopes, and Sandra Galheigo coined the term "social occupational therapy" at the end of the 1990s. They aimed to designate a specific field of intervention, with a specific methodological framework and professional knowledge directed at specific populations for the accomplishment of occupational-therapeutic practice (Barros et al., 2005; Barros et al., 2007; Barros, Ghiradi, & Lopes, 2002). Their construction of social occupational therapy is rooted in a defense of the specificity and distinct nature of this a field.

The concept of the scientific field proposed by Bourdieu (1986) is here employed to consider intervention fields in occupational therapy and defend *social* occupational therapy as a field that falls under the larger umbrella of the knowledge and actions associated with occupational therapy. According to Bourdieu, the scientific field can be defined as a network or a configuration of objective relationships between positions that disputes spaces and legitimacy, dialoguing with the capital and relations of power involved. Thus, defending social occupational therapy as a subarea of occupational therapy means defending a field of knowledge and practices and disputing its recognition within occupational therapy. However, this process involves questioning of the hegemonic orders and struggle for power within the profession.

Defending social occupational therapy as a field within occupational therapy means establishing a specialty of its own, with actions aimed at the social inclusion of people whose central disadvantage is the socioeconomic factors that hinder and/or preclude their social participation and inclusion. This work demands from the professionals the development of specific assistance technologies focused on the social dimension of life. To this end, it is necessary to engage in a dialogue with the human and social sciences, to inform the development of a theoretical-methodological framework that focuses centrally on the social dimension. Social occupational therapy is

> a field of reflection and intervention defined sociologically as assistance to social groups experiencing processes of disruption to their social support networks. . . . [We] seek links capable of accounting for the occupational therapy practice that has been forming outside the health-disease structuring axis.
>
> (Barros et al., 2002, p. 95)

In the multiplicity of theoretical-methodological approaches that social occupational therapy has been implementing in Brazil, two related principles stand out: the *collective perspective of understanding the reality of population groups* and the *articulation between the micro- and macro-social aspects*. The *collective perspective of understanding the reality of population groups* refers to a reading of reality that extrapolates from the individual elements; it understands that the individual manifestations denote social problems, with each carrying subjective characteristics. Kleinman, Das, and Lock (1997) propose the concept of social suffering, pointing out the collective and class origins that many questions assume, to theoretically address contemporary themes associated with violence, gender, and the marks they make on the life histories of individuals. They consider social suffering to be the problems that arise from a collective condition. Coping with social suffering involves understanding social inequalities and avoiding the individualization of explanations for social phenomena. Thus, for instance, it is not possible to understand the homeless people through the life history of just one person and the discussion of the presence or absence of alcohol abuse in his or her trajectory. It is not possible to discuss offense only by explaining the paths traveled by one family or to address drug use exclusively by the addiction or dependence patterns of one individual. These are among many examples related to contemporary life. From the perspective of social occupational therapy, intervention with the homeless people, for example, presupposes action articulated through the policies and services available in the assistance network, including the macro-social questions, seeking action toward the people as well as the

collectives of this population. Intervention with young offenders should include understanding the structure of inequality, questioning the origin of these youths and their collective possibilities of access to social services and goods, and then jointly plotting strategies involving their options and potential courses of action. The structuring of services and assistance for drug addicts is necessarily permeated by a discussion of social organization, illegality, and prohibition, which is articulated through actions directed to the access of these groups to their social rights and the autonomous exercise of their lives. With this array of situations, we assume a clear posture contrary to the individualizing perspectives of the interpretation of social problems; there is no sense in conducting actions that focus only on decontextualized individuals, blaming them for the structural inequalities of which they are victims. Only through a collective approach to population groups can we discuss social occupational therapy.

The second principle is the *articulation between the micro- and macro-social aspects*. As previously argued, under the prism of the collective scope of the social situation of different population groups, articulation between a life history and the macro-structural elements is essential to discuss any action undertaken toward these people and groups. Once again relying on Kleinman et al. (1997), it is considered that the critical moments of social suffering experienced by people are reflexes of the macro-social aspects that determine their lives. Based on this assumption, professional intervention will occur for the expansion of social support networks, individual and social, as described by Castel (2003). In the individual sphere, strategies will be developed to assist people with finding support for their social inclusion and participation, respecting their choices and autonomy. As for the collective sphere, practice is connected to social policies and action in public spaces aimed at the maintenance and/or extension of the social recognition of certain needs, intervening in the expansion of services and other spaces that allow access to the rights of this group. It thus comprises the arduous task of articulating individual and collective actions—of a personalized and individualized work that is, at the same time—integrated with political actions. It is necessary to consider life histories, trajectories, moments, portraits, and explanatory flashes of reality that are linked to collective actions of different demands, with a multiplicity of social actors involved, to be able to approach social issues.

Therefore, the *collective perspective of understanding the reality of population groups* refers to a reading of the reality that always contextualizes the individual within a collective condition of the social life, and so professional action that specifically promotes the *articulation between micro- and macro-social aspects* is required. Based on these principles, we illustrate the possibilities of two approaches, very present in the experiences of occupational therapy in Brazil. One of them is the focus on the *cotidiano* (everyday life) of people. *Cotidiano* is a word of Latin origin widely used in Brazilian occupational therapy that does not translate satisfactorily into English. It is not restricted to everyday life, routine, or a mechanical or automatic idea of life reproduction. It involves politics, social condition, and culture: that is, the collective elements that constitute people. Thus, from now on, the term *everyday life* will be used in italics, referring to *cotidiano*. As advocated by Galheigo (2020), *everyday life* is not distinct from social life, and its concept is very advanced in the proposal of activities of daily living and instrumental activities of daily living that underlie and support some paradigms in occupational therapy. Including *everyday life* as a central element in the creation of intervention strategies in occupational therapy implies work that is rooted in context, in the personal, social, and territorial resources of people's lives. In social occupational therapy, this is named "Articulation of Resources in the Social Field" (Lopes, Malfitano, Silva, & Borba, 2014, p. 598). To consider *everyday life* as the work *locus* of social occupational therapy refers to a dedication to approaching multiple ways of life, to understanding them, and, finally, to jointly undertaking actions with the people involved.

The second principle chosen to be highlighted here is the *promotion of spaces of living together*, which aims to facilitate the approach of professionals to people and the mediation of demands for access to social goods. Designing work methodologies that foster the creation of spaces of living together for different population groups is in tune with the perspective of constituting spaces for collective experiences that may interest different people who choose to be there and collectively address certain issues of their lives. Such spaces may or may not be permeated by activities, and occupational therapists are professionals trained for the creation/improvement of spaces that lead to coexistence. This principle refers to the construction of spaces where people can talk, listen, express themselves, meet, and be with others in similar situations. To this end, the activity can be a medium for the accomplishment of this coexistence, a prerequisite for the encounter, or an artifact for collective organization. It means being open to what is meaningful to the other and to how occupational therapists can work with people to design strategies that facilitate living together, being together, and the coexistence of the relationships occurring in this space.

While it can be argued that social occupational therapy's focus on the social context is not different from that of occupational therapy in general, social occupational therapy seems to create a specific area for itself. Its specificity is associated with its actions with population groups for whom the socioeconomic question is central to their lives. It implements actions based on the precepts of human and social sciences and operates in different social policy centers (governmental and nongovernmental organizations): social assistance, education, culture, justice, and, depending on the approach, health. Through the inseparability of the macro- and micro-structures, social occupational therapy plans individual and collective actions that seek to mediate situations that may foster greater social participation and inclusion for people in situations of social inequality.

Individualization and the Medicalization of Social Life

In the final section of this chapter, I highlight a discussion that has been tangential to social occupational therapy: the contemporary trend toward an individualized understanding of the social phenomena and the offer of medicalization responses to social problems. I believe that there is a contemporary tendency associated with the individualization of life in which the health sector has embraced social demands without creating connections with the social sector. It creates responses, often intentionally, that go against the propositions of inclusion and assistance, in what is called iatrogenesis (Illich, 1970), that is, the creation of illnesses based on social problems, and healthism (Crawford, 2006), that is, biomedical contributions that obscure social determinants.

The theme of medicalization is quite old and has previously attracted the interest of academics seeking to understand social life. Ivan Illich introduced the concept of iatrogenesis, the creation of nonexistent diseases that are in fact rooted in social background, as early as the 1970s (Illich, 1974). In the context of Brazilian occupational therapy, Denise Barros discussed health medical organizations in the social area in the early 1990s (Barros, 1990), which demonstrates both how old and how current this theme is.

Didier Fassin (1998) shows that, in Western society, *urban figures* narrate social situations that gain a place of intervention in health services but that have economic causes. He goes on to discuss that "the figure is, on the one hand, the external form of a body, like an appearance, seen as a more precise resignation, the aspect of the person, which is expressed in its characteristics; on the other hand, it is the visual representation of the thing that is situated in the world of art or in the field of rhetoric" (Fassin, 1998, p. 10). Thus, looking only at the "visual representation of the thing," we have difficulty in seeing people, making it necessary to approach people from a collective perspective and understanding the individual elements of life stories as macro-social representatives of particular situations. Hence, the individual perspective gains strength and the iatrogenic illnesses appear as a consequence to social medicalization.

Instead of looking at people in relation to their collective social inclusion, we prioritize an individualizing explanation about the problems they experience, which often implies the culpability of these people. When we associate these people with *urban figures*, visible forms that do not represent real people but visual situations of what affects the world, the responses are standardized and cataloged to the individual explanations, which end up being understood as health problems. Thus, medicalization serves as an easy response to complex contemporary urban figures with whom it is difficult to engage. With the same critique, Chiara Pussetti (2010) describes the increase in diagnoses of mental health problems in immigrants in Europe, notably in Portugal, through the designation of "immigrant depression." She points out that there are growing cases that disregard the complex social situation the people are experiencing, pervaded by the precariousness of effective socioeconomic conditions for life, resulting in a medical diagnosis whose solution is the individual administration of medicines.

Rather than focusing on iatrogenesis and the medicalization of life, social policies implemented in the social area seek creative methodologies to work with the suffering other and understand the causes of that suffering.

As argued by Castel, looking for "the weaknesses of the individuals that cause or are the bases of the catastrophic situations they are experiencing" is the great risk that we take in responding to social problems only through the clinical sector in health, or in a reductionist way. In Castel's words:

I am concerned with the trend to psychologize or pathologize the problems; however, it is legitimate to think and have practices that try to correspond to the effects of objective processes of precariousness on the general psychic condition of individuals. And it is perceived that there may be certain rationality in thinking that someone who does not have the objective conditions of their social independence has problems of suffering and, indisputably, of pure and simple pathology. It seems to me that moving in this direction constitutes a necessary extension of the problem, and the risk is to reduce problems to psychologization and look for the weaknesses of individuals that cause or are the bases of the catastrophic situations they are experiencing. But it is clear to me that the conditions of non-social independence have psychic repercussions in terms of suffering or pathology. If people do not have conditions for their social independence, they may fall into a limited state.

(Castel, 2005, p. 157)

The dissociation of contexts, causes, and implications present in contemporary society can result in little or no effective progress and unassisted problems in the scope of social policies. The *new* demands that have been included in the social arena and become a topic of public debate present challenges for social policies, with their different inherent interfaces and intersectoralities, to implement modifications of paradigms, models, and intervention methods that respect the expression of multiple ways of life.

Occupational therapists often act as reproducers of actions of medicalization of social life, contributing to iatrogenic and/or healthist diagnoses and approaches. The challenge has been launched for professionals to engage in critical thinking that does not reduce social problems to health problems. Social occupational therapy contributes to the critique of this contemporary phenomenon and delimits specific actions for the social field, with its own methodologies, in the composition of an interdisciplinary, intersectorial, and interfaced field, acting against demands of medicalization to social problems. Social occupational therapy must effectively seek resources for action that aim at social inclusion and participation, always considering the structural limits of the unequal society in which we live. Moving in this direction, guided by the principles of social rights and working from a perspective committed to expanding access to social goods for all by means of technical, ethical, and political action, we will certainly witness the development and growth of occupational therapy in the social field.

REFERENCES

Almeida, M. C., Soares, C. R. S., Barros, D. D., & Galvani, D. (2012). Processos e práticas de formalização da Terapia Ocupacional na Assistência Social: alguns marcos e desafios [Formalization processes and practices of occupational therapy in social assistance: Landmarks and challenges]. *Cadernos de Terapia Ocupacional da UFSCar, 20*(1), 33–41. doi:10.4322/cto.2012.004

Barros, D. D. (1990). Operadores da saúde na área social [Health operators in the social field]. *Revista de Terapia Ocupacional da Universidade de São Paulo, 1*(1), 11–16.

Barros, D. D. (2004). Terapia ocupacional social: o caminho se faz ao caminhar [Notes for a social occupational therapy: The way is done by the way we go]. *Revista de Terapia Ocupacional da Universidade de São Paulo, 15*(3), 90–97. doi:10.11606/issn.2238-6149.v15i3p90-97

Barros, D. D., Galvani, D., Almeida, M. C., & Soares, C. R. S. (2013). Cultura, economia, política e saber como espaços de significação na Terapia Ocupacional Social: Reflexões sobre a experiência do Ponto de Encontro e Cultura [Culture, economics, politics and knowledge as meaning-spaces in social occupational therapy: Reflections on the experience of "Ponto de Encontro e Cultura"]. *Cadernos de Terapia Ocupacional da UFSCar, 21*, 583–594. doi:http://dx.doi.org/10.4322/cto.2013.060

Barros, D. D., Ghirardi, M. I. G., & Lopes, R. E. (1999). Terapia ocupacional e sociedade [Occupational therapy and society]. *Revista de Terapia Ocupacional da Universidade de São Paulo, 10*(2/3), 71–76.

Barros, D. D., Ghirardi, M. I. G., & Lopes, R. E. (2005). Terapia ocupacional social [Social occupational therapy]. *Revista de Terapia Ocupacional da Universidade de São Paulo, 13*(3), 95–103. doi:10.11606/issn.2238-6149.v13i3p95-103

Barros, D. D., Lopes, R. E., & Galheigo, S. M. (2007). Novos espaços, novos sujeitos: a terapia ocupacional no trabalho territorial e comunitário [New places, new people: Occupational therapy in the territorial and communitarian work]. In A. Cavalcanti & C. Galvão (Eds.), *Terapia ocupacional - fundamentação & prática* [Occupational therapy: Fundamentals and practices] (pp. 354–363). Rio de Janeiro: Guanabara Koogan.

Basaglia, F., & Ongaro-Basaglia, F. (1977). *Los crimines de la paz: investigación sobre los intelectuales y los técnicos como servidores de la oppression* [The crimes of the peace: Investigation about intellectuals and practitioners as oppression servers]. Madrid: Siglo XXI.

Borba, P. L. O., & Lopes, R. E. (2010). Organizações Não Governamentais, Jovens Pobres e Educadores Sociais nas Cidades [Non governmental organizations, poor youngsters and social educators in cities]. *Eccos Revista Científica, 12*(2), 437–452. doi:10.5585/eccos.n2.1904

Bourdieu, P. (1983). *Questões de sociologia [Sociological issues].* Rio de Janeiro: Ed. Marco Zero, 1983.

Bourdieu, P. (1986). *Distinction: A social critique of the judgement of taste.* London: Routledge.

Castel, R. (2003). *From Manual Workers to Wage Laborers: Transformation of the Social Question,* (Richard Boyd, Ed. & Translation). New York, NY: Routledge.

Castel, R. (2005). Risques, insécurité sociale et psychiatrie: Entretien [Risk, insecurity and psychiatry: Conversation]. In M. Joubert & C. Louzoun (Eds.), *Répondre à la souffrance sociale: la psychiatrie et l'action sociale en cause* [Answers to social suffering: The psychiatry and the social action on debate] (pp. 147–162). Paris: Edition Erès.

Castel, R., & Duvoux, N. (2013). *L'avenir de la solidarité* [The future of the solidarity]. Paris: La vie des idées, Presses Universitaires de France - PUF.

Crawford, R. (2006). Health as a meaningful social practice. *Health (London, England: 1997), 10*, 401–420. doi:10.1177/1363459306067310

Dagnino, E. (2000). Cultura, cidadania e democracia: a transformação dos discursos e práticas na esquerda latino-americana [Culture, citizenship and democracy: Transformation of discourses and practices in Latin-American left]. In S. E. Alvarez, E. Dagnino, & A. Escobar (Eds.), *Cultura e política nos movimentos sociais latino-americanos: novas leituras* [Culture and politics in social movements in Latin-America: new readings] (pp. 61–102). Belo Horizonte: Ed. da Universidade Federal de Minas Gerais (UFMG).

Dorneles, P. S., & Lopes, R. E. (2016). Cidadania e diversidade cultural na pauta das políticas culturais [Citizenship and cultural diversity in agenda of cultural policies]. *Brazilian Journal of Occupational Therapy, 24*(1), 173–183. doi:10.4322/0104-4931.ctoARF0669

Fassin, D. (Ed.). (1998). *Les figures urbaines de la santé publique* [The urban figure of the public health]. Paris: La Découverte, 1998.

Fassin, D., & Lézé, S. (2013). *La question morale: une anthologie critique* [The moral question: A critique anthropology]. Paris: Presses Universitaires de France - PUF.

Galheigo, S. M. (1997). Da adaptação psicossocial à construção ao coletivo: a cidadania enquanto eixo.[From psychosocial adaptation to construction to the collective: citizenship as center line] *Revista de Ciências Médicas PUCCAMP, 6*(2/3), 105–108.

Galheigo, S. M. (2020). Occupational therapy, everyday life and the fabric of life: theoretical-conceptual contributions for the construction of critical and emancipatory perspectives. *Brazilian Journalof Occupational Therapy, 28*(1), 5–25. https://doi.org/10.4322/2526-8910.ctoao2590.

Gerlach, A. J., Teachman, G., Laliberte-Rudman, D., Aldrich, R. M., & Huot, S. (2018). Expanding beyond individualism: Engaging critical perspectives on occupation. *Scandinavian Journal of Occupational Therapy, 25*(1), 35–43. doi:10.1080/11038128.2017.1327616

Ghirardi, M. I. G. (2012). Terapia Ocupacional em processos econômico-sociais [Socioeconomic processes in occupational therapy]. *Cadernos de Terapia Ocupacional da UFSCar, 20*(1), 17–20. doi:http://doi.editoracubo.com.br/10.4322/cto.2012.002

Gramsci, A. (1971). *Selections from the prison notebooks.* New York, NY: International Publishers.

Heller, A. (1984). *Everyday life.* London: Routledge.

Ilich, I. (1974). *Medical nemesis.* London: Calder & Boyars.

Kappel, V. B., Gontijo, D. T., & Alves, H. C. (2014). As ações do terapeuta ocupacional na rede de atenção aos adolescentes em conflito com a lei [The occupational therapist in the care network for young offenders]. *Revista Brasileira Adolescência e Conflitualidade, 10*, 61–86. doi:10.17921/2176-5626.n10p%25p

Kleinman, A., Das, V., & Lock, M. (Eds.). (1997). *Social suffering.* Berkeley, CA: University of California Press.

Leca, J. (2004). Etat [State]. In L. Boussaguet, S. Jacquot, & P. Ravinet (Eds.), *Dictionnaire des politiques publiques* [Dictionary of the public policies] (pp. 180–190). Paris: Presse de la Fondation Nationale des Sciences Politiques.

Lenhardt, G., & Offe, C. (1984). Social policy and the theory of the state. In C. Offe (Ed.), *Contradictions of welfare state* (pp. 88–118). Cambridge, MA: MIT Press.

Lopes, R. E. (2013). No pó da estrada [On the road]. *Cadernos de Terapia Ocupacional da UFSCar, 21*(1), 171–186. doi:10.4322/cto.2013.022

Lopes, R. E., Malfitano, A. P. S., Silva, C. R., & Borba, P. L. O. (2014). Recursos e tecnologias em Terapia Ocupacional Social: ações com jovens pobres na cidade [Resources and technologies in social occupational therapy: Actions with the poor youth in town]. *Cadernos de Terapia Ocupacional da UFSCar, 22*(3), 591–602. doi:10.4322/cto.2014.081

Malfitano, A. P. S. (2005). Campos e núcleos de intervenção na terapia ocupacional social [Intervention fields and cores in social occupational therapy]. *Revista de Terapia Ocupacional da Universidade de São Paulo, 16*(1), 1–8. doi:10.11606/issn.2238-6149.v16i1p1-8

Morais, AC, Malfitano, APS (2014). Medidas socioeducativas em São Paulo: os serviços e os técnicos. [Socio educational measures in São Paulo: services and technicians]. *Psicologia & Sociedade, 26*(3), 613-621. https://doi.org/10.1590/S0102-71822014000300010

Offe, C. (1974). Structural problems of the capitalist state. Class rule and the political system. *German Political Studies, 1*, 31–57.

Oliver, F. C., Pimentel, A., Uchoa-Figueiredo, L. R., & Nicolau, S. M. (2012). Formação do terapeuta ocupacional para o trabalho na Atenção primária à Saúde (APS): contribuições para o debate [Training of occupational therapists for primary health care (PHC): Contributions to the debate]. *Cadernos de Terapia Ocupacional da UFSCar, 20*(3), 327–340. doi:10.4322/cto.2012.033

Pussetti, C. G. (2010). Ethnographies of new clinical encounters. Immigrant's emotional struggles and transcultural psychiatry in Portugal. *Etnográfica, 14*(1), 115–133. Retrieved from http://www.scielo.mec.pt/scielo.php?script=sci_arttext&pid=S0873-65612010000100006&lng=en&tlng=en

Telles, V. S. (1990). Espaço público e espaço privado na constituição do social: notas sobre o pensamento de Hannah Arendt [Public space and private space building the social: Notes about Hannah Arendt thoughts]. *Tempo Social, 2*(1), 23–48.

Townsend, E. A. (1993). Muriel Driver Memorial Lecture: Occupational therapy's social vision. *Canadian Journal of Occupational Therapy, 60*, 174–184. doi:10.1177%2F000841749306000403

Universidade de São Paulo (USP). (1997). Definição de Terapia Ocupacional [Definition of occupational therapy]. Mimeo.

Whiteford, G., & Pereira, R. (2012). Occupation, inclusion and participation. In G. Whiteford & C. Hoking (Eds.), *Occupational science: Society, inclusion, participation* (pp. 187–208). West Susexx, UK: Whiley-Blackwell.

Whiteford, G., & Townsend, E. (2011). Participatory Occupational Justice Framework (POJF 2010): Enabling occupational participation and inclusion. In F. Kronenberg, N. Pollard, & D. Sakellariou (Eds.), *Occupational therapy without borders* (Vol. 2): *Towards an ecology of occupation-based practices* (pp. 65–84). Edinburgh, UK: Elsevier.

Wilcock, A., & Townsend, E. (2000). Occupational terminology interactive dialogue. *Journal of Occupational Science, 7*(2), 84–86. doi:10.1080/14427591.2000.9686470

World Federation of Occupational Therapists (WFOT). (2012). *Statement on occupational therapy*. Retrieved August 10, 2020, from https://www.wfot.org/about/about-occupational-therapy Access on August 10th, 2020

6

Occupational Therapy in the Context of Social Protection Expansion

Luciana Assis Costa

INTRODUCTION

Occupational therapy's application in the social field should be understood in association with the changes undergone by Brazilian Social Assistance, which resulted in the expansion of social policies as a right of citizens and a duty of the state. Therefore, this field cannot be dissociated from the context of the transformations that occurred in the political system and societal organization of the country, which resulted from the democratic opening up that led to the inclusion of social inequality and poverty in the political agenda as a matter for the state and legislation, no longer restricted to the liberal charitable scope or welfare models. Through the Brazilian redemocratization process, which featured the action of several social movements and a transformation in the relationship between the state and society, public policy frameworks were reconstructed based on the principles of social inclusion and the expansion of social rights, as expressed in the Constitution of the Federative Republic of Brazil of 1988 (Brasil, 2004). Social rights are outlined in Article no. 6 of the constitution of 1988 as those related to education, health, food, work, housing, leisure, safety, social security, protection of childhood and motherhood, and assistance for all (Brasil, 2012).

The expansion of occupational therapy practices addressing social issues arose in a paradoxical context alongside the redemocratization process. That process included the expansion of citizenship rights, especially within the social and political contexts, in the face of a developmental trajectory of the state imbued with strong liberal characteristics, marked by a historical social debt, and supported by inequality and extreme poverty—a pattern of Brazilian society practically unchanged until the mid-1990s. In the second half of the 1990s, with the expansion of public policies and social programs and given the complexity of Brazil's problems, new spaces for interdisciplinary practices were created for professionals in the social field, such

as occupational therapists, who were then at a fertile and challenging moment to consolidate epistemic and methodological strategies that could contribute actions aimed at a significant portion of the population deprived of basic social rights.

Based on this, and with a focus on the theme of social occupational therapy, this chapter is divided into five sections. The first section, the introduction, presents a general discussion of the social political context, in which poverty and social exclusion are major elements, and concludes with a brief case report that illustrates the possible contributions of occupational therapy to the social field. The second section briefly addresses the characteristics of Brazilian Social Assistance and the transformations that occurred after the redemocratization process with respect to the upsurge in social occupational therapy as it directly relates to the consolidation of social rights and the expansion of public policies in Brazil. The third section discusses the inclusion and professionalization of occupational therapy within social policies, particularly concerning the social security system. Considering the complexity of the phenomenon of poverty and social inequality, the fourth section analyzes some basic concepts of the social sciences, particularly in the field of social policies, identifying theoretical frameworks that may contribute to analytical reflection on social occupational therapy, considering that the phenomenon investigated is common to both areas. Finally, the fifth section presents an occupational therapy intervention in the social protection system in the form of a case report based on the follow-up of a young woman.

THE WELFARE STATE'S FUNCTION IN MITIGATING THE EXCLUDING EFFECTS OF THE CAPITALIST SYSTEM

The welfare state is a phenomenon that emerged in industrialized countries in the 20th century and was consolidated during the postwar period and, later, in developing countries. It is aimed at providing social services as a right guaranteed by the state to significant strata of the population, covering various forms of individual and collective risks. The welfare state acts as a compensation mechanism balancing the inequalities resulting from the capitalist system through the institution of a system of rights and social policies to avoid conflict and social disruption. "If the production and exclusion of social surpluses are a natural component of the market dynamics, the welfare state constitutes the appropriate social regulation of advanced capitalism" (Draibe, 1997, p. 6).

Nevertheless, social welfare provision and social policies can only be understood when analyzed with an understanding of the existing models of states, which establish different levels and forms of intervention concerning the delivery of social services. Regardless of the political system adopted, it is a duty of the state, in a more or less interventional way and with greater or lesser representation of the public interests, to confront the trends of social exclusion and fragmentation, protecting the collective order from their disruptive effects and providing national societies with minimum standards of social integration to preserve democratic life and economic participation (Draibe, 1997). This means that expansion of the state and the scope of assistance vary according to the political matrices of each country.

The classic definition by Esping-Andersen (1991) of the three ideal types of welfare state regimes—liberal, conservative, and social democratic—expresses the different conceptions of welfare state. In the liberal welfare state, assistance is predominantly provided to proven low-income recipients, or those with reduced rights or modest social security plans. Benefits are targeted mainly at the low-income population, the working class, or those relying on the government. In this model, the progress of social reform is severely limited by the traditional and liberal rules of labor ethics: the perceived drawback of the welfare state is the possibility of people opting for social benefits rather than working. The conservative welfare state, a historical legacy of state corporatism, is intended to assist the new postindustrial class structure. In this model, the preservation of differences in status is predominant; rights are thus associated with class and status. The social democratic welfare state, which occurs in the smallest number of countries, is adopted by nations where the principles of decommodification and universalism of social rights have also reached the new middle classes. Instead of abiding by a dualism between state and market, between the working class and the middle class, the social democrats aspire to a welfare state that promotes equality of the highest standards of quality of life, opposing the idea of equality of minimal needs, which is adopted everywhere else (Esping-Andersen, 1991).

Marked by dictatorial and authoritarian governments, Brazil accomplished the construction of a basic social protection system during the 1960s and 1970s. The context in which such a structure was built was a hybrid state with liberal and corporative features, classified as of a meritocratic-particularistic nature (Nunes, 2010). This model, characterized by institutional fragmentation, high levels of centralization, corporatism, selectivity, and patronage and associated with an underdeveloped economic system, partially explains the continuity of the high level of social exclusion and inequality in Brazil.

It is worth mentioning that the expansion of the social rights in Brazil occurred inversely to the Marshall model of citizenship (Marshall, 1967), because social benefits were provided during periods of severe restriction of individual liberties and denial of political rights. Marshall defines citizenship as the full participation of the individual in the political community and makes a distinction between three types of rights: civil rights, which guarantee individual liberties; political rights, which ensure participation in the exercise of political power; and social rights, which ensure access to a minimum material welfare. Marshall's argument is based on the logic that once civil rights are guaranteed, people will fight for political rights and will eventually achieve social rights (Marshall, 1967).

Access to goods and social services in Brazil until the 1970s depended almost exclusively on a person's formal participation in the labor market and, thus, on the condition of being a consumer and a taxpayer. Those on the margins of the labor market had to rely on philanthropic initiatives mostly of a religious or charitable nature. In the 1980s, the democratization process paved the way for the incorporation of social protection systems into the state reform agenda. In the case of Brazil, which had emerged from an autocratic regime, the idea was strengthened that political democracy would be followed by social democracy—established on the expansion of social rights, with higher levels of universalism; the expansion of the coverage of the programs; and the enhanced effectiveness of social expenditure (Draibe, 2003). Since then, social policy principles such as universality, integrality, decentralization, and democratization through participation channels have been established and have become the guide to the implementation and, consequently, the actions of professionals linked to these policies and programs (Brasil, 2004). The constitution of 1988 ratified the new restructuring principles of the social policy system, with social rights forming the basis of the policy, integrating taxpayers' rights into citizens' rights (Faria, 2005). In the early 1990s, a significant reduction in the social programs took place as a result of a strong neoliberal trend, fiscal adjustments, and a financial crisis. Only as of 1993 has the reform of social protection systems become evident. These initiatives emanated from the decentralization of the policies, articulation between the various programs, and the partnership between the government and social movements. Such trends specially affected the social and health assistance policy reforms, which have been considered social rights under the principle of universal free access to the public services since 1988.

In Brazil, social policies can be categorized for analysis within four thematic groups: (1) policies regarding labor and employment, which include social security and support to workers; (2) policies in the Social Assistance and Poverty Tackling Axis, which consist of social assistance, food security, and cash transfer; (3) policies in the Unconditional Rights to Social Citizenship Axis, such as health and education; and (4) policies in the Social Infrastructure Axis, especially those concerning housing and sanitation (Cardoso & Jaccoud, 2005).

The progress and expansion of Brazilian social services that took place between 1990 and 2010 cannot be denied, especially concerning access to health, social assistance, and cash transfer programs. However, one of the key criticisms of the current system is that state intervention is strongly oriented toward emergency policies and programs, lacking consistency of robust investments in social actions that are effectively redistributive, universal, and committed to the reduction of social inequalities. It is unquestionable that the need for focused and emergency actions developed, above all, as a result of policies that failed to consistently provide social assistance and tackle poverty. Occupational therapists have sought to contribute to the development of policies that transcend the necessity of urgent actions to address the most basic needs, aiming to lessen inherited inequalities and neutralize or reduce the distortive market dynamic effects of the capitalist system, which is the ultimate purpose of the welfare state (Reis, 2005).

EXPANSION OF OCCUPATIONAL THERAPY PRACTICE WITHIN THE SOCIAL SECURITY SYSTEM

From the normative point of view, the constitution of 1988 transformed the contributive perspective of the social insurance model into a conception of social security understood as "an integrated set of actions from the public powers and society aimed at assuring the population of rights to health, social security, and social assistance" (Brasil, 2012). The inclusion of health, social security, and social assistance as the tripod of social welfare introduced

the notion of universal social rights as a condition of citizenship, which was previously restricted to recipients of the social security system. Nonetheless, the Brazilian social protection system does not distinguish contribution-based rights from non–contribution-based ones, as in the case of social security, which, despite operating under the contributory logic, has increased its base of redistributive coverage through cash transfer programs such as rural retirement. As for health, once recognized as a universal right and a duty of the state, a social security medicine model was transformed into a national health model. Later, having acquired the status of public policy, social assistance began to break its links with the welfarist legacy (Monnerat & Souza, 2011).

In this chapter, attention is drawn to two of the policies that compose the social security tripod—health and social assistance—and to the inclusion of occupational therapists in this context of expansion of social policies. The growth of occupational therapy practice in the social field follows new demands generated by social programs and services resulting especially from the health policy that consolidated, in 1990, the Brazilian Unified Health System (SUS) and, later, implemented the Unified Social Assistance System (SUAS). Traditionally, the inclusion of occupational therapy in the context of social services was influenced by welfarist and philanthropic trends characteristic of the assistance provided to socially vulnerable populations.

To a certain extent, since 1970, occupational therapy has been included in philanthropic initiatives of a social nature that were historically responsible for providing assistance to the vulnerable and the poor in nursing homes for the elderly, the State Foundation for Well-Being of Minors (FEBEM), child day care centers, and shelters (Galheigo, 2003). It is important to stress that in that scenario, occupational therapy intervention with socially marginalized people was anchored in the health clinic logic, influenced by the concept of social pathology or deviation. After the 1990s, with the expansion of public social policies, the phenomenon of poverty was included in the dimension of social rights, making it a duty of the state to intervene in what used to be the responsibility of philanthropic organizations. Given its enhanced scope, occupational therapy intervention has been expanding and becoming more established both in the health area, with an increased number of positions in the public health department, and in the social assistance and social protection fields (Federal Council of Physical Therapy and Occupational Therapy [COFITO], 2014).

It is worth emphasizing that occupational therapy practice in the social security system, both in health and in social assistance, arose mainly from a political and academic positioning of the practitioners, either in the scope of societal organization, through the association with social movements during the 1970s, or in the epistemic and professional field, through questioning the role, methods, and theoretical framework of occupational therapy. In view of the complexity and multiple dimensions of Brazil's social issues, it is important to incorporate interdisciplinary, integrality, and intersectoral approach guidelines into the sectorial policies, combined with the social concepts of territoriality and networking. In the epistemological scope, it is important to propose inter- and multidisciplinary interventions associated with occupational therapy actions and, therefore, provoke new questions about the approach and intervention methods of the professionals linked to the social field. In the social field, it is important to stress that the focus of intervention remains on the relationship between individuals and their doing or their occupations. However, to form an understanding of the restrictions and interruptions to the everyday activities of individuals resulting from social exclusion, it is also necessary to understand the social relations and structures in which they are included.

The condition of exclusion hinders even the most ordinary daily activities not only at home but also in public spaces. Occupational therapists act as mediators when the occupational activities between individuals and their routines have been interrupted and they require the intervention of social policies and programs to gain access to goods or services. To widen the range of opportunities and choices for individuals who are in conditions of social exclusion and vulnerability, a minimum guarantee of access to social goods and services through social policies is necessary. In other words, providing citizenship patterns makes it possible to address the disadvantaged situations of these individuals. Therefore, social occupational therapy is intimately attached to the provision of social policies, which justifies a more comprehensive discussion on the phenomenon of poverty and social exclusion, as well as on how to tackle it through the guarantee of basic social rights.

The Brazilian literature addressing social policies, poverty, and social exclusion demonstrates concern about the inefficiency of public programs, whether governmental or philanthropic, which face sectorial fragmentation, low investment in structural policies, and a large portion of the population still living in vulnerable social conditions (Draibe, 2003; Faria, 2005; Bronzo, 2007; Filgueiras, 2004). In the current Brazilian context, characterized by the expansion of social rights and the perpetuation of poverty and social exclusion, some studies on this theme have sought to analyze the multiple factors that determine social marginality in order to combine the macro-social determiners of poverty with a micro-social analysis that may contribute to more effective intervention. Considering that social occupational therapy addresses individuals living in

socially vulnerable and disadvantaged conditions, it seems sensible to turn to social science discussions to contribute to the theoretical framework of this field.

Multidimensional Nature of Poverty and Social Exclusion: Contributions of Social Science to Social Occupational Therapy

Traditionally, occupational therapy practice has been associated with the physical or psychological conception of individuals, which tended to restrict individual attributes to knowledge about the processes of becoming sick and healing, as well as of social adaptation and reintegration. Not only in the natural sciences but also, above all, in the political and economic sciences, the individualistic approach to methodology has supported arguments that every individual bears sole responsibility for their own life; that is, each individual makes choices regardless of social constrictions, habits, and external aspirations. However, when we consider social inequality and social vulnerability, it becomes evident that while poverty and marginality are experienced on an individual and familial basis, their causes and remedies can never be understood as being restricted to one's personal sphere. This inversion of the traditional paradigm may be the biggest challenge faced by occupational therapists within their role as an articulator in society, which means they must intervene in the personal scope but take into consideration strategies and methodologies that affect social relations and structures. This means that isolated and enclosed actions, guided only by one individual, one program, or even one particular policy, tend to neglect the multiple factors that lead to conditions of vulnerability and social exclusion. For that matter, it is fundamentally important to comprehend the phenomenon in which one is intending to intervene so that occupational therapists or other professionals in this area do not make the mistake of transferring the problem of social poverty and misery onto the individual level.

With this in mind, we have sought theoretical studies that could be useful in the analysis and intervention of social occupational therapy. The proposed approaches have in common an attempt to combine, for the understanding of human behavior, relational elements from the concepts of social networks, space, and territory associated with structural contexts, especially those regarding the system of production and social protection that directly affect the phenomenon of poverty and social marginality.

Castel's work, as described in the specific literature on social occupational therapy, undeniably contributes to an understanding of the exclusion involved in the phenomenon of poverty and social inequality, associating the societal context within the capitalist system (Castel, 1998).

Castel goes beyond the usual binary understanding of the inclusion/exclusion relationship, instead understanding it as a dynamic and multifaceted process. From the combination of these two interdependent and dynamic processes, Castel suggests four types of "zones" where individuals may be distributed: (1) "integration" zone, where individuals are provided with the guarantee of stable work and are immersed in solid social relationships; (2) "vulnerability" zone, in which individuals experience a situation of precarious work relations and weakening of social connections; (3) "assistance" zone, which is the public sphere that has the goal of avoiding social rupture among individuals experiencing precarious work and fragile familial bonds; and (4) "disaffiliation" zone, where in addition to being unemployed, individuals have broken with the primary and secondary social ties that had been created in the labor environment, the neighborhood, the close vicinity, and so forth (Castel, 1998).

Castel defines social cohesion, within a dialectical relation with disaffiliation, as the capacity that a society has to coexist as a group formed by interdependency links based on two integration axes: economic, concerning the relationship between capital and work, and social or interactive, related to social and familial bonds. In the economic dimension, employment stability coexists with several work modalities that range from precarious situations to unemployment. Concerning the societal perspective, inclusion in social networks such as family, neighborhood, and community may deteriorate from solid relationships to situations of retraction and strain. From this dynamic and multifactorial understanding, it is possible to highlight at least three suppositions associated with the concept of *social exclusion* that are pillars of the theoretical and interventional formulations of social occupational therapy. Social exclusion:

1. is a multifactorial and multidimensional phenomenon linked to micro- and macro-social aspects that cannot be explained by individual attributes despite reflecting directly on the construction of the individuals' subjectivities;
2. encompasses poverty but is not restricted to material goods or to economic-occupational issues because it is also linked to the impossibility, or difficulty, of accessing mechanisms of social and community inclusion and protection systems;
3. is associated with failures of social cohesion mechanisms and the rupture of ties or integration principles, which result in isolation experiences, anonymity, crises in social connections, negative self-image, and disturbance to the sense of social belonging (Filgueiras, 2004).

It is possible to infer that the concept of social exclusion previously outlined—in addition to complementing an understanding of poverty, since it does not restrict its concept of social disadvantage to material elements—not only evidences the social function of the state concerning the *decommodification* of access to social rights but also evokes social cohesion mechanisms as an element that must be considered in the formulation, evaluation, and intervention of social policies.

Additionally, and still with an eye to integrating the micro- and macro-social analyses to understand social poverty and exclusion, the theme of territory has been acquiring the position of a relevant analytical category in this field of study. The territory issue emerges out of recognition of the heterogeneity of the poverty phenomenon, with the confirmation of a diversity of forms of its manifestation that arise from the combination of various vectors of exclusion that interact locally (Torres & Marques, 2004). There are questions related to the pertinence and legitimacy of the territorial approach as a strategy for reducing poverty, as focusing on this dimension would obscure the causes of inequality (Filgueiras, 2004). However, it is worth highlighting that focusing on territory to tackle poverty does not mean, a priori, holding a naive point of view that ignores the macro-structural causes of the phenomenon but allows the assertion that, given its geographically concentrated form, adopting such an approach to social policies has to do not only with the existence of strong negative external factors related to extremely poor neighborhoods but also with the local sociability potential that tends to minimize social deficits (Torres & Marques, 2004). One can observe a social dislocation process occurring within weakened social segments, which manifests in progressive isolation and retreat to familial relations. In contrast, at a local level, given the proximity and the geographical contiguities, possible social and mobility networks may be the anchor underpinning a collective identity construction, establishing a set of practices that become evident in "reciprocal regular services (shopping, childcare, administrative issues, sickness assistance, etc.)" (Paugam, 2003, p. 34).

In line with the idea that human existence is structured on the dimensions of historicity, sociability, and space, Lefebvre's (1994) notion of social space also suggests the dynamic potential of the concept of territory when it highlights space not only as a product of social relations but also as a means and condition of the (re)production of such relations. According to Lefebvre, social space involves many overlapping and interactive dimensions: the material spatial practices that are part of everyday life, the symbolic practices related to representations, and the imaginary spaces developed on utopian constructions, literature, and other forms.

The potential associated with territorialized socialization is described in the study by Cantor Magnani, where the author coins the notion of "part" as the spatial dimension that anchors the concepts of sociability and social networking development. In his words, "it is on the 'part' that the everyday fabric is woven: everyday life, leisure, exchange of information and small services, inevitable conflicts, participation in neighboring activities" (Magnani, 1982, p. 68). Magnani stresses the importance of social networking, especially for groups that are vulnerable to market oscillations or difficulties related to access to urban devices and social policies, which reflects an everyday life not yet characterized by concrete, comprehensive access to social rights (Brazil, 2004). In keeping with this line of thought, Koga presents the concept of territory as the concrete floor of every life, public policies, and citizenship, acting as a potential catalyst for "political and social refounding," where "the right to have rights is expressed, or denied, renounced, or claimed from concrete places: living, studying, working, leisure, healthy living, moving about, expressing opinions, participating" (Koga, 2003, p. 33).

According to Bronzo (2007), cited in the studies by Richardson and Munford, the category of *social infrastructure*, despite not evoking a new element for discussion, reiterates the articulation between the geographical (place) and community spaces concerning the understanding of poverty and social exclusion, stressing two empirical dimensions for investigation: (1) access to social goods and services and (2) societal aspects. The first refers to services and facilities present at the local level, such as housing, access to credit, education, health, social assistance, environment, and transportation; the latter involves the existence and quality of friendship networks, small informal groups, and performance of the social control mechanisms, such as collectively shared rules and regulations.

Aiming to qualify the community or social organization aspect foreseen in the concept of *social infrastructure*, Elias and Scotson (2000) take a figurative approach to offer a consistent analytical perspective to understand the social aspects of the exclusion phenomenon, according to their figurative form of established individuals and *outsiders*. They look beyond the dimension of class in their analysis of the *outsiders*, or *marginal individuals*, pointing out the difference in the organization of the individuals, evaluated according to the level of group cohesion, social control, and collective identification, and to communal regulations capable not only of constituting a consciousness of belonging but also of defining social positions with different levels of inclusion. Through this approach, the concept of exclusion or *outsider* is operationalized within the following dimensions: the ways individuals belong to local institutions (religious, leisure, educational, community spaces, etc.); the cohesion level among the residents; and the uniformity of regulations and beliefs, as well as their

concomitant external and internal discipline (Elias & Scotson, 2000). They also highlight that social marginality is produced within the group's interrelations and in the establishment of power positions and stress that social stigma tends to penetrate the marginalized individual's self-image, causing an even greater weakness. Stigmatization is less likely to occur when the existing sources of power are altered. Nonetheless, it is not possible to analyze relationship networks if they are disconnected from opportunities of access to goods and services. In that case, an informal social network of control and regulations may be reconstructed, as they are necessary to the social organization.

Still concerning social networks, Granovetter (1973) provides an important theoretical contribution, stating that, as with the term "exclusion," the concept of social network comes with a range of interpretations that end up compromising its analytical potential. In this study, Granovetter's concept of social network was chosen, which discusses the open or diverse social network as structures typical of modern society that generate social density. The interaction between individuals in society depends, to a certain extent, on the *weak ties* established between people, which transcend the most intimate circles (primary groups) and enable intergroup connections. These weak ties play a relevant role in individual mobility, because their potentialities lead to increased information circulation and labor market inclusion via interaction with different groups (Granovetter, 1973). Understanding the range of weak ties that compose individuals' social bonds may reveal their potential for sociability and demonstrate the influence of such interactions on social mobility and inclusion. Bearing in mind that social exclusion and poverty are the bases of this study, it is worth mentioning that collective mobilization is less evident where the establishment of weak ties is scarce. This occurs in the disadvantaged social economic classes because the homogeneity of the economic conditions limits exchanges and opportunities to access resources and information. However, the societal and relational factors should be considered in the process of diagnosis and in the interventions of policies and social programs, as an issue to be raised in the local sphere, if added to more complex social problems that associate the sociability potential with the access to material goods and services to facilitate the understanding and tackling of poverty and social vulnerability.

Faced with the variety of dimensions in which poverty and social exclusion are expressed, it would be naive not to problematize the fact that a *social status* of inferiority and devaluation marks the identities of those who experience poverty, compromising the development of social bonds and the collective claim for better living conditions (Paugam, 2003). This diminishing self-image, which results from the regular experiencing of extreme deprivation conditions, can only be overcome through the construction of new social networks mediated by the expansion of opportunities and guarantee to citizenship rights.

Notes on the Possible Contributions of Social Occupational Therapy

Some theoretical and empirical studies present consensus in the current literature about the scope of social occupational therapy, whose main focus is to assist people who have been deprived of material, symbolic, and social goods (Galheigo, 2003). In this context, Barros, Ghirardi, and Lopes (2002) identify four assumptions that support the need for occupational therapy to overcome the clinically oriented paradigm with the intention of addressing the phenomenon of social disadvantage that affects the everyday life of individuals, groups, and communities, limiting their opportunities, choices, and occupational perspectives. The study shows that occupational therapy remains focused on intervening in the relationship established between people and their activities and/or occupations. The fundamental change observed regards the origin of the factors that interfere with the everyday lives of this population, factors that are predominantly social in nature and therefore cannot be explained through biological, psychological, or functional approaches, although poverty and social exclusion are symbolically and subjectively experienced at the individual level. Thus, it must be understood that moving away from the clinical approach does not mean ignoring the singularities of individuals, since the experience of exclusion and marginality present personal particularities in spite of the common *leitmotif* (Lopes et al., 2005). Having said that, this study aims to discuss each assumption raised by Barros et al. (2002) that guides the practice of social occupational therapy according to the theoretical framework discussed in the previous section.

The first argument refers to "decentralizing the technical knowledge and moving to the idea of plural knowledge when facing social issues" (Barros et al., 2002, p. 100). This principle corroborates the previous discussion on the multidimensional nature of poverty and social exclusion, since social disadvantage is not restricted to material or personal aspects. Given the complexity of this phenomenon, it is necessary to expand from specialized knowledge to plural knowledge, which justifies the adoption of interdisciplinary and intersectoral guidelines concerning occupational therapy practices within social policies and programs.

Two other assumptions found in Barros et al. (2002)—decentralization of the individuals' actions to the collective sphere and decentralization of the setting actions to the context of everyday life—can be analyzed together because they regard changes in the conception and understanding of human behavior and their repercussions on the objective of occupational therapy intervention (Barros et al., 2002).

From an explanation provided in the natural and psychological sciences, from which individuals are a source of understanding of the processes of becoming sick and social exclusion, a relational conception was sought aiming at the inseparability between individual action and the surrounding social relationships and structures. If the phenomenon of social exclusion cannot be explained by the individual, tackling it should necessarily consider the social and institutional relationships in which the individual is involved, and in this case, the importance of occupational therapists transposing "the action of the setting to the spaces of everyday life" is reiterated.

In examining literature for this study, concepts were sought that could assist with understanding everyday life spaces for occupational therapy intervention aiming at dialogue about the connection between macro realms (such as the social inequalities) and micro realms (such as daily occupations). The definition of territory, which involves communitarian or social cohesion dimensions addressed in the concepts of *social networks*, *part*, and *social space* and in the *established-outsiders* configuration associated with access to social goods and services, as indicated in the term "social infrastructure" and in the conceptualization of integration and disaffiliation, offers an applicable theoretical framework to support occupational therapy interventions in the social field. From this point of view, not only can the material dimensions experienced in everyday life be expressed by occupational activities (study, leisure, work, art, self-care, domestic activities, etc.) but also the symbolic or representational (beliefs, social codes, regulations, social control, etc.) and subjective activities should also be taken into account when understanding the intervention of social occupational therapy. As a result, "decentralizing the concept of activity from a solely individual process to a historical and cultural process" (Barros et al., 2002) may be the nodal point for social occupational therapy's contribution, given the challenge of transposing the analytical understanding of the phenomenon of social exclusion to intervention strategies.

In view of the complexity of the social problem and the social debt that the state has with a significant part of the population, which still lacks basic social rights, how can occupational therapists contribute to the effective transformation of the current scenario? First, it seems fundamental that the professional be linked, directly or indirectly, to social policies and programs, especially those aimed at tackling poverty and social inequality. Only with the support of public policies can occupational therapy be enabled to formally contribute to the social field, considering that this problem is connected to the disruption of social and citizenship rights and ought to be addressed by the welfare state system. The relationship with individuals under vulnerable conditions should be understood from this context, bearing in mind at least four dynamic and interdependent dimensions that influence occupations: (1) quality access to the basic social services available in the region; (2) strong working relations and access to income for individuals and their families; (3) level of social cohesion, belonging, and self-image constructed by the individuals based on the group codes into which they are included; and (4) the possibility of exchanging and accessing resources and information that arise from the weak ties established between groups. Only through this set of information will occupational therapists, in an interdisciplinary way, be able to outline intervention strategies, individual or collective, that contribute to tackling the issues previously described. In light of this reflection, it can be clearly stated that "occupational therapists feel challenged when realizing that their praxis is part of a historical process, and that it presents inseparable technical and political dimensions" (Barros et al., 2002, p. 96).

The systematic needs faced by people who live in conditions of marginality tend to limit personal choices and opportunities, often resulting in progressive isolation, lack of perspectives and life projects, and a retreat to the sphere of domestic relationships. Therefore, to act as an articulator in society, before the complexity of the determinants of social exclusion, occupational therapists should deconstruct the myths around the concept of activity/occupation, regarding the naturalization of their therapeutic value that results from an abstract interpretation, lacking a concrete sense to the individual (Galheigo, 2003).

In the social field, the relationship between the individual and the activity should be understood through experience and everyday practices, intermingled with societal (relational) and structural elements that directly affect the individual's actions, choices, desires, and life projects. This means that the space of occupational therapy intervention is built on the reality experienced by the assisted population, that is, from the individual or collective that resides, lives, and moves about a certain social space (territory) in which the daily life fabric is woven: everyday life, leisure, exchange of small services and information, inevitable conflicts, and participation in neighborhood activities, thus a space where construction of new personal experiences is possible (Magnani, 1982). Based on the conceptual understanding that the individual is constituted from the interdependency of social and historical relationships, occupational therapists will be able to contribute as mediators in the creation of alternatives that seek to modify occupational patterns marked by limitations stemming from inadequate schooling or early exclusion

from educational institutions, precarious labor relations or unemployment, and a lack of leisure, arts, culture, and sports collective spaces, often expressed by feelings of social disqualification, lack of perspective, and low self-esteem (Paugam, 2003).

A possible contribution of social occupational therapists would be to identify, unravel, and potentialize personal interests and abilities and, simultaneously, present and arouse new possibilities and desires that may expand and diversify not only the occupations that are part of the everyday lives of these individuals but also, above all, the construction of new social bonds and roles.

In keeping with this line of thought, the concept of the social network defined by Granovetter (1973) is relevant in thinking about intervention strategies in social occupational therapy, considering that access or restriction to everyday life activities—leisure, education, work, communal, religious, and so forth—is directly associated with the possibility of exchanging information and resources that enable choices and life projects. There is a reciprocal effect between the expansion of opportunities and occupational activities offered and the expansion of social ties between groups (social network), consequently increasing individuals' chances of social inclusion. The expansion and enhancement of the social network, understood as strengthening the weak ties, and the expansion of the range of everyday activities are two dimensions that should be contemplated by occupational therapy intervention proposals, with the main objective of expanding the social and civic participation of those who are in socially vulnerable conditions. Therefore, the opportunities and choices depend, concomitantly, on access to social goods and services, as well as personal involvement and motivation, stressing the fact that occupational therapists cannot ignore the structural dimensions and causes of inequality or the social function of the state to provide such goods and services. Thus, the practice of occupational therapy should be interdisciplinary and intersectoral, making use of existing social policies and programs—such as education, social assistance, health, safety, food security, cash transference programs, housing, culture, leisure, and labor—to effectively enable the expansion of the opportunities and choices of the population living in vulnerable conditions.

What follows is the presentation of a brief case report to exemplify one possible social occupational therapy practice. The intervention was conducted within the public security policy and targeted young women who were incarcerated in a so-called socioeducational institution.

Case Report

Since 2012, the Department of Occupational Therapy of the Federal University of Minas Gerais (UFMG), in partnership with the state secretary of social defense of the state of Minas Gerais, Brazil, has been constructing learning spaces and experiences for young offenders. The secretary is responsible for formulating and implementing processes of restriction to freedom for young offenders in Minas Gerais.

In Brazil, protection and assistance policies for children and adolescents have gone through changes since the federal constitution of 1988, which recognized the rights of these populations. The Brazilian Child and Adolescent Statute (CAS) establishes childhood and adolescence as the periods between 0 and 12 and 12 and 18 years of age, respectively. The CAS conceives children and adolescents as individuals under special conditions of development. Article 2013 of the CAS defines "offense" as a crime or misdemeanor (Brasil, 1990). Young offenders are subjected to social-educational measures regulated by the National System of Socioeducational Care (Sinase), which aims to identify the offender, encourage social integration, and guarantee social and individual rights. The measures are classified into six categories, applied according to the seriousness of the offense: warning, obligation to repair damage, community service, assisted freedom, secure detention, and secure confinement (Brasil, 1990). Secure confinement is the most severe measure because it deprives the adolescent of freedom, and it is applied in cases of serious crime or threat to the community (according to the CAS). During secure confinement, the CAS establishes that certain rights are compulsory, such as activities dedicated to education, health, social assistance, culture, sports, and qualification for work. The period of confinement is not set by a court ruling; instead, maintenance of confinement is assessed every 6 months, and the maximum period of the measure is 3 years (Brasil, 1990).

Two distinct ideas concerning secure confinement can be identified: coercion and socialization. The service must deal with coercion to maintain order and guarantee the establishment of routine, uniformity, and discipline. On the other hand, socialization and the reconstruction of values, identities, and attitudes need to be considered, as they are the basis for social educational measures. Although social integration is the main purpose of these measures, there is a high level of recidivism. Studies show that young offenders return to the centers 6 months after release on average. Given this problem, occupational therapists proposed follow-up work with adolescents in the final period of their confinement, aiming to support them in their return to community life. To this end, undergraduate students of the UFMG occupational therapy program, doing placement in the social field, followed the release process of some adolescents, aiming to mediate their return to community life. The purpose was to assist with access to

public services (education, leisure, social assistance, etc.), identify and expand support networks, and expand occupational opportunities that could transform life histories marked by deprivation and lack of opportunities in various areas of life. The following case report details the follow-up of an adolescent called Dandara in a youth detention center for women.

First, the adolescent's social occupational background was surveyed through the formal records of the service, conversation with the adolescent herself, and the use of manual and expressive activities (drawing and writing). The interns identified a history of social and economic vulnerability throughout Dandara's life, with a consequent lack of opportunities. However, once the interns got closer to her, they learned that activities involving music and arts were an interesting possibility for her.

In one of the first interventions with Dandara, she was asked to freely name "people, places, and ideas" that referred to some kind of affective, resource, or assistance support on which she would be able to rely after being released. It was then possible to identify interests connected to leisure, professional, artistic, and spiritual activities, in addition to social networks and emotional and reliance bonds that composed her social relations. Dandara wrote her name in the center of a sheet of paper and expressed, in words, family, aspects related to personal care, religion, sports, schooling, and digital media resources. The last ones seemed to be written in a very random way. On the back of the sheet, she wrote words that at first seemed inarticulate but made sense when she composed a rap. The song was about the idea that she was "no longer under secure confinement." It also mentioned the period during which she was confined in the youth detention center, as well as her life history.

Lyrics of the rap "Project I'm Off":

I'm off drugs / I'm off brawl / no matter the purpose / I'm off / freedom is the goal / patience is the key / I had to go to jail / to find the truth / this is awesome / children growing up / teenagers at school. . .

The interventions that followed provided knowledge about her family relationships, her fragile bond with school, her precarious inclusion in the labor market, her interest in collective sports, and her need for having a profession. However, some of the most frequently highlighted interests, needs, and demands were connected to musical activities, especially to funk, her favorite kind of music, which was often present in her particular way of expressing her experiences and thus was the lead topic of the first interventions. Once her familiarity with music was discovered, partnerships with music schools were sought and DJ lessons were provided. In seizing this opportunity, she eagerly expressed the importance of formally learning music. In this opportunity, she highlighted the fact that obtaining the DJ certificate meant fulfilling a dream and gaining new professional perspectives. In the following lyrics, Dandara expressed how much the opportunity to attend a DJ course made sense to her. In addition, she offered a more comprehensive reflection on some desires and obstacles she had to face in her everyday life:

> *Whether I would be able to get there, I don't know*
>
> *Now I have the opportunity to be a DJ*
>
> *My name is Dandara and my brother's name is Luciano*
>
> *My nickname is Dara and his is MC Jordan*
>
> *I didn't have a mind, but I have evolved*
>
> *I'm going to become a DJ and he is going to become an MC*
>
> *Before, I couldn't focus to think*
>
> *Now, what I really want is to study and work*
>
> *I have dreamed of being a police officer or a doctor*
>
> *But I'm afraid of the ENEM*
>
> *But one day I will try*
>
> *I'm going to stop here and slow down*
>
> *"Xia, xia" lessons!!! (Dandara)*

In the institutional sphere, her experience with the Youth Detention Center's multiprofessional team, with its social workers and security officers, produced an understanding of the occupational therapists' work, which facilitated the planning of external activities with her, such as the DJ course and visits to the university, in addition to weekly meetings with the occupational therapist. Aiming to map a social support network that would assist her during her return to community life, the occupational therapist contacted some members of social movements and nongovernmental organizations focused on young people, such as the Observatório do Funk (Funk Observatory) and the Youth Reference Center. The Funk Observatory is a cultural political collective created in 2017, formed by lawyers, journalists, and cultural producers of the Aglomerado da Serra, one of the largest groups of favelas in Latin America, composed of six villages with approximately 80,000 inhabitants. It seeks better ways to hold funk concerts in the city, in addition to promoting activities such as the Funk Incubator, which conducts workshops and debates on funk music. The Youth Reference Center of Belo Horizonte, state of Minas Gerais, is the first public organization specifically aimed at youth, with the objective of promoting culture, leisure, sports, education, and professional training activities directed to the population aged 15 to 29.

All interventions took place in the 4-month period that preceded her release. Notwithstanding her confinement, it was possible to articulate and mediate her access to social services and other organizations in her community that would provide opportunities and perspectives after her release and still consolidate the support that is essential to all successful social interventions. Intervention in a closed institution presents real limits concerning the curtailment imposed on young women's daily lives due to their restriction of freedom. However, assisting them while they are being released from the youth detention center enables the mobilization of support networks, whether affective or of services, which increases the chances of a successful return to community life. Taking into consideration the wide range of vulnerability factors that act on the lives of these young women, social occupational therapy does not neglect the structural dimension, especially the socioeconomic one, that restricts choices and opportunities. Conversely, the professionals act to create new spaces of leisure, arts, sports, education, and interaction experiences that may arouse new interests and perspectives that were not previously part of their lives. Thus, it is essential that occupational therapists become familiarized with the territories and the social networks that are part of those young women's lives so that the intervention can, in fact, provide them with a wider range of opportunities. This is one of the approaches of occupational therapy practice in dealing with populations living in vulnerable conditions and deprived of basic social rights. Interaction with public policies, especially the social ones, is one of the ways of amplifying opportunities of occupational experiences among this population, aiming at the support of citizenship rights.

In short, considering the multiple challenges inherent to the field, professionals ought to establish a constant dialogue between the everyday actions of the target population and the macro-structural dimensions and how they can directly influence their life conditions (Malfitano, 2005). It is expected that the professionals present a political attitude to stimulate, along with the assisted population, a critical and active attitude regarding the search for answers to social needs and demands.

FINAL REMARKS

In view of the expansion of social programs and policies in Brazil and the possibility of social occupational therapy's contribution, professional practice in this field should be constantly mindful of the multiple dimensions that make up/construct poverty and social exclusion. Thus, occupational therapy's contributions to this field should involve actions that encompass not only the personal, subjective dimension of the social connections but also structural issues, especially those regarding the provision of social services and goods. Therefore, all variables and explanatory mechanisms that can support social occupational therapy within the selected theoretical framework should be exhausted. The presented literature, however, contemplates the dialogue between the micro- and macro-social elements that influence the relationships of individuals with everyday life. Thus, this brief case report illustrates, though on a small scale, a perspective for social occupational therapy practice with youths under vulnerable conditions based on the theoretical framework herein presented.

Finally, occupational therapists are only one part of this social mechanism, playing the role of mitigators of human miseries. If their actions are limited, given the multiple dimensions of the problem presented, they should consider the complexity of the phenomenon so that their practice is, in fact, able to cause transformation and reflect, in a comprehensive way, on the struggle to guarantee social rights and citizenship.

REFERENCES

Barros, D. D., Ghirardi, M. I. G., & Lopes, R. E. (2002). Terapia Ocupacional Social [Social occupational therapy]. *Revista de Terapia Ocupacional da Universidade de São Paulo, 13*(13), 95–103. doi:10.11606

Brasil (1990). The Brazilian Child an Adolescent Statute (CAS). Retrieved from http://www.planalto.gov.br/ccivil_03/leis/l8069.htm

Brazil, F. P. D. (2004). Território e territorialidade nas políticas sociais [Territory and territoriality in social policies]. In C. Bronzo & B. Costa. (Eds.), *Gestão Social: o que há de novo?* (pp. 45–66). Belo Horizonte: Fundação João Pinheiro.

Brasil. (2012). *Constitution of the Federative Republic of Brazil of 1988.* Retrieved from http://www.planalto.gov.br/ccivil_03/constituicao/constituicao.htm

Bronzo, C. (2007). Território como categoria de análise e como unidade de intervenção nas políticas públicas [Territory as a category of analysis and as a unit of intervention in public policies]. In M. Fahel & J. A. B. Neves (Eds.), *Gestão avançada de políticas sociais no Brasil* [Advanced social policy management in Brazil] (pp. 91–114). Belo Horizonte: Editora PucMinas.

Cardoso Jr., J. C., & Jaccoud, L. (2005). Políticas Sociais no Brasil: organização, abrangência tensões da ação estatal [Social policies in Brazil: Organization, comprehensiveness, tensions of state action]. In L. Jaccoud (Ed.), *Questão Social e políticas sociais no Brasil contemporâneo* (pp. 181–260). Brasília: IPEA.

Castel, R. (1998). *As metamorfoses da questão social: uma crônica do salário* [The metamorphoses of the social question: a chronicle of wages]. Petrópolis: Vozes.

Draibe, S. (1997) Uma nova institucionalização das políticas sociais? Reflexões a propósito da experiência latino-americana recente de reformas dos programas sociais [A new institutionality of social politics? Reflections on experience recent Latin American reforms of social programs]. *São Paulo em perspectiva, São Paulo, 11*(4), 3–15.

Draibe, S. (2003). A política social no tempo de FHC e o sistema de proteção social [Social policy in the FHC period and the social protection system]. *Tempo Social, São Paulo, 15*(2), 63–101. doi:10.1590/S0103-20702003000200004

Elias, N., & Scotson, J. (2000). *Os estabelecidos e os outsiders* [The established and the outsiders]. Rio de Janeiro: Zahar.

Esping-Andersen, G. (1991). As três economias políticas do Welfare State [The three political economies of the welfare state]. *Lua Nova: Revista de Cultura e Política, São Paulo, 24*, 85–116. doi:10.1590/S0102-64451991000200006

Faria, C. A. P. (2005). O gato de Alice e as agendas da política social brasileira [Alice's cat and the agendas of Brazilian social policy]. *Teoria e Sociedade*, n. esp. 6, 56–67 (série fora de série).

Federal Council of Physical Therapy and Occupational Therapy (COFITO). (2014). Resolution n.383 December 22nd 2010 [It defines the competences of the occupational therapist in the social context and presents other measures]. Retrieved from http://www.coffito.org.br

Filgueiras, C. A. C. (2004). Exclusão, risco e vulnerabilidade: desafios para a política social [Exclusion, risk and vulnerability: Challenges for social policy]. In C. Bronzo & B. Costa (Eds.), Gestão Social: o que há de Novo? [Social management: what's new?] (pp. 25–34). Belo Horizonte: Fundação João Pinheiro.

Galheigo, S. M. (2003). O social: idas e vindas de um campo de ação em terapia ocupacional [The social: Comings and goings of a field of action in occupational therapy]. In E. M. Pádua & L. V. Magalhães (Eds.), *Terapia ocupacional: teoria e prática* [Occupational Therapy: theory and practice] (pp. 29–46). Campinas: Papirus.

Granovetter, M. (1973). The strength of weak ties. *American Journal of Sociology, 78*(6), 1360–1380.

Koga, D. (2003). *Medidas de cidades: entre territórios de vida e territórios vividos* [Measures of cities: Between living territories and lived territories]. São Paulo: Cortez.

Lefebvre, H. (1994). *The production of space.* Oxford: Blackwell.

Lopes, R., Palma, A., & Reis, T. (2005). A experimentação teórico-prática do aluno de Terapia Ocupacional no campo social: uma vivência com a população em situação de rua [The theoretical-practical experimentation of an Occupational Therapy student in social field: an experience with homeless people] . Revista de Terapia Ocupacional da Universidade de São Paulo, 16(2), 54–61. https://doi.org/10.11606/issn.2238-6149.v16i2p54-61

Magnani, J. G. C. (1982). Os pedaços da cidade [Periphery and downtown: Sociability and uses of the urban areas]. *Espaços e Debates, São Paulo, 2*(5) 67–80. doi:10.11606/2179-0892.ra.1992.111360

Malfitano, A. P. S. (2005). Campos e núcleos de intervenção [Intervention fields and cores in social occupational therapy]. *Revista de Terapia Ocupacional da Universidade de São Paulo, 16*(1), 1–8. doi:10.11606/issn.2238-6149.v16i1p1-8

Marshall, T. H. (1967). *Cidadania, classe social e status* [Citizenship, social class and status]. Rio de Janeiro: Zahar.

Monnerat, G. L., & Souza, R. G. (2011). Da seguridade social à intersetorialidade: reflexões sobre a integração das políticas sociais no Brasil [From social security to "intersectoriality": Reflections on the integration of social policies in Brazil]. *Revista Katálysis, Florianópolis, 14*(1), 41–49.

Nunes, E. (2010). *A gramática política do Brasil: clientelismo, corporativismo e insulamento burocrático* [The political grammar of Brazil: Clientelism, corporatism and bureaucratic insulation]. Rio de Janeiro: Garamond.

Paugam, S. (2003). *Desqualificação social: ensaio sobre a nova pobreza* [Social disqualification: Essay on the new poverty]. São Paulo: Cortez.

Reis, F. W. (2005). Política, democracia e questão social [Politics, democracy and social issues]. *Teoria e Sociedade,* n. esp. (6), 24–43 (série fora de série).

Torres, H. G., & Marques, E. (2004). Políticas sociais e território; uma abordagem metropolitana [Social policies and territory: A metropolitan approach]. *Revista São Paulo em Perspectiva, São Paulo, 18*(4), 28–38.

7

Occupational Therapy and Social Assistance: Building a Critical Thinking about the Field

Marta Carvalho de Almeida and Carla Regina Silva Soares

A systemized reflection on the action of occupational therapy in social assistance in Brazil is a proposal that opens an array of possibilities if the challenge is to advance the debate on professional interventions in this field. It is worth noting that in 2011, Brazilian legislation (resolution no. 17, 2011) formally recognized occupational therapists as professionals qualified to compose teams and assume management functions as part of Brazil's social assistance services. It was a moment when the legislative understanding of occupational therapists broadened beyond perceiving them exclusively as health professionals. This fact raised many questions about where occupational therapists practice, gaining academic and professional relevance.

However, discussion guided only by the instrumental and technical character of professional practice should be avoided. Thus, this chapter prioritizes the gathering of aspects that enable incursion through some social processes that lead the professional actions in the social field in general, and in Brazil in particular. This chapter will begin by introducing social assistance as a historical phenomenon and, consequently, as a set of practices inseparable from the general scope of political, economic, and cultural development. This led to the emergence and development of social policies within the framework of capitalist socioeconomic formations, that is, marked by the contradictions of this mode of production. Occupational therapy—a profession that has also emerged within these contradictions and in the context of the sociotechnical division of labor—was approached as a sphere of construction and validation of notions connected to the set of interpretations and responses historically produced to cope with social problems.

SOCIAL POLICIES AND THEIR RELATION TO SOCIOECONOMIC DEVELOPMENT

Social policies have been studied by different areas of knowledge. Usually, they are described as principles, legislation, and actions that affect the well-being of members of a society through shaping the distribution of and access to goods and resources in that society. They range, therefore, from protection against particular life cycle circumstances, such as childhood and old age, to adverse situations such as poverty, deprivation, accidents, unemployment, and diseases (Viana & Levcovitz, 2005; Behring & Boschetti, 2011).

Similarly to Behring and Boschetti (2011), this text affirms, based on a critical-dialectical perspective, that social policies reflect the process and result of complex and contradictory relationships between the state and society, which occur in the context of struggles between the different interests that exist in capitalist society (capital–labor relations). These interests are commonly expressed by social collectives politically constituted and organized, and the difference between their interests lies in the fact that individuals, depending on their social class and social groups, occupy unequal positions in the social scene. In other words, they don't have the same opportunities to gain protection or to access and enjoy collectively produced goods to meet their various needs (Behring & Boschetti, 2011; Faleiros, 2012). From this standpoint, social policies neither are definitive solutions to ensure social justice and well-being (since they do not change the origin of inequalities) nor merely function to increase capitalist accumulation, although they certainly play an important role in reducing workforce reproduction costs for employers, helping to maintain high productivity and consumer demand.

A historical-critical interpretation of social policies leads us to consider their multi-causality, their contradictory role in society, and their different dimensions—historical, economic, political, and cultural—in an articulated and imbricated way. Thus, the existence of social policies is closely associated with the achievements of different groups in the sense that they have their needs and interests legitimized and guaranteed by the state, depending on the decisions enacted by the ruling political forces at a given historical moment. Nevertheless, they also depend on structural economic issues, which assign a given configuration to capitalism.

Based on this theoretical-methodological perspective, it is necessary to look at the development of social policies—and more specifically that of the Brazilian social assistance policy—as an expression of the social question. Equally, it is important to consider the social conflict that originates and maintains the dispute between different social projects, each composed of different social actors organized as forces that act in the defense of specific interests. It is in this process and in the arenas where these disputes occur, whether institutional or otherwise, that individuals and collectives are constructed. It is also during this process that Brazilian occupational therapy and occupational therapists work, assuming a position and intervening in the social field.

Social Policies: Origins

It is worth remembering that social policies were born in the 19th century, in the context of capital-labor struggles, in the scenario of consolidated industrial capitalism in Western Europe. They resulted from the new social relations that were inherent to the formation process of modern states, to the establishment of the fundamentals of the market, and to industrialization. It was during this period that, according to Polanyi (2011), social protection became one of the organizing principles of society, with the working class representing the interests associated with the most vital need of protection. However, we must go a little further in history, underlining important aspects of the institutionalization of protection and assistance. To this end, we will take the work of the French sociologist Robert Castel as reference, particularly his book, *From Manual Workers to Wage Laborers: Transformation of the Social Question* (Castel, 1998). The author recalls that the transition from the feudal mode of production to the capitalist mode occurred between the 12th and 15th centuries and was marked by the association between the extreme exploitation of the human labor force and the dissolution of traditional ties present in feudal society. In addition to perpetuating inequalities between the socially stratified estates, the social relations typical of feudalism maintained the cohesion of the social fabric within the limits of a rigid system of rights

and obligations that involved protection for needy and dependent individuals. In feudal society, security was defined by a protection established by coexistence in the same community, based on networks that, to avoid external aggression, remained strongly united.[1]

However, the changes that occurred in the late Middle Ages, especially land transactions, triggered the migration of large masses from the countryside to cities, which, anchored in trade and in the process of the formation of the bourgeoisie, attracted peasants expelled from their territory in search of means of earning a living; therefore, these changes brought the disruption of known ways of collective life. It is in this period that Castel situates the emergence of *social supports*. He defines social supports as assisting individuals unfit for work shifts from a condition under which there was no formal mediation—that is, assistance was assumed by the community and its resources—to a condition under which the assistance of hospitals and orphanages, as well as of units of organized distribution of alms, begins to evidence "specialized" institutional practices that constitute what Castel calls "social-assistance." It is the historical emergence of the intervention of society in itself, with a protective and integrative function. Castel considers that the structuring of assistance as a field organized to create protection occurred long before the term "social question" was used for the first time in 1830 to designate awareness of the poverty experienced by those who were agents and victims of the Industrial Revolution.[2] Although this was a time at which the social question gained new contours, the author states that "social" already existed before "invention of social"; that is, there were systems of nonmarket regulation that were instituted to try to fill the gap between the political organization and

---

[1]Castel describes these societies as those in which individuals are included since birth into a network of obligations, reproducing the injunctions of tradition and custom. Ancestral rules are imposed, generating stable relationships that accompany social roles in the family, the neighborhood, and the division of labor. They are strict social organizations marked by the sacralization of the past and linked to relationships of dependence and interdependence built through blood ties and lineages. It should be emphasized that Castel classifies them as "societies without social," insofar as he understands that "social," unlike "societal"—a term applicable to any form of collective existence—is a specific configuration of practices found in all human collectivities.

[2]As clarified by Netto (2001), the "social question" is not univocal, and there are many meanings attributed to the term. Netto argues that, historically, poverty only started to be designated as a "social question" after the reactions and protests of the poor against the bourgeois order, when the impoverished masses started to be seen as threats; after that, the term entered the vocabulary of conservative thinking.

the economic system, seeking to reestablish their ties. To establish this position, Castel goes back in particular to the historical facts that show that, as of the 14th century, the cities of Western Europe lost their relative abundance of work, unlike in the previous period, which was a time of trade expansion. Thus, the peasants attracted to the city were not integrated, creating a mass of indigents that, in Castel's view, were "disaffiliated." In his opinion, the "vagabonds"—as these individuals were called at that time—were not "predators roaming the margins of the social order, living off robberies, and threatening the possessions and safety of people" (Castel, 1998, p. 128), but rather were meek people affected by a process of disaffiliation that was fueled by the precariousness of their relationship with work and the fragility of their social networks. They had lost the sociofamilial ties that provided them with protection and security, they could not enjoy the social supports available to those unfit for work because they did not fall into this classification, and, moreover, they did not find ways to live off work. In medieval Western Europe, this type of hardship constituted a new phenomenon different from the poverty that had hitherto occurred, when only those who were considered unable to meet their needs by their own means fell into this category. The situation of poverty began to include those who, although able to work, could not do it.

Systematic modes of interaction sprang from this poverty, such as repression of "vagabondage," an obligation to work, and control of the circulation of labor. In these modes, political power played a role both in maintaining the organization of work and in regulating the mobility of workers. Assistance is included in municipal policies to the extent that municipal power acts on urban indigence and makes it a central issue for the organization of social life. According to Castel (1998), therefore, a clear organization of assistance, which ceases to be a clerical monopoly and becomes a target of the local governments, emerges in the 14th century. Together with the Catholic Church, confraternities of notable gentlemen and wealthy bourgeois, now imbued with the responsibility for the good government of the city, served the function of financing social assistance. Thus, at the beginning of the 16th century, generally considered a time of emergence of new forms of intervention in the social field, nothing new was actually observed, but rather the systematization of a movement already in progress since the 14th century. This process was strengthened by the accentuation of the social disintegration factors of the period, such as population growth, the subsistence crises, and the consequences of the Great Plague, which also nourished a broad public debate on poverty, also influenced by Renaissance and reformist ideas.

In this context, the 16th century was marked by the establishment of principles governing the relationship between *municipal power* and "vagabondage," such as the expulsion of foreigners from the cities, the prohibition of begging, and the classification of the needy, and also due to the fact that certain categories of needy individuals, even if fit for work, began being assisted by sheltering and assistance institutions that had the function of social control. The Poor Laws, which made charity compulsory, were developed in this century and were aimed at the recollection and sheltering of the poor population. They emerged as local laws but were subsequently disseminated nationally in several European countries. However, the transformations that occurred in the late 17th century and throughout the 18th century were even more profound, leading to essential changes concerning assistance. As is known, this period was marked by the process of transition from mercantile capitalism to industrial capitalism, including the bourgeois revolutions and the Industrial Revolution in the last decades of the 18th century. It was a moment of profound changes to the foundations of the social order.

Transition to Industrial Capitalism and the New Contours of the Social Question

Given that poverty and inequality were not new facts, the significant change that occurred in the 18th century was the perception and concern about the vulnerability of the masses—that is, about the precarious living conditions that, at that time, also involved the workers. Vulnerability became the "collective dimension of the popular condition" (Castel, 1998, p. 222). The economic upturn had produced a decrease in the number of destitute people but also a larger number of poor individuals who were permanently at risk of becoming destitute.

At the same time, the evident relation between work and the production of social wealth generated an important change: labor began being organized through the adoption of the principles of the new political economy based on the notion of a need for rational use of the workforce to produce wealth. Adam Smith, David Ricardo, and Thomas Malthus, as exponents of the liberalization of the economy, largely defended the impossibility of coexistence of the capitalist order, for which self-regulation of the market was conceivable (including with regard to assistance), with a system of wages and assistance subsidized by public funds, which demanded a strong state. According to such principles, it was necessary to tackle poverty by reorganizing labor. Thus, Castel (1998) states that the emergence of the "wage society" was also a result of the discovery of the need to liberate labor, that is, the idea that men should sell their labor freely, which is an essential element for the maintenance of the capitalist order. Hospitals—places of confinement and forced labor of the destitute—started to be criticized for nullifying the power of the human labor force. Therefore, in the late 18th century, the social question was at the center of political debate guided by a new social order focused on labor. However, the first decades of the 19th century witnessed, with the growth of savage industrialization, not the social balance preconized by liberal thought, but rather an aggravation of the scenario of misery, injustice, exploitation, and social degradation. This unprecedented scenario confronted the foundations of liberal thought in the 18th century because poverty was not the result of lack of work as had been thought, but of the *new form of labor organization*. It thus associated industrialization with the risk of social disintegration and disruption of the social order. Poverty grew at the same rate as the social capacity to generate wealth.

In the last decades of the 19th century, in a context in which social actors such as workers' organizations began to emerge in some countries such as England and Germany, the intense mobilization and strong protests of workers against their precarious working and survival conditions became events essential to the emergence of the first measures that led to the founding of the so-called social policies. At that time, workers had a daily workload of up to 16 hours, received very low salaries, and did not have weekly paid days off, vacations, safety, or protection in situations in which they could not work. Children worked under the same conditions as adults and received even lower wages. The factory environment was notoriously unhealthy, and work-related accidents were frequent. In this scenario, the creation of "social insurance" played the role of introducing some protections through contracts that involved the financial resources of employees, employers, and the state. Under this system, the workers began to contribute financially in advance for events or circumstances that could take away their possibility of working. Their security would be proportional to their contribution.

Initially employed in Germany in the 1880s, social insurance emerged in the form of laws that required insurance for sickness, work-related accidents, and the guarantee of pensions based on age (Vianna, 2002). This model of social protection rapidly expanded to other European countries in the 20th century, involving a larger number of workers. Associated with the expansion of capitalism, the intervention of the state, and social struggles and their demands, social protection measures began with the regulation of labor and gradually came to encompass other spheres of life and guarantees, such as the right to education and health. However, it was only after the end of World War II (1939–1945), with the great sociopolitical changes that involved the process of reconstruction of the economies of advanced capitalism, that true *social protection systems* were structured. With more comprehensive and national coverage, these systems were based on the idea that the state was responsible for ensuring its citizens the opportunities of access to services and benefits that generate well-being that characterized the "golden age of the capitalism," that is, great economic expansion with distribution of welfare by the state (Fiori, 1997); thus, a conception different from the liberal ideas of the past that advocated a minimal and nonintervening state with reserved functions. The universality of social rights entered the picture.

These ideas integrated the creation of comprehensive protection systems in Western Europe, which characterized the welfare states (Fiori, 1997; Draibe & Henriques, 1988; Draibe, 2007). These systems were first consolidated in England, where they were supported by the "Report on Social Insurance and Allied Services of 1942," known as the Beveridge Report after its author, William Beveridge. The report resumed and applied John Maynard Keynes' notions on income redistribution, that is, the advocacy that social protection systems be structured so that they directly interfere with access to material and social goods to favor the cycles of production and consumption. Keynes, an English economist, had postulated the adoption of state strategies to support the balance between production and consumption in his General Theory of 1936. He argued in favor of the investment of public resources in the control of the economy and the market, considering that maintaining the consumption capacity of the masses is essential to facing economic crises and threats of social rupture (Fiori, 1997). The Beveridge Report proposed social reforms involving society and the state in a form of organization founded on social rights conceived to guarantee the basic needs of the population. It was considered a new paradigm since it proposed the financing of social protection by the state budget and not based on a contractual relationship with the beneficiary (Fiori, 1997). According to Keynesian economics, public financing of social protection is a fundamental element to maintain the mode of production. It advocates strong articulation between social policies, economic processes, and capitalist development, assigning them a role in maintaining labor and stimulating the demand for goods and services.

Social Policies and Neoliberalism

Due to the major changes in international capitalism that occurred in the last decades of the 20th century, the welfare states succumbed. Although a total and widespread dismantling of social protection systems has not occurred worldwide, legitimate welfare states came to be considered an old-fashioned phenomenon after the many reforms and setbacks in the guarantee of protections (Draibe &

Henriques, 1988). The crisis of the welfare states has been studied by several authors who have highlighted their economic, technical-organizational, and philosophical components (Draibe, 2007). Draibe and Henriques (1988), like others, consider that from a political standpoint, the crisis developed through a process in which the typical postwar, social democratic consensus—based on full employment, redistributive policies, and strong participation of political parties and trade unions in the social pacts—was replaced by the neoliberal consensus and its restrictive policies.

Perry Anderson (1995), when analyzing the impact of neoliberalism, recalls that it began as a doctrine in Europe and also North America shortly after World War II. It was born as a critique of the welfare state and Keynesian economics. At that time, although not very influential, its advocates such as Milton Friedman and Ludwig von Mises argued that inequality was a positive value that maintains an essential relationship with freedom and free competition, which are vital to Western societies. However, it was only with the great global economic crisis of 1973, which linked high inflation rates to low rates of economic growth, that neoliberal ideas ascended and manifested in the reduction of public social expenditures, the withdrawal of protections and rights, and interventions aimed at maintaining an unemployment rate capable of breaking the strength of trade unions and labor movements. The hegemony of these ideas, therefore, did not occur all at once, but throughout the 1970s, as shown by Anderson (1995). In 1979, when Margaret Thatcher assumed leadership of the United Kingdom, the main opportunity to put these ideas into practice occurred. Thereafter, the same process spread throughout Germany and several countries in northern Western Europe, supported by the wave of new right-wing governments (Anderson, 1995). Put another way, Anderson describes that what initially seemed to be a practice restricted to governments identified as extreme right wing started to be employed also by the so-called Social Democrats and even by leftist governments.

Studies and discussions addressing the consequences of neoliberalism on various planes and in different continents have been of great importance. Draibe and Riesco (2011) reported extensive literature recording the socially adverse outcomes of globalization and neoliberalism in Latin America (late in relation to Europe), emphasizing the changes in the production structure, the low growth rates, and the growing levels of poverty, inequality, unemployment, and informal work. They also discuss what they consider to be the structural and historical meanings of the changes experienced under the aegis of neoliberalism, and it seems opportune to mention those that refer to the plane of values. First, however, it is worth remembering that social policies have been an important part of the institutionalization of values and norms of collective life, because by defining governmental guidelines on certain collective problems, they significantly contribute to the construction of how they are understood by the whole society (Lobato, 2009).

According to Draibe and Riesco (2011), under the influence of neoliberal thought, new cognitive and evaluative maps of the state, economy, freedom, and social justice, and of the desirable roles and relations between the state, economy, and population, emerged in society. These established the distancing of the popular masses from conservative ways of seeing and thinking inherent in agrarian-based communitarianism, instead favoring liberal and cosmopolitan, but above all individualistic and competitive values. Anti-statist values spread among the elites and the middle class, which would have contaminated the very legitimacy of public institutions decisive for the maintenance and the expansion of social cohesion. However, the great financial crisis of 2008–2009 profoundly unsettled the global economic and political scenario. During this critical period, many doubts about the economic future of the world were brought into the discussion, including those directly concerning social policies. The collapse of Wall Street was interpreted, across a broad political and intellectual spectrum, as a terminal moment for neoliberal policies (Peck, Theodore, & Brenner, 2012).

Nevertheless, we have not witnessed the end of neoliberal policies in recent years. Mainly in countries with dependent capitalism, such as Brazil, a deepening of the association between the political reforms that operate restriction of the rights of the population and the reduction of state financing for social policies is observed, consecrating the primacy of fiscal adjustment policies. Recent data show that this has particularly affected users of social services, which is the reason a "significant impact is projected in the coming years on both the increased demand for income guarantee assistance benefits and the whole set of services offered by the Unified Social Assistance System (SUAS)" (Instituto de Pesquisa Econômica Aplicada [IPEA], 2018, p. 55).

SOCIAL PROTECTION, SOCIAL ASSISTANCE, AND SOCIAL RIGHTS IN BRAZIL

Reflecting on social assistance in contemporary Brazil requires, initially, that emphasis be placed on the existence of a challenge that has been in course since the promulgation of the Constitution of the Federative Republic of Brazil in 1988. It is a matter of implementing at the practical level the *universalization of rights* predicted at the normative level.

Among the changes introduced by the constitution is the principle of universally instituted social assistance as a right for all who need it (Couto, 2010). This moment was a historical milestone in the country, in which legal changes in the field of Brazilian social protection were guided by the principles of the welfare state. In this way, these changes assigned responsibility to the state and legally consolidated Brazilian social security (integrating the rights to health, social security, and social assistance) (Couto, 2010). However, policies of a neoliberal nature—that is, restrictive to public expenditures—began to be implemented in Brazil as of the 1990s, meaning that, in practice, there would be a restricted role of the Brazilian state in effectively ensuring social rights. As discussed by Sposati (2002), the opposition between these two trends created a peculiar scenario. She adopted the term *late social regulation* to undertake her analysis, noting that it involves a set of characteristics that mark the countries, especially those in Latin America, in which social rights were legally validated only in the last quarter of the 20th century, after long struggles against military dictatorships that violated human and social rights. In these countries, as in Brazil, social rights were registered in the legislation but were neither institutionalized nor given a place in public budgets soon after their validation (Sposati, 2002). Therefore, Sposati (2002) affirms that the effects of neoliberal measures on social policies are characterized neither by *social disintegration* nor by a reduction in social expenditures, as in some welfare states. They occurred because, prior to these measures, there was not a broad and consolidated system of social protection. In a scenario of greater complexity owing to the combination of these opposing conditions and their nuances, neoliberal policies promoted the construction of a new and specific mode of state regulation for the social field in Brazil. According to Sposati, such a scenario moved away from the universalization of labor rights and the centrality of full employment, moving, although incipiently, toward the achievement of human rights.

Thus, constitutional innovations regarding the Brazilian protection system—the centrality of the state's responsibility in the regulation, standardization, proposition, and implementation of public policies, as well as the proposal to decentralize the management and participation of society in the control of social policies—emerge in opposition to the transformations occurring in the international economic order. The redistributive design of Brazilian social protection was born amid the process of diminishing national autonomy. It was defined by the pressure coming from the Washington consensus and the consequent demands of international financial organizations, which provided for the reduction of public expenditure and liberalization of the economy, that is, the opening of national markets to the interests of capital, especially of foreign origin (Yazbeck, 2012). That is the reason that, in the 1990s,

which was marked by the reorganization of conservative forces, Brazil witnessed the subordination of social policies to economic adjustment policies. The universalistic orientation soon clashed with the focused and privatizing trends, with reduction of social expenditures and channeling of resources to the poorest segments of the population, as shown in the studies mentioned by Yazbeck (2012). In this context, the implementation of a social assistance policy based on constitutional principles was delayed and only became possible through much effort as of 2004, with the promulgation of the National Social Assistance Policy (Brasil, 2005).

However, in addition to the financial problem, other challenges are imposed on Brazilian social assistance so that it can achieve its mission of expanding rights. Yazbeck (2012) discussed the central necessity to change the logic that supports the daily practices of social assistance institutions and services. According to her, there is a need to break with the traditions of discontinuity, welfarism, clientelism, and the lack of professionalization that marked the charitable and philanthropic approaches to the social questions in Brazil. Because this is a sensitive theme of the Brazilian reality, it is worth remembering that the development of social assistance in Brazil reflected the historical and social formation of the country, which was marked by a long period of dependence relationships and agro-export economy based on slave labor, favoring the rooting of authoritarian traits in the approach to dealing with social inequality. Until the end of the 19th century, social and philanthropic works prevailed in the Brazilian assistance setting, which was managed mainly by religious orders that established and enforced a charitable model in which shelter, meals, and some material aid were offered to the poor, orphans, and sick using donations. Combining basic aid and repression, hospitals and nursing homes were the only institutionalized strands of assistance for many years (Yazbeck, 2012).

It was only at the beginning of the 20th century, with the formation process of the Brazilian industrial economy and the emergence of the working class and its struggles for better living conditions,[3] that social protection gained new contours. Considered a structural milestone, the law that established the obligation to create the Retirement and Pension Funds of 1923 inaugurated the presence of the Brazilian state in the sphere of labor regulation (Behring &

---

[3]The Brazilian labor movement experienced important moments in the early 20th century, both with regard to its organization and the confrontations it experienced. Between 1917 and 1920, major strikes were launched in the main Brazilian cities. In São Paulo, for instance, approximately 70,000 textile workers were involved in plant shutdowns in 1917, and the government repressed the movement intensely (Carone, 1979).

Boschetti, 2011). These organizations relied on the contributory capacity of the expanding working class and began implementing the social insurance model in Brazil, which was in force until the Constitution of the Federative Republic of Brazil of 1988.

In the decades following the implementation of social insurance, there was a growing development of the Brazilian proletariat, and the action of the state on capital–labor relations expanded. Particularly under the government of Getúlio Vargas, the state legislated a minimum wage, the regulation of the working day, the right to a paid weekly day off, and the health of insured workers—that is, taxpayers and their dependents—among other developments. Although these were important achievements, Getúlio Vargas promoted the cooptation of the working class and, either through repression or by the charismatic domination typical of populism, impaired its capacity for mobilization and its demanding force. In this way, he benefited politically from the visibility he was able to attribute to the so-called social issues and from the strategies he developed to reconcile the interests of capital and workers (Behring & Boschetti, 2011).

In 1942, the Brazilian Legion of Assistance (LBA) was created, with activities initially dedicated to assisting Brazilian soldiers fighting in World War II, then later extended to the social segments not included in the social insurance model, such as individuals with disabilities, the elderly, pregnant women without health care coverage, and children and youths from poor families, among others. From 1942 to 1995, the LBA was supported by the combination of an extensive network of female volunteers and agreements with philanthropic institutions. The main characteristic of the LBA was the emergency and compensatory nature of its actions (Sposati & Falcão, 1989); it was closed in 1995. According to Mestriner (2005) and Couto (2010), this institution exemplifies the historical relationship between the Brazilian social assistance and charity and philanthropy, having acted to perpetuate welfarist traditions opposed to the principles of social justice. This state of affairs did not change during the military dictatorship (1964–1984). On the contrary, the authoritarian regime stimulated and supported the profitability of the private sector in the provision of social protection, especially in the area of health; abolished the possibility of workers' participation in decisions and control of public spending; and did not change the philanthropic approach to those who could not pay for social protection in the form of insurance, who were blamed for their own misfortune and treated as vagabonds or "marginal" (Behring & Boschetti, 2011). In 1988, during the Brazilian redemocratization process, that model was widely criticized for having left unprotected the informal, rural, and domestic workers; the unemployed; and the poor, who were always numerous in Brazil. For these, the only possibility was to be subordinate to the logic of benevolence and receive assistance as "the needy" from philanthropic institutions. From this point on, the primacy of the state's responsibility for social assistance was proposed. The scenario was complex and required enormous changes, both from the point of view of the assistance offered and from the political and economic standpoint, which did not occur for several years.

Thus, the approval of the National Policy on Social Assistance (Brasil, 2005) in 2004 in consonance with the constitutional principles and its definition as a right of Brazilian citizens represented an important innovation. Through this policy, the guidelines and objectives of social assistance for the entire country were established, in addition to defining the three levels of social protection (basic, medium, and high complexity) with their respective assistance units and services organized in the form of a network, that is, with integrated operation. Thus, the concepts and the organizational basis of the Unified Social Assistance System (SUAS) were established and started to be implemented in 2005, adopting a decentralized and participatory management model through which Brazilian municipalities play a central role in the execution of social assistance actions.

Among the conceptual axes around which the SUAS is articulated, the territorialization of the social assistance network and the sociofamilial matrix are intended to generate a relevant impact on the configuration of assistance actions: the first, because it directs the offer of services based on the incidence of vulnerability and risks based on the logic of proximity of the user; the latter, because it focuses as a priority on the family and its members as a unit of intervention, with the purpose of strengthening social ties and preventing the breakdown of bonds of affection and social belonging (Teixeira, 2009). In this process, as of 2005, the Social Assistance Reference Centers (CRAS) and the Social Assistance Special Reference Centers (CREAS) were implemented; both are public welfare units of municipal characteristics distributed according to the vulnerability and risk analysis of the territories. Their functions include not only the direct offer of actions but also the integration of all services that compose the social assistance network aiming to comply with the guidelines of the SUAS. This requires monitoring of the private nonprofit units that act in the assistance but that now must be associated with the public power and meet the conceptual and operative norms of the policy. Currently, the CRAS and CREAS units are present nationwide and make up the fundamental structure for the ramification of the policy (Couto, Yazbeck, Silva, & Raichelis, 2014).

Although significant progress has been observed in the implementation of this policy, based on social rights, the process has evidenced the continued presence of serious obstacles to its full consolidation, as well as the predominance of investments in cash transfer programs. Analyzing experiences that have materialized in Brazil, Silva, Yazbeck, and Giovanni (2012) stated that if, on the one hand, these programs represented the only concrete possibility of obtaining income, albeit low, for many families, then, on the other hand, the opportunities to access services that meet other social needs are not occurring satisfactorily.

OCCUPATIONAL THERAPISTS IN SOCIAL ASSISTANCE: BUILDING PROPOSALS, REAFFIRMING FOUNDATIONS

As previously shown, the contemporary challenges of social assistance in Brazil are many, and they add to a sociopolitical scenario of structural and conjectural contradictions. In this context, occupational therapists have been working at all levels of social protection of the SUAS and as important parts of the different types of assistance units that compose it. In 2016, 1,323 professionals were working at the SUAS, representing 7.56% of Brazil's occupational therapists (Almeida & Soares, 2018). Although insertion in different care units has demanded sets of specific knowledge, some general questions can be addressed here.

Occupational therapists who are committed to building a fair, egalitarian society (World Federation of Occupational Therapists [WFOT], 2006) that cultivates diversity as a value (WFOT, 2010) should integrate processes that aim to prepare, create, assess, and improve new ways of intervening on social problems, in a dialogical process with the population that experiences them (Barros, Ghirardi, & Lopes, 1999; Barros, Lopes, & Ghirardi, 2002; Lopes, 2016). In other words, it is necessary to implement what Paulo Freire has demonstrated to be a way of opposing domination and passivity and enabling the construction of knowledge in communion mediated by the real, everyday world (Freire, 2005). According to Freire, the word is also praxis, and true dialogue—the encounter—establishes the dimensions of action and reflection on real life.

It is through the development of this process, assumed as the work methodology in the scope of Brazilian social occupational therapy (Barros, 2004; Barros, Ghirardi, & Lopes, 2005; Lopes, 2016), that occupational therapists can better intervene in social issues. It is important considering that in Brazil they express complex relationships historically constituted in the sense of invalidating individuals and their needs, rights, and powers. It is necessary, above all, to recognize that products of social inequality have repercussions at various levels of human experience, penetrating the great and small movements and actions of everyday life in an incisive and destructive way. Situations of vulnerability and violation of rights result in the impediment or difficulty (systematic or temporary) of individuals or social groups to autonomously conduct activities that are meaningful for themselves and their social environment and which enable them to recognize their condition as individuals with rights who participate in society on equal terms. These processes nullify the possibilities of today and the plans for tomorrow. However, sometimes these experiences of suffering and the paralysis that is inherent to them are silenced before the predefined and standardized responses of programs, services, and professionals. It is thus necessary to disrupt these determinations.

Occupational therapists working with individuals, families, groups, or communities in social assistance should seek to prevent or change an often sterile and devastated reality by rescuing and exercising, in principle, the right to participate in activities that represent real opportunities for living with dignity, engaging in social exchanges, prospering, developing potential and projects in different paths of life, and finding fulfillment in line with their cultures and beliefs (WFOT, 2006). This participation should be the concrete representation of the exercise of social rights. It should produce expansion, enlargement, and openness to new fields through which complete human beings can transit with their powers and limits.

It should be remembered that the presence of the state and the fulfillment of its responsibilities are crucial factors in the field of social protection. Autonomy cannot be treated as synonymous with "self-sufficiency," which ultimately releases the state from the obligation to protect and defend human life. Therefore, it is the responsibility of occupational therapists who work in social assistance, especially in a country with high unemployment and poverty rates such as Brazil, to contribute to the offer of public actions compatible with a view of society in solidarity, in which the state plays a fundamental role in improving the living conditions of the population.

Because there are no ready-made proposals for specific demands, occupational therapists support and explore ever unique processes whose essence involves the agency of the participants in activities that are treated as instruments for the mediation of the individual's transforming action over the real world. Therefore, action and production of knowledge, meanings, support networks, coexistence, and life projects—even if they are elementary in their apparent content—are interconnected to support people to recognize themselves as individuals with rights and to advance in their individual and collective capacity for action/transformation. It is under this perspective that occupational therapists are currently working with people who are living through, or at risk of experiencing, processes of disruption of social support networks, of disorganization of the bases of coexistence and social belonging, and of violation of rights. In the course of monitoring inherent to social occupational therapy, a dialogue is an essential aspect of methodology guiding this practice, operating as the mechanism that enables the validation of the "other." The attitude of the professionals before the individuals who require their work, in turn, shows the central character of what they seek to produce: it either perpetuates domination or creates opportunities for gains of autonomy and agency. Thus, overcoming the immediacy of actions and their low impact on human emancipation and identifying their boundaries are permanent tasks of occupational therapists in the field of social assistance.

Reflecting on Pathways

In Brazil, occupational therapy has been included in the field of social assistance since the 1970s, when it integrated teams of coercive programs, developed by closed institutions, with youths considered "marginal." In addition, it was present in nursing homes for the elderly and community programs for children and adolescents of low-income families (Galheigo, 2016). It is important that this history is remembered; however, it should always be accompanied by the perception that the profession has changed since then, as has the Brazilian social reality.

Among these changes, resolution no. 17 of the National Social Assistance Council of 2011 can be considered a fundamental component of the implementation of the SUAS (Brasil, 2006), as well as of the process of professionalization of social work (Ferreira, 2011), because it defined and recognized a delimited set of professional categories qualified to act in the system. The process of defining these categories involved a comprehensive debate between workers of the SUAS from all regions of Brazil and the main management bodies of the system in 2009 and 2010. The collaborators, including occupational therapists, discussed the conditions and training for work in the SUAS, the interdisciplinarity and political organization, among other topics whose synthesis was brought to the National Meeting of Workers of the SUAS held in 2011. By formalizing the professional work of occupational therapists within the scope of social assistance, resolution no. 17/CNAS generated an expectation of the expansion of the work of these professionals at the SUAS (Almeida, Soares, Barros, & Galvani, 2012), which in fact seems to be occurring (Almeida & Soares, 2018). With this, the challenges of the profession to improve the quality of their interventions become more evident.

In this sense, it should be emphasized that the implementation of a social assistance policy that universalizes social rights depends deeply on the professionals who work in it, since they can bring about essential changes so that the new model can be effective and improved. Given the historical conformations of this field, it is not an exaggeration to suppose that the professional multiplicity—as well as the adequate training of these professionals—has a strategic function in the transformation of ethical-political guidelines into daily professional action in the assistance units.

Finally, the teaching and professional education of occupational therapists must adapt to the enormous responsibility that fell on this profession when it was institutionalized in social assistance. The challenge of educated professionals qualified for social intervention must be vigorously met, always considering the need to open spaces for the construction of a critical perspective of the current reality.

REFERENCES

Almeida, M. C., & Soares, C. R. S. (2018). *Social assistance: Field of professional activities and challenges for occupational therapists in Brazil.* WFOT Congress 2018, Cape Town, South Africa.

Almeida, M. C., Soares, C. R. S., Barros, D. D., & Galvani, D. (2012). Processos e práticas de formalização da Terapia Ocupacional na Assistência Social: alguns marcos e desafios [Formalization processes and practices of occupational therapy in social assistance: landmarks and challenges]. *Brazilian Journal of Occupational Therapy, 20*(1), 33–41. doi:10.4322/cto.2012.004

Anderson, P. (1995). Balanço do neoliberalismo [Balance of neoliberalism]. In E. Sader & P. Gentili (Eds.), *Pós neoliberalismo: as políticas sociais e o Estado democrático* [Post neoliberalism: Social policies and the democratic state] (pp. 9–23). Rio de Janeiro: Paz e Terra.

Barros, D. D. (2004). Terapia Ocupacional Social: o caminho se faz ao caminhar [Notes for a social occupational therapy: The way is done by the way we go]. *Revista de Terapia Ocupacional da Universidade de São Paulo, 15*(3), 90–97. doi:10.11606/issn.2238-6149.v15i3p90-97

Barros, D. D., Ghirardi, M. I. G., & Lopes, R. E. (1999). Terapia ocupacional e sociedade [Occupational therapy and society]. *Revista de Terapia Ocupacional da Universidade de São Paulo, 10*(2/3), 69–74.

Barros, D. D., Lopes, R. E., & Ghirardi, M. I. G. (2002). Terapia Ocupacional Social [Social occupational therapy]. *Revista de Terapia Ocupacional da Universidade de São Paulo, 13*(3), 95–103. doi:10.11606/issn.2238-6149.v13i3p95-103

Barros, D. D., Ghirardi, M. I. G., & Lopes, R. E. (2005). Social occupational therapy: A socio-historical perspective. In F. Kronenberg, S. Simó Algado, & N. Pollard (Eds.), *Occupational therapy without borders: Learning from the spirit of survivors* (pp. 140–151). Londres: Elsevier Science - Churchill Livingstone.

Behring, E., & Boschetti, I. (2011). *Política social: fundamentos e história* [Social policy: Fundamentals and history]. São Paulo: Cortez.

Brasil. (2006). *Ministério do Desenvolvimento Social e Combate à Fome, Norma Operacional Básica de Recursos Humanos do NOB-RH/SUAS.* Brasília: Author.

Brasil. Ministério do Desenvolvimento Social e Combate à Fome. (2005). *Política Nacional de Assistência Social PNAS/2004 e Norma Operacional Básica NOB/SUAS.* Brasília: Author.

Carone, E. (1979). *Movimento operário no Brasil. 1877–1944* [Labor movement in Brazil. 1877–1944]. São Paulo: Difel.

Castel, R. (1998). *As metamorfoses da questão social: Uma crônica do salário* [From manual workers to wage laborers: Transformation of the social question]. Petrópolis: Vozes.

Couto, B. R. (2010). *O direito social e a assistência social na sociedade brasileira: uma equação possível?* [Social law and social assistance in Brazilian society: A possible equation?] São Paulo: Cortez.

Couto, B. R., Yazbeck, M. C., Silva, M. O. S., & Raichelis, R. (2014). *O Sistema Único de Assistência Social: uma realidade em movimento* [The system of social assistance in Brazil: A reality in movement]. São Paulo: Cortez.

Draibe, S. M. (2007). Estado de Bem-Estar, Desenvolvimento Econômico e Cidadania: algumas lições da literatura contemporânea [Welfare state, economic development and citizenship: Some lessons from contemporary literature]. In G. Hochman, M. Arretche, & E. Marques (Eds.), *Políticas Públicas no Brasil* [Public policies in Brazil] (pp. 27–64). Rio de Janeiro: Fiocruz.

Draibe, S. M., & Henriques, W. (1988). Welfare State, crise e gestão da crise: um balanço da literatura internacional [Welfare state, crisis and crisis management: An international literature review]. *Revista Brasileira de Ciências Sociais, 3*(6). Retrieved from http://www.anpocs.org.br/portal/publicacoes/rbcs_00_06/rbcs06_04.htm

Draibe, S. M., & Riesco, M. (2011). Estados de Bem-Estar Social e estratégias de desenvolvimento na América Latina. Um novo desenvolvimento em gestação? [Welfare state and development strategies in Latin America: A new developmentalism in gestation?]. *Sociologias, 13*(27), 220–254. doi:10.1590/S1517-45222011000200009

Faleiros, V. P. (2012). *A Política Social do Estado Capitalista* [The social policy of the capitalist state]. São Paulo: Cortez.

Ferreira, S. S. (2011). *NOB-RH Anotada e Comentada.* Brasília: Secretaria Nacional de Assistência Social.

Fiori, J. L. (1997). Estado de Bem-estar Social: padrões e crises [Welfare state: Patterns and crisis]. *Physys: Revista de Saúde Coletiva, 7*(2), 129–147.

Freire, P. (2005). *Pedagogia do Oprimido* [Pedagogy of the oppressed] (42nd ed.). Rio de Janeiro: Paz e Terra.

Galheigo, S. M. (2016). Terapia ocupaiconal social: uma síntese histórica acerca da constituição de um campo de saber e de prática [Occupational social therapy: A historical synthesis about the constitution of a field of knowledge and practice]. In R. E. Lopes & A. P. S. Malfitano (Eds.), *Terapia Ocupacional Social: desenhos teóricos e contornos práticos* [Social occupational therapy: Theoretical drawings and practical fields] (pp. 49–68). São Carlos: EdUFSCar.

Instituto de Pesquisa Econômica Aplicada (IPEA). (2018). *Boletim de Políticas Sociais: monitoramento e análise* [Social policies bulletin: Monitoring and analysis]. 25. Brasília: Author.

Lobato, L. V. C. (2009). Dilemas da institucionalização de políticas sociais em vinte anos da Constituição de 1988 [Dilemmas of the institucionalization of social policies in twenty years of the 1988 Constitution]. *Ciência & Saúde Coletiva, 14*(3), 721–730. doi:10.1590/S1413-81232009000300008

Lopes, R. E. (2016). Cidadania, direitos e terapia ocupacional social [Citizenship, rights and occupational social therapy]. In R. E. Lopes & A. P. S. Malfitano (Eds.), *Terapia Ocupacional Social: desenhos teóricos e contornos práticos* [Social occupational therapy: Theoretical drawings and practical fields] (pp. 29–48). São Carlos: EdUFSCar.

Mestriner, M. L. (2005). *O Estado entre a filantropia e a assistência social* [The state between philanthropy and social assistance]. São Paulo: Cortez.

Netto, J. P. (2001). Cinco notas a propósito da "questão social" [Five notes on the "social issue"].. In J. P. Netto (Ed.), *Capitalismo Monopolista e Serviço Social* [Monopoly capitalism and social work] (pp. 151–176). São Paulo: Cortez.

Peck, J., Theodore, N., & Brenner, N. (2012). Mal estar Pós-neoliberalismo [Post-neoliberalism malaise]. *Novos Estud.–CEBRAP, 92*, 59–78. doi:10.1590/S0101-33002012000100005

Polanyi, K. (2011). *A Grande Transformação* [The great transformation]. Rio de Janeiro: Elsevier – Campus.

Silva, M. O. S., Yazbek, C., & Giovanni, G. (2012). *A Política Social Brasileira no Século XXI: a prevalência dos programas de transferência de renda* [The Brazilian social policy in the 21st century: The prevalence of income transfer programs]. São Paulo: Cortez.

Sposati, A. (2002). Regulação Social Tardia: características das políticas sociais latino americanas na passagem entre o segundo e o terceiro milênio [Late social regulation: Characteristics of Latin American social policies in the passage between the second and third millennium]. *Proceedings of the VII Congreso Internacional del CLAD sobre la Reforma del Estado y de la Administración Pública*, Lisboa, Portugal, 8–11. Retrieved from http://www1.londrina.pr.gov.br/dados/images/stories/Storage/sec_assistencia/pdf/Regulacao_social_tardia_Aldaisa.pdf

Sposati, A., & Falcão, M. C. (Eds.). (1989). *LBA: identidade e efetividade das ações no enfrentamento da pobreza brasileira* [LBA: Identity and effectiveness of actions in facing Brazilian poverty]. São Paulo: EDUC.

Teixeira, S. M. (2009). Família na política de Assistência Social: avanços e retrocessos com a matricialidade sociofamiliar [Families in the social assistance policy: Advances and setbacks within the familiar social matrix]. *Revista de Políticas Públicas São Luis, 13*(2), 255–264. Retrieved from http://www.periodicoseletronicos.ufma.br/index.php/rppublica/article/view/4769/2787

Viana, A. L. d'Á., & Levcovitz, E. (2005). Proteção Social: introduzindo o debate [Social protection: Introducing the debate].

In A. L. d´Á. Viana, P. E. M. Elias, & N. Ibañez (Eds.), *Proteção Social: Dilemas e Desafios* [Social protection: Dilemmas and challenges] (pp. 15–60). São Paulo: Hucitec.

Vianna, M. L. W. (2002). *Em torno do conceito de política social: notas introdutórias* [Around the concept of social policy: Introductory notes]. Rio de janeiro: [s.n.]. Retrieved from http:,www.unerj.br/ead/ead/20052/curso_sequencial/up_cidadania/arquivos/Em_torno_do_conceito_de_politica_social.pdf

World Federation of Occupational Therapists. (2006). World Federation of Occupational Therapists position statement on human rights. *World Federation of Occupational Therapists Bulletin, 59*(1), 5. doi:10.1179/otb.2009.59.1.002

World Federation of Occupational Therapists. (2010). World Federation of Occupational Therapists position statement on diversity and culture. England: London. Retrieved from http://www.wfot.org/ResourceCentre.aspx

Yazbeck, M. C. (2012). Pobreza no Brasil contemporâneo e formas de seu enfrentamento [Poverty in Brazil in the contemporary time and ways to confront it]. *Serviço Social & Sociedade, 110*, 288–322. doi:10.1590/S0101-66282012000200005

The Theory of Communicative Action: A Theoretical-Methodological Contribution to Social Occupational Therapy

Regina Célia Fiorati

INTRODUCTION

The 1980s were a very important period for both Brazil and the profession of occupational therapy. During that decade, social relations and the institutions of Brazilian society underwent major transformations stemming from social movements geared toward the political and social redemocratization of the country. In addition to the struggle to end the military dictatorship, in the health field—specifically in mental health—two important reforms triggered social policies and processes of conceptual and practical changes during those years: health reform and psychiatric reform. Both of these reforms, which originated in the struggle for Brazil's redemocratization, established new models of action in health and mental health based on de-hospitalization, psychiatric de-hospitalization, the conception of primary health care as a reorganizer of the universal health system, recognition of health as a right of citizens and a duty of the state, and the creation of the Unified Health System (SUS), the public national health policy that guarantees universal access to all citizens. The engagement of occupational therapists in social and health movements triggered a process critical of the political alienation present in professional practice and of reductionist practices that, by relying on conceptions immersed in positivism, reflected uncritical and ahistorical views of the world, life, society, health, and disease. In addition, an important reflection on the political-social role of the technical professional was developed (Drummond, 2007).

As a result of this critical-reflexive process, different methodologies emerged in the professional practice of occupational therapy. This process also fostered the production of corresponding knowledge, which opened up new fields of practice, and the abandonment of practices centered on institutions to focus instead on actions carried out with groups and communities within different territories. Regarding social practice in particular, there was also an important technical-methodological reorientation that questioned the previous approaches to practice, which were implemented during the military dictatorship and that were institutionalized and centered on a methodological framework originating in clinical practices. This reorientation proposed a practice in the social field based on new standards (Barros, Lopes, & Galheigo, 2007).

Theoretical frameworks such as those by Robert Castel, Karl Marx, Antonio Gramsci, Franco Basaglia, Michel Foucault, Erving Goffman, and Paulo Freire, among others, provided a new methodological approach to social occupational therapy. This new approach decentralizes the clinical field, instead proposing a social and political analysis of the sociocultural contexts generated in a society dominated by political-economic orientation. This approach recognizes the immense social inequalities and the social exclusion of population segments with respect to access to goods, services, income, housing, education, health, information, safety, civil rights, and citizenship. In addition, it enables an analysis that overcomes functionalist interpretations of social reality, which transform social problems into clinical matters, and place social problems within the scope of the individual such that people are conceived as social deviants or misfits. In this new approach, social problems are recognized as resulting from processes of social dynamics related to power dynamics and conflicts of interest among various orders that intervene in the social context, thus producing a constant sociopolitical transformation of reality (Barros et al., 2007).

The sociopolitical analysis that underlies the new social practice in Brazilian occupational therapy is based on global economic-political events resulting from the decline of the welfare state. The welfare state was most relevantly developed in industrialized European countries after World War II, coinciding with considerable economic growth at that time. The aim of the welfare state is to ensure minimum levels of quality of life or to distribute resources through social policies that provide the working classes with access to material and symbolic goods and with public opportunities and services such as health systems, education, housing, social security, and so forth (Domingues, 2005).

With the decline of the welfare state and the rise of neoliberal economic and political orientations, social protection systems have been compromised worldwide. These systems intended, through negotiated strategies, to lead the interested social poles to accept mutual objectives and commitments that would ensure the stability of the social system through distributive social policies and the maintenance of stable working relations. However, under neoliberalism, social security is no longer an obligation of the state, and the crisis of the welfare state has caused a crisis of solidarity and social cohesion, which is amplified by the transformation of relations between the economy and society (the labor crisis) and of the modes of constitution of individual and collective identities (Sorj & Martuccelli, 2008).

According to Castel (2001), this scenario generates transformations in the world of work that are at the root of a societal wage crisis, characterized by the emergence of unemployment and the precariousness of labor relations. Thus, an increasing number of people become victims of structural unemployment, forming segments of the population that are irremediably out of the labor market. The centrality of work as the axis of social relations and the crisis of the de-structuring of these forms of sociability generate a growth of mass vulnerability, considering that even workers who remain integrated are vulnerable to disintegration (described later) due to the threat of unemployment. Disintegration is the condition in which population segments are found in a situation of social "disaffiliation," meaning they have experienced a rupture in their belonging and the societal bond. People in this condition of social disaffiliation, in addition to having insufficient material resources due to structural unemployment and the lack of means to generate income, are also weakened by the instability of the relational context. Consequently, these individuals begin to experience, in addition to the precariousness of the labor relations, a process of vulnerability within family, kinship, and community relations, in which their participation begins to lose meaning because their identity was created through work.

Although a welfare state was not properly constituted in Latin America, including Brazil, some social policies, such as the Unified Health System (SUS), were developed in

Brazil in the 1990s as a result of the struggle for the country's political redemocratization that occurred in the 1980s. Nevertheless, also in the 1990s, a neoliberal political-economic orientation was initiated in Brazil, whereby public policies underwent a process of reducing the government's responsibility for providing a minimum safety net. As a result of this political-economic orientation, a decrease in distributive policies was observed simultaneously with weakened regulatory capacities of political power (which came about as a result of popular will) in relation to the effects caused by a line of economic action. Following the emergence of this reduction in government responsibility, the social problems historically constituted in Brazil were accentuated, and so were the degradation of labor relations and the mechanisms of social protection. This generated growth in the number of social groups and individuals living in a state of social exclusion, characterized by the inaccessibility of the labor market and compromises to social support networks, housing, education, cultural goods, and facilities (Sawaia, 2007).

Debate about the exclusion of large masses of workers, according to a structuralist-historical framework developed by the previously mentioned authors, became part of the reorientation of social occupational therapy, mainly during the 1990s. Social occupational therapy then began a process of conceiving of a methodology, beyond the scope of previous theoretical-methodological perspectives, focused on practice in the social field. From the social occupational therapy perspective, action was directed to these populations and groups to seek the creation of social support networks as a means to foster emancipation and social-political autonomy. The development of the body of knowledge and practice around social occupational therapy has centered on disciplinary-specific knowledge with interdisciplinary interfaces in a larger social field (Malfitano, 2005).

Thus, a methodology of practice in the social field began to be outlined, its goals being the universalization of the right to citizenship, the production and expansion of social networks to support population groups, and the construction of instruments capable of interpreting reality from interfaces between subjectivities, social contexts, and culture. The aim of these instruments is to foster the understanding of relationships between individuals and among groups, communities, and society and to produce the possibility of reconstituting histories and contexts, enabling the formation of criteria for community and territorial participation and action, the construction of social projects, and the analysis and preparation of public policies (Barros et al., 2007).

In the Brazilian context of public policies, occupational therapy was formally included in the Unified Social

Assistance System (SUAS, the national public social assistance policy) in 2011. Consistent with the guidelines of this policy, occupational therapy has affirmed its commitment to the inclusion and effective social participation of socially vulnerable individuals and groups, to denouncing the violation of the social rights of these groups and individuals, and to creating mechanisms to encourage full recognition of human rights and recovery of citizenship. Thereafter, it became necessary to qualify the intervention of occupational therapists who work in the social field (Almeida, Soares, Barros, & Galvani, 2012). From this perspective, a philosophical framework that can contribute to the construction of a methodology for social action in occupational therapy was developed drawing on the work of Jürgen Habermas' (1988) theory of communicative action.

Three dimensions of Habermasian social theory are highlighted in this chapter. The first concerns critical reflection based on his theory of communicative action and on communicative reason superimposing on strategic action and instrumental reason, as a rational basis for the development of consensus building as a device for coordinating social, economic, and democratic projects and practices. The second dimension is associated with the concept that develops the so-called lifeworld, providing a relevant analysis for the interpretation of relations between cultural, social, and subjective worlds. The third dimension involves the contribution of his most recent works (Habermas, 2012, 2014), in which the philosopher explores the urgent and necessary prioritization of the struggle for commitments to solidarity and social cohesion, which are expressed in the charter of the Universal Declaration of Human Rights and calls for the unconditional defense of human dignity. In these studies, the author also defends the guarantee of full democratic processes through the direct inclusion of people, as organized social individuals, in decision-making processes and decision-making bodies with respect to political-economic and financial concerns. This approach surpasses the current model of representative democracy, in which a deliberate centralization is observed in the election or appointment of politically powerful bodies. Hereafter, these concepts are developed in an attempt to better understand this philosophical contribution to social occupational therapy.

COMMUNICATIVE ACTION, DIALOGUE, INTERSUBJECTIVITY, DEMOCRACY, AND EMANCIPATION

Before beginning the theoretical discussion, it is important to distinguish between Reason and reason—terms that will be used in this section of the text. The term "Reason"

(capitalized) will be used to refer to the general faculty of knowing, judging, and reflecting that characterizes human beings, whereas "reason" (in lowercase) will refer to a specific way of using human rationality (e.g., the Enlightenment reason, the postmodern reason, etc.) (Japiassu & Marcondes, 2006).

Jürgen Habermas is a contemporary philosopher who has developed a theory of society and modernity and performed a critical diagnosis of the present time. Indeed, the purpose of conducting a critical diagnosis of the current moment and of always updating it according to historical transformations is a legacy that Habermas inherited from his initial intellectual formation and his association with the Frankfurt school and critical theory, centrally represented by the philosophers Max Horkheimer, Theodor Adorno, Walter Benjamin, and Herbert Marcuse. However, over time, it is possible to glimpse Habermas' criticism of these thinkers, especially with regard to the question of Reason and its relation to human emancipation.

In "Dialectic of Enlightenment,"[1] Adorno and Horkheimer radically criticize the Enlightenment reason, which is understood as a source for domination of some human beings over others, a source that transforms knowledge of reality as well as social relations in a process of complete human alienation. Marcuse (as cited in Habermas, 1987) would later deepen this critique, evolving toward the concept of a society of total administration, in which science and technology become productive forces to the detriment of human forces and constitute pervasive ideologies. In this way, conceiving of Reason as an emancipatory possibility as a mere illusion, Adorno (1951) argues that art is the way to abolish the Reason of illustration, whereas for Horkheimer (2002), this can occur through religion. Habermas (1987) shares this critique of modern reason but does not agree with the course of action proposed by Adorno, Horkheimer, and Marcuse, instead warning against the path of what he views as a dangerous "irrationalism" implied in the thought of these members of the Frankfurt school of critical theory.

---

[1]Adorno and Horkheimer (1984). Written in 1947, *Dialectic of Enlightenment* is a seminal work of the first generation of the Frankfurt school of critical theory. Adorno and Horkheimer criticize the process of "enlightenment" that constitutes a series of modern phenomena such as the process of rationalization, the demythologization of the world, and the mathematization of knowledge. They argue that the process imprisons human beings within the rational logic of modern science and transforms knowledge into a device of political and economic domination, making human beings hostage to technique, and irremediably leading to the general alienation of individuals and the total reification of the world.

Habermas' reflection begins from a fierce criticism of positivism as a theoretical reference of modernity that induces the elimination of the individual, intersubjectivity, values, norms, history, and knowledge in the name of a mathematical, objectified, universalized, and superficial interpretation of the world. In this sense, the philosopher deepens an analysis that proposes that the crisis and decadence of the Enlightenment reason of modernity is due to the fact that it is incorporated into an instrumental autonomous reason. He argues that the latter, by dominating modernity's project of truth, as based solely on science and technique as forms of legitimation, does not fulfill the emancipatory principles of liberty, equality, and fraternity but, on the contrary, consolidates itself as a force of domination and exploitation of human beings over themselves. Nevertheless, he argues that there is a path that leads to Reason: the submission of instrumental reason to communicative reason and the reestablishment of democratic processes founded in consensus building and supported by radical dialogue and intersubjectivity, directed toward the coordination of social practices.

Habermas partially endorses Marcusian theory[2] with regard to science and technology becoming the main productive and ideological forces in late capitalism. The autonomous progress of science and technique will determine the development of social life. The state absorbs the specific logic of technical and scientific reason and begins to guide its decisions not by practice, but by technical rationality. Technocratic ideology supports a worldview that affirms the necessarily technical nature of the state's action. This ideology proposes a perspective according to which the development of the social system is determined by the logic of technical-scientific progress, whose immediate effect is the depoliticization of the masses and the concealment of the real interests that underlie this social functioning and prevent the public from expressing critical opinions. This occurs because to the extent that the

foundations of technocratic functioning respond only to the imperatives of a technical rationality, they become immune to any challenge. Furthermore, insofar as the technocratic ideology presents practical questions in the form of technical questions, it excludes the themes significant to praxis from public debate and produces an even more serious result: the invalidation of the distinction between instrumental action and communicative action in the consciousness of human beings. Human beings begin to self-objectify themselves under the exclusive perspective of instrumental action and the consequent adaptive behavior, and communicative action is consequently absorbed by instrumental action (Fiorati & Saeki, 2011, 2012).

Habermas, however, proposes an alternative concerning Marcuse's critique of society and culture, without defending what he views as the dangerous path of irrationality or the invalidation of scientific and technological knowledge. In the 1970s, Habermas' thinking invoked a linguistic turn, abandoning the paradigm of consciousness, which held that Reason was possible through subjective reflexive activity and focused instead on the paradigm of language, believing that it is through language that we gain access to Reason, rationality, and the activity of interpreting reality.

The Habermasian critique emphasizes that the only way possible for the authors of *Dialectic of Enlightenment* (Adorno & Horkheimer, 1984) was irrationalism, because they were tied to the paradigm of consciousness when they critically analyzed the reality, which took them to an analysis centered on the individual as the bearer of Reason, and thus to a monological and egocentric rationality, making the way to a more comprehensive and deeper analysis of the lifeworld inaccessible. By affirming language as a way to access thought and knowledge of the reality and social universe of human beings, Habermas provides an interpretation of the real and human relations through a rationality no longer centered on the individual but intersubjective, and thus no longer monological, but rather dialogical.

Habermas (1988) defines human interaction as the process by which human beings solve their problems and coordinate among themselves for the preparation and execution of action plans as social actors within a field of play of possible choices, contingencies, and conflicts, given an intertwining of themes and actions in social spaces and historical epochs. He distinguishes between two dimensions present in human interaction: communicative action and strategic action. He contends that these two types of action are linguistically mediated. For Habermas, strategic action is a dimension of human action that aims at a teleological action with purposes determined for practical success and, to this end, it uses language as a means of information, whereas communicative action aims at mutual understanding between the speakers about something in

---

[2]Based on the concepts established by Max Weber that modern society undergoes a process of increasing rationalization as technique and science invade its institutional spheres and the old legitimations fall apart, leading to secularization and disenchantment of worldviews, and inaugurating a growing rationalization of social actions, Marcuse indicates that, with technical-scientific development, the productive forces enter a new constellation with the relations of production: they no longer work in favor of political awareness as the foundation of critique of the existing legitimations, but they themselves, as well as technique and science, become the basis of legitimation. Thus, he proposes that there is a "fusion" between technique and science and forms of domination, which exercise their own mechanisms within a rationality of oppression.

the lifeworld, and thus the use of language is directed toward understanding and requires a scope of cooperation for the coordination of action plans between people. Strategic action, by sending linguistic information aimed at the private interests of the actors who pursue a certain functional success, does not require dialogue. Communicative action requires the use of intersubjectively shared language, leading the actors to abandon self-centered orientations guided by the rational end of their own success, and to submit to the public criteria of rationality of understanding.

Communicative action aims at social integration, is commanded by communicative reason, necessarily presupposes dialogue and intersubjectivity, and grounds the political action of human beings, because here the interest is public and aims at the coordination of social action for a collective good. Strategic action entails teleological action directed by instrumental reason, uses language as a means to influence the opinion and behavior of the other, and seeks technical success based on private interests.

From this perspective, Habermas proposes that, through communicative action, human beings can understand matters in the lifeworld and develop a well-founded consensus to ground their actions and projects of social action. The mutual consensus is provisional, current, and contextual and focuses on the understanding between social actors for the coordination of their actions. Nonetheless, to be achieved, there is need for what Habermas refers to as an ideal speech situation in which all participants have equal opportunities of expression and decision making, symmetry of positions, and equal values for each of the utterances. Only under these conditions is there a "dialogue," that is, a truly intersubjective relation, without coercion to the utterances and discourses under discussion. These are the propositions that Habermas proposes as central to the radical exercise of democracy.

According to Souza (2005), democracy for Habermas is understood within his pretension to make it normative, that is, a radical democratic behavior that endures beyond the contingency dimensions and that ethically guides the relations between human beings in any society. Habermas (1993), however, presents three models of democracy: liberal, republican, and deliberative, with the last being the version that is proposed to overcome the weaknesses of the first two. The liberal model mediates society and the state through a system structured according to market laws and private interests, and the state submits its decision to interests of the economy, characterizing itself as an apparatus of public administration. The republican model advances in the democratic process by presenting the need for the formation of public opinion, popular will, and social solidarity that result from reflection and awareness of free and

equal actors. However, Habermas argues that it is with the deliberative model that democracy achieves its full meaning: shared decision-making power and decision making radically extended to civil society. For Habermas, society is organized in parallel deliberative forums, including those constituted by elected representatives as well as members of civil society that overcome the concentration of power in small privileged groups, to constitute a form of socialized sharing of power in the deliberative model. After this brief conceptualization of democracy according to Habermas' perspective, let us resume the question of the value of dialogue for this philosopher.

Habermas (1988) contends that dialogue is a form of true consensus because it moves through understanding and does not aim to suppress dissent but instead advocates that all conflicting positions should have full force and equal chances and opportunities of expression—this is what he calls argumentative speech. Therefore, in addition to presenting a theory of society through the theory of communicative action, Habermas does so without prescinding Reason. Similarly, moving Reason from the axis it occupied during modernity (as an autonomous instrumental reason) to a new guiding axis represented by language allows him to affirm communicative rationality as the reason that reconstructs the emancipatory potential that the former perspective has left unfinished.

Nevertheless, there is an important contextualization about communicative rationality that deserves to be outlined because it involves a relevant discussion about situations in which communication can be distorted. For Habermas, an ideal speech situation is often disturbed by human interests, by operations of power, and through deception. In these cases, a false consensus is established because the dialogue has been corrupted and ceased to exist in that communicative process, and it is no longer aimed at mutual understanding but guided by private rather than public interests. False consensus may occur because of mistakes, deceptions, or corruption that deviates and perverts the true objectives that led a group of individuals to gather to coordinate their actions. This pseudo-consensus is termed "systematically distorted communication" (Habermas, 1994, p. 193).

According to Habermas, systematically distorted communication can generate three situations: (1) communicative action is transformed into strategic action, from which the communicative process becomes vulnerable to situations of power and coercion, oriented by private interests, and thus the situation of systematically distorted communication imposes itself; (2) there may be disruptions, as the process of negotiation and debate is interrupted and efforts to achieve solutions to problems are frustrated; or (3) communicative action can be resumed through the reestablishment of argumentative action, generating mutual consensus. According to Habermas, the likelihood that possibilities 1 and 2 are removed or controlled and possibility 3 is enacted is due to the systematic denunciation of distorted communication by participants, who move to unveil pretension regarding the sincerity validity in participants' objections.

Another important field of Habermas' thinking is the concept of "lifeworld," which is understood as the entire human existential dimension: the intersection of the physical and symbolic worlds of human creations, the social world, and the subjective world. It is composed of human creations that involve the world of things and their pragmatic contexts that constitute the manipulation of things and events; the social world, jointly constituted, formed by historical groups, institutional and normative orders, and the interactive relation between people, which constitute the governing communities of cooperation and language; and the subjective world, which consists of experiences with the body itself, as well as internal nature, feelings, aesthetic expressions and experiences, moral representations, and so forth (Habermas, 1990).

The lifeworld, symbolically structured, is society and culture, and it is through these two dimensions that it becomes real. Thus, for Habermas, lifeworld is the spatial-temporal-symbolic dimension in which culture, society, and personality intertwine through language. Culture is the storehouse of knowledge, from which participants of communication extract interpretations when they understand each other about something. Society is composed of legitimate orders by which participants of communication regulate their belonging to social groups and ensure solidarity and social cohesion. The personality structures that compose the subjective world are formed by the motives and skills that enable individuals to speak and act and that guarantee their identity. In short, the components of the lifeworld—culture, society, and personality structures—form complex and communicating sets of meaning: cultural knowledge is embodied in symbolic forms; society is constituted in institutional orders, norms of law, or normatively regulated practices and customs; and finally, personality structures are realized by means of all human subjective expressions, which personalize in an identity through the process of socialization.

Therefore, the lifeworld is structured through cultural traditions, institutional orders, and identities created by the processes of socialization. It constitutes the territory in which networks of interaction among groups more or less integrated in the social field, more or less cohesively united, are formed and understood communicatively to coordinate their social actions. Lifeworld is a concept that Habermas has borrowed from Husserl's phenomenology and has

developed on the basis of his theory of communicative action as the spatial-temporal-symbolic dimension in which elements of the cultural, social, and subjective worlds are intertwined, forming cross-structures that generate the world of everyday life, where social and intersubjective production occurs and is symbolically mediated by language.

This composition that intertwines and intersects the various dimensions of physical and symbolic, social, and subjective/intersubjective life allows an interpretation of reality that abandons forms of knowledge based solely on cognitive-positivist rationality—which separates subjectivity and symbolism from knowledge—to enable a process of knowledge production of the real through a hermeneutic, interpretative, and reconstructive approach.

According to Habermas (1990), it is in the lifeworld that the foundations necessary for a self-determination capable of conducting an emancipatory project based on Reason and communicative action must occur. They demand the integration of daily social life, through engagement of civil society through political participation, voluntary associations, social movements, and civil disobedience, in the process of seeking mutual understanding in validity judgments. It is precisely in this conceptual articulation of a communicative-discursive level and a sociopolitical level of coordinated action, as inseparable levels of intersubjective practical life, that Habermas manages to rethink the democratic exercise from the perspective of daily social life.

It is important to consider, however, the Habermasian diagnosis of the *colonization of the lifeworld by the imperatives of the system*, driven by the increasing technocratic instrumentalization of society. For Habermas, the lifeworld contrasts and conflicts with the world of systems. On one hand, the philosopher defines the world of systems as composed of economic and public administrations that undergo systemic functional rationalizations; on the other hand, he defines the dimension of the symbolic reproduction of the world, which moves through a communicative rationalization, and this is the dimension of the lifeworld. The situations in which the dynamics of money (characteristic of the economic system) and power (characteristic of the government system) invade activities and structures of the lifeworld are termed by Habermas as "colonies of the lifeworld" and are designated by the author as the main "pathologies" of communication and intersubjective relations to which modern societies are exposed (Habermas, 1994, p. 193).

According to this diagnosis, the communicative domains of society are constantly exposed to the risk of being "invaded" or "colonized" by the functional domains—a process that overlaps the technical instrumental and communicative dimensions and suppresses the political debate of the lifeworld. Habermas confronts instrumental and technocratic rationality as a form of colonization that controls the social structure, with a defensive strategy that recognizes that the lifeworld places limits on the action of systems (Habermas, 2000).

The third dimension of Habermasian thought is emphasized in his more recent works (Habermas, 2012, 2014), in which the philosopher discusses the process of European unification, focusing his concern on the inability of the polity to control the economy, the loss of meaning and legitimacy of politics itself in the eyes of the citizens, and the need to redress people's democratic participation, both in transnational decision-making processes and in the management of economic and financial policies. Habermas (2012) addresses two themes associated with this discussion: the role played by the concept of human dignity in the justification and practice of human rights and a proposal of global institutional reform aimed at creating a fairer society not only for the purpose of guaranteeing basic liberties but also for ensuring more equality and equity in a fairer and more dignified life for all human beings.

Habermas (2012) claims that the process of European unification must move toward a "transnational democracy"—instead of simply being constituted in a "post-democratic executive federalism" (p. 40) as observed in some current trends in Europe—in which global society can project itself into geopolitical and multicultural constellations organized by transnational democracies. To this end, effective mechanisms need to be established so that decisions relating to the sphere of economics and finance, as well as political decisions, can be submitted to the scrutiny of a democratic public opinion. Perhaps this is another historical reconstruction of Habermas to affirm, in other words, the need for communicative reason of reciprocal understanding and mutual consensus, and hence for its political sphere in which communicative action is manifested, to submit and command the instrumental sphere and technique of human action. Even without ignoring the structural difficulties imposed on the proposal for direct inclusion of citizens in decision-making processes, and not only on the basis of representativeness criteria, Habermas insists that consensus must be guided by the unquestionable horizon of human dignity above all other aspects. The philosopher also argues that popular sovereignty cannot be accomplished without the existence of a public sphere capable of extending the decision-making process beyond governing councils and parliaments and equally stresses the need for the decision-making process to become transparent and open to discussion, influenced by public opinion and not by organized private interests. Habermas (2014) deepens the idea of crisis and the need to overcome the model of representative democracy, a liberal political model characteristic of the capitalist mode of social organization. In this sense, he draws attention to the dilemma of political parties and their inability to represent contemporary social and political-institutional needs, as well as proposing a participatory democratic model as a response to the misery of a fragmented and iniquitous world society under the integration of capitalism.

It is worth emphasizing that, utopian or achievable, Habermasian thinking directly implies a struggle for a radical democratic process; for the realization of the unfinished project of modernity regarding equality, liberty, justice, and solidarity among people; for overcoming a highly stratified world society in which goods and opportunities are unbearably unevenly shared; and for the creation, under a contemporary perspective, of an articulated and democratically organized multicultural global society.

CONTRIBUTION OF HABERMASIAN THINKING TO SOCIAL OCCUPATIONAL THERAPY

Social occupational therapy, as it was conceived in Brazil in the 1990s and has been developing up to the present, is fundamentally concerned with social questions related to human segments, groups, and communities that are on the margin of access to goods, services, income, and vital opportunities or that are undergoing processes of social disintegration for being vulnerable or excluded in relation to social support networks—populations that are also currently growing in the global context (Lopes et al., 2008). To address these problems, social occupational therapy has sought methodologies, technologies, and strategies of action aimed at such populations who are experiencing social vulnerability or excluded from the public spheres of production of social relations (Barros et al., 2007).

Therefore, the concern for developing actions in and with communities that contribute to the discussion of problems and their organization in collective spaces that form consensus for social action is an important issue for social occupational therapy. Another is the concern for creating spaces and mechanisms of democratic expansion for popular participation in decision-making forums and preparation of public policies for social well-being (Lopes, Borba, & Cappellaro, 2011). These questions are also at the core of the discussions and aspirations of the Habermasian philosophical framework approach, such as his theory of communicative action.

In this context, two fields of social occupational therapy that could immediately benefit from the Habermasian theoretical framework are highlighted. The first field regards the constitution of a methodology for the construction of social projects and the coordination of the actions of groups and communities in pursuit of their demands, as well as in the organization of sectors of civil society and administration for the preparation, implementation, and management of public policies. This area bases the action of occupational therapists on social practice as social articulators/mediators not only in the community sphere and the territory but also in the suprastructural spheres of the technical and popular forums where the preparation and implementation of social policies take place. The second scope refers to the methodological field to operationalize action based on a theoretical framework that can contribute to an analysis of the social field that binds to and is realized in the interface between culture, society, and personal dimensions.

The perspective of responding to questions regarding the immense social inequalities and the lack of dignified living conditions and full citizenship experienced by groups and communities living in conditions of social vulnerability presents social occupational therapy with two primary tasks: (1) to organize social actions and projects of citizenship together with these communities based on activities developed in the local territories and (2) to ensure that these social projects, prepared and claimed by the assisted groups, gain space for expression and enter the agenda of administrative bodies and managers in all spheres of government, local and national.

To this end, the possibilities of social occupational therapy action, in addition to the creation of discussion groups and the preparation of strategies to cope with problems directly with the populations and communities assisted, include a practice focused on the organization of intersectoral discussion/debate forums. Ideally, these forums would generate consensus for the preparation of public policies and strategies aimed at eradicating poverty and social inequalities, which are represented by disparities in access to social rights and the universalization of rights and full citizenship, as well as at the level of implementation of public policies that ensure human rights and dignity.

Given the complexity, multidimensionality, and polysemy of contemporary social issues, current debates and political decisions present the compelling imperatives for interdisciplinarity and intersectoriality. In a world with global flows of wealth, power, and images, the search for identity, collective or individual, and the guarantee of elementary rights of human dignity, among other issues, become the primary source of multiple social meanings, which necessarily impose many views and interpretations. Therefore, this multiple and polysemic global trajectory will only be able to be unraveled through interdisciplinarity of knowledge. Similarly, making decisions today

requires multisectoral initiatives that not only include specific administrative sectors (social assistance, health, education, legal, culture, etc.) but also coordinate actions between various sectors of political management of the governmental spheres, as well as civil society organizations (Castells, 2011).

The challenge of interdisciplinarity and intersectoriality requires dialogue *par excellence* as a starting point and in its procedural development. Moreover, it demands the construction of consensus for the implementation of coordinated actions. Although consensus is confronted with immense manifestations of private powers and interests, they are needed so that some agreements on the implementation of actions to address these issues are minimally guaranteed—hence the importance of creating social forums for the preparation of proposals and the development of action plans and for ensuring that debate can be conducted without coercion and with appreciation and symmetry of all discourses without restrictions, with systematic denunciation when the dialogue is confronted with private interests over public interests.

In this sense, it is worth recalling the importance of Habermas' theory of communicative action, not only regarding the formation of consensus for decision making grounded in discussion and debate of the issues involved but also with respect to the disturbances that may occur, and often do, in these communicative processes, and which are the basis of the constitution of intersectoral and interdisciplinary forums aimed at the construction of social action projects.

As an example, an experience occurred in a municipality in the state of Sao Paulo, Brazil, in 2012. It refers to a transfer of financial resources from the federal government to municipal governments to be applied in local projects aimed at coping with problems associated with abusive consumption of alcohol and other drugs. This transfer of funds was agreed upon between the presidency of the republic and the mayors of municipalities as part of the actions foreseen by Decree 7799, of May 20, 2010, which established the Integrated Plan to Combat Crack and Other Drugs. This municipality had discussed where to invest the funding. Because our group develops teaching, research, and extension activities (related to projects in partnership between the university and communities) in this municipality, we participated in this process. We understand that the issue of drugs is not only a matter of health care but also of culture, education, and other issues, and therefore we outlined a proposal to direct the funding to a psychosocial care network rooted in intersectoral strategies. However, the municipality instead focused efforts on the construction or expansion of local hospitals and approved compulsory hospitalization for street users, favoring a process of the psychiatrization of poverty. In this sense, there is urgent need to shift from highly centralized and fragmented sectoral governance to decentralized management, with actions and policies integrated intersectorally and with the participation of the communities. This is a current issue in the global context; that is, there is a need for intersectoral and decentralized governance at the planetary level in the face of increasingly complex international matters.

In another experience that occurred in the same Brazilian municipality, a forum was formed by different administrative and professional sectors involving professionals and managers of the health, social assistance, education, and legal areas, including occupational therapists. In regular meetings held to discuss and prepare intersectoral strategies, the members of this forum tried to approve initiatives and actions aimed at the population that uses alcohol and other drugs based on the harm reduction approach, putting forth proposals to create interdisciplinary teams of physicians to assist at street offices and other initiatives to address street users of alcohol and other drugs. Nonetheless, these intersectoral strategies must contend discursively throughout the social space with prejudiced (distorted) conceptions of society, with the private interests of individuals and groups that profit from hospitalization, and with the interests of government representatives who must also seek to captivate the electorate and who may use the public machinery for their own benefit, fragmenting the negotiated powers into sectors. The path to intersectoriality and forums for building democratic consensus is winding and arduous, but these forums are presented as a current necessity worldwide, given the worsening of highly complex social problems that demand transversal actions involving different actors of government and civil society. Although they have many disparities, these forums exist and resist. These examples show that the Habermasian framework is present once again; that is, the practice of denunciation when forums are put together to constitute democratic-founded consensus is confronted with all types of distortions, mainly from the sector and private powers of small groups against social interests, as well as the constant struggle of community members, motivated by public interest based on the principle of the discursive validity of sincerity and dialogue, to maintain the democratic debate with a view to forming a mutual consensus for the coordination of social action.

Social occupational therapy is inserted into contexts such as these, into communities, and works with the aim of contributing to the organization of socially vulnerable groups, reinforcing their social support networks, working with them to solve their problems, and opening expanded deliberative spaces to include people from these communities

and from other social sectors. Social occupational therapy also works in intersectoral collective spaces to prepare public policies focused on social issues (Lopes, Borba, Silva, & Malfitano, 2012).

This chapter presents the relevant contribution of the Habermasian theory to a social occupational therapy methodology; as such, two propositions for action are proposed. The first is the creation of groups of activities and discussion with the assisted communities to achieve some consensus on their problems and guidelines to be claimed. The second is the proposition of creating intersectoral and interdisciplinary forums, formed by technicians, managers, and civil society, to discuss and implement strategies, programs, and social policies of citizenship.

However, to participate in decision-making forums, discern social problems, and act in local spaces, as well as in suprastructural interstices, there is a need for a social theory that serves as a basis for experimenting with different concepts and articulating them within a frame of knowledge that is consistent with the field of practice. In this context, another challenge posed for social occupational therapy, as Barros et al. (2007) propose, is the need to outline a theoretical approach that provides tools for interpreting reality in the articulation between single experiences and culture and understanding the relationships between individuals, groups, community, and society. In a complementary sense, according to Malfitano (2005), it is necessary to read the contexts that interfere with micro- and macro-social structures. To such concerns, it is suggested that the Habermasian concept of lifeworld presents a useful contribution.

According to this perspective, the Habermasian theory of lifeworld contributes by establishing a coherent connection between the dimensions of the physical and cultural worlds, society, and the subjective world, enabling a social analysis that integrates constitutive elements of social reality such as individuals, groups, and communities, as well as fostering the relation between the local structures of a community and the social superstructures.

When emphasis is placed on the actions of social articulation in the communities and social articulation to create intersectoral forums that form consensus for the coordination of social action, there is no intention to minimize other equally important lines of social occupational therapy action, such as the strengthening and construction of social support networks, the creation of income-generating devices, activation of initiatives through a solidarity economy, social articulation based on culture, school–community articulation, and so forth. These two domains of social occupational therapy were highlighted because it is through them that the contribution of the Habermasian philosophical framework can be most clearly and immediately perceived, although it can also be applied to actions in small groups.

Finally, this chapter resumes consideration of the third point of Habermas' theory and the proposal of his more recent works on the direct inclusion of people of civil society in the decision-making processes of the state, both at the level of economic decisions and in the scope of political decisions. Habermas (2012, p. 111) states that "to put away the neoliberal agenda and the whole program of unscrupulous subordination of the lifeworld to the imperatives of the market" and simultaneously repair the effects of this political-economic orientation of social injustice imposed on vulnerable social groups, an agenda of democratization of public opinion is needed, and it should be directly involved and included in decision-making bodies with power over political and economic directions. Therefore, it is necessary to include civil society in the decision-making processes directly in the spheres of government.

Habermas (2014), however, deepened these reflections even further and proposed that, in the wake of technocracy, the globalized capitalist organization has led to the fragmentation of world society and established immense economic inequalities, generating geographically identified social inequities. Thus, from the perspective of fighting capitalism itself, a radical democratic model must be established: deliberative democracy, in which civil society is definitively inserted into the decision-making spheres of political power as a whole.

Civil society, historically understood as the sphere of political constitution as a counterpoint to the imperatives and determination of the market and exploratory economy over the life of the people, must be reorganized around citizen issues, which, according to Habermas (2000), is the organization of society based on rights and guided by freedom of thought and free communication between individuals. Unlike the state, which is guided by the logic of power underpinned by institutionalized violence and the market, civil society envisages the possibility of building an ethical and communicative rationality focused on social justice. It is worth noting that, according to Avritzer (1993), the contemporary idea of social movement and civil society is strongly present and pervades the whole theoretical formulation of Habermas' theory of communicative action.

These propositions integrate relevant parameters of the field of knowledge and constitute the central themes of reflection for social occupational therapy. It is in the communities, and with civil society, that social practice can establish and construct instruments of action aimed at the emancipation of groups and populations in positions of social vulnerability.

The conception of deliberative democracy advocated by Habermas acquires here a solid foundation to establish a social practice for occupational therapy. While respecting the role of the state as coordinator in the formulation of a redistributive social policy, there is need for political-institutional and organizational reforms of government and of their relation with society and the operations of power. The proposal is based on the need to include segments of the population in the decision-making, political, financial, social, environmental, and developmental spheres and increasing social representativeness, control, and participation in decision making and sharing of power in all sectors.

Thus, the perspective of expanding democratic spaces for individuals, groups, and communities with which social occupational therapy works, in addition to developing instruments and technologies for operationalizing it, becomes a challenge for the insertion of social occupational therapy into this discussion.

REFERENCES

Adorno, T. W. (1951). *Minima moralia*. Lisboa: Edições 70.

Adorno, T. W., & Horkheimer, M. (1984). *Dialética do esclarecimento* [Dialectic of enlightenment]. Rio de Janeiro: Jorge Zahar Editor.

Almeida, M. C., Soares, C. R. S., Barros, D. D., & Galvani, D. (2012). Processos e práticas de formalização da terapia ocupacional na assistência social: alguns marcos e desafios [Formalization processes and practices of occupational therapy in social assistance: Landmarks and challenges]. *Cadernos de Terapia Ocupacional da UFSCar, 20*(1), 33–41.

Avritzer, L. (1993). Além da dicotomia estado-mercado: Habermas, Cohen e Arato [Beyond the state-market dichotomy: Habermas, Cohen, and Arato]. *Novos Estudos, 5*(36), 213–222.

Barros, D. D., Lopes, R. E., & Gualheigo, S. M. (2007). Terapia ocupacional social: concepções e perspectivas [Social occupational therapy: Concepts and perspectives] in A. Cavalcanti & C. Galvão (Eds.), *Terapia ocupacional: fundamentação & prática* [Occupational therapy: Grounding and practice] (pp. 347–353). Rio de Janeiro: Guanabara/Koogan.

Castel, R. (2001). *As metamorfoses da questão social: uma crônica do salário* [The metamorphosis of the social question. A chronicle of the wage] (3rd ed.). Petrópolis: Editora Vozes.

Castells, M. (2011). *A sociedade em rede* [The network society]. São Paulo: Editora Paz e Terra.

Domingues, L. H. (2005). *Políticas sociais em mudança: o estado, as empresas, e a intervenção social* [Changing social policies: The state, enterprises, and social intervention]. Lisboa: Universidade Técnica de Lisboa. Instituto Superior de Ciências Sociais e Políticas.

Drummond, A. (2007). Fundamentos da terapia ocupacional [Occupational therapy: Grounding and practice]. In

A. Cavalcanti & C. Galvão (Eds.), *Terapia ocupacional: fundamentação & prática* [Occupational therapy: Grounding and practice] (pp. 10–17). Rio de Janeiro: Guanabara/Koogan.

Fiorati, R. C., & Saeki, T. (2011). A inserção da reabilitação psicossocial nos serviços extra-hospitalares de saúde mental: o conflito entre racionalidade instrumental e racionalidade prática [The inclusion of psychosocial rehabilitation in outpatient mental health services: The conflict between instrumental rationality and practical rationality]. *Revista de Terapia Ocupacional da Universidade de São Paulo, 22*(1), 76–84.

Fiorati, R. C., & Saeki, T. (2012). As atividades terapêuticas em dois serviços extra-hospitalares de saúde mental: a inserção das ações psicossociais [Therapeutic activities in mental health extra-hospital services: The inclusion of psychosocial actions]. *Cadernos de Terapia Ocupacional da UFSCar, 20*(2), 207–215.

Habermas, J. (1987). *Técnica e ciência como ideologia* [Technology and science as ideology]. Lisboa: Edições 70.

Habermas, J. (1988). *Teoría de la acción comunicativa* [The theory of communicative action]. Madrid: Taurus.

Habermas, J. (1990). *Pensamento pós metafísico: estudos filosóficos* [Postmetaphysical thinking: Philosophical essays]. Rio de Janeiro: Tempo Brasileiro.

Habermas, J. (1993). Três modelos de democracia [Three models of democracy]. Sobre El concepto de uma política deliberativa. [About the concept of deliberative politics] (G. Cohn & A. de Vita, Trans.). *El ojo del Huracán* [The eye of the hurricane], 4, 14–15. Paper presented at Seminário "Teoría da democracia" at Universidade de Valência.

Habermas, J. (1994). *Teoría de La acción comunicativa: complementos y estúdios prévios* [The theory of communicative action: Complements and previous studies]. Madrid: Ediciones Cátedra.

Habermas, J. (2000). *O discurso filosófico da modernidade: doze lições* [The philosophical discourse of modernity: Twelve lectures]. São Paulo: Martins Fontes.

Habermas, J. (2012). *Sobre a constituição da Europa: um ensaio* [On Europe's constitution: An essay] (D. L. Werle, L. Repa, & R. Melo, Trans.). São Paulo: Editora UNESP.

Habermas, J. (2014). *Na esteira da tecnocracia: pequenos escritos políticos XII* [The lure of technocracy: Short political writings XII]. São Paulo: Editora UNESP.

Horkheimer, M. (2002). *Eclipse da razão* [Eclipse of reason] (S. U. Leite, Trans.). São Paulo: Centauro.

Japiassu, H., & Marcondes, D. (2006). *Dicionário básico de filosofia* [Basic dictionary of philosophy]. Rio de Janeiro: Jorge Zahar Editor.

Lopes, R. E., Adorno, R. C. F., Malfitano, A. P. S., Takeiti, B. A., Silva, C. R., & Borba, P. L. O. (2008). Juventude pobre, violência e cidadania [Poor youth, violence and citizenship]. *Saúde e Sociedade, 17*(3), 63–76.

Lopes, R. E., Borba, P. L. O., & Cappellaro, M. (2011). Acompanhamento individual e articulação de recursos em terapia ocupacional social: compartilhando uma experiência [Individual support and resources articulation in social occupational therapy: Sharing an experience]. *O Mundo da Saúde, 35*(2), 233–238.

Lopes, R. E., Borba, P. L. O., Silva, C. R., & Malfitano, A. P. S. (2012). Terapia ocupacional social no Brasil e na América Latina: panorama, tensões e reflexões a partir de práticas profissionais [The social field of occupational therapy in Brazil and Latin America: Overview, tensions and reflections from professional]. *Cadernos de Terapia Ocupacional da UFSCar, 20*(1), 21–32.

Malfitano, A. P. S. (2005). Campos e núcleos de intervenção na terapia ocupacional social [Intervention fields and cores in social occupational therapy]. *Revista de Terapia Ocupacional da Universidade de São Paulo, 16*(1), 1–8.

Sawaia, B. (2007). *As artimanhas da exclusão: análise psicossocial e ética da desigualdade social* [The twists of exclusion: A psychosocial and ethical analysis of social inequality]. Petrópolis: Vozes.

Sorj, B., & Martuccelli, D. (2008). *O desafio latino-americano: coesão social e democracia* [The Latin American challenge: Social cohesion and democracy]. Rio de Janeiro: Civilização Brasileira.

Souza, J. C. (Ed.). (2005). *Filosofia, racionalidade, democracia: os debates Rorty & Habermas* [Philosophy, rationality, democracy: The debates Rorty & Habermas]. São Paulo: Editora UNESP.

9

Citizenship and Cultural Diversity in Management of Cultural Policies[1]

Patricia Silva Dorneles and Roseli Esquerdo Lopes

INTRODUCTION

Cultural diversity and cultural citizenship are diffuse concepts still under construction that permeate the current guidelines on cultural policy in Brazil. As indicators of a cultural policy's democratic nature, these concepts bear responsibility for representing paradigms and cultural actions capable of breaking both with the processes of exclusion that result from the traditional Eurocentric and elitist views of art and culture and with the assimilationist political practices associated with neoliberal globalization. With a view to fostering and ensuring respect for all people's cultures, the concepts of cultural diversity (in an extended way) and cultural citizenship (in a more localized way) establish commitments and efforts among public managers of culture at different levels by reorganizing their investment and promotion guidelines in the field of Brazilian political culture. In Brazil, the concepts and guidelines on citizenship and cultural diversity were included at the federal level in the national culture policy during President Lula's administration (2003–2010). This chapter aims to contextualize the subject of cultural public policies within the guidelines of citizenship and cultural diversity by reflecting on the possibilities of occupational therapy action in the cultural field associated with current paradigms, leading us to propositions that have been adopted through social occupational therapy (Barros, Ghiradi, & Lopes, 2005).

[1]This theoretical reflection is part of the postdoctoral study "In Favor of Occupational Therapy in the Management and Actions of Cultural Policies," which was developed by the first author between 2014 and 2015 at the Post-Graduate Program in Occupational Therapy, Federal University of Sao Carlos (UFSCar), advised by Roseli Esquerdo Lopes, funded by the Coordination for the Improvement of Higher Education Personnel, CAPES, Brazil.

ON CULTURAL POLICIES

Although Brazil has become a model with respect to the application of the current paradigms of public cultural policies, according to the guidelines of international organizations, there is still much to be done for the democratization of production and the right to cultural enjoyment and dissemination. This remains a challenge for Brazil, and it has become more difficult to overcome since the beginning (2018) of the current federal administration. Studies on cultural policies are a relatively recent development. In Brazil, a movement of researchers and intellectuals interested in systematizing and reflecting on this theme began just over 10 years ago. The new cultural public policy model of the federal government, which began to be implemented during the administration of Culture Minister Gilberto Gil (2003–2007), has been the subject of much academic research. Prior to this, there were a number of studies in the 1930s and 1940s addressing the state's action on culture, but as Calabre (2008) emphasizes, in most of them, such actions were not necessarily treated as cultural policies.

The subject of cultural policy has been developed within the framework of cultural studies since it emerged in England in the 1950s. The Center for Contemporary Cultural Studies was founded by Richard Hoggart and included Raymond Williams and Edward Palmer Thompson as members, with Stuart Hall joining later. The first writings of this group of thinkers addressed working-class culture and the impact of mass media. In Latin America, cultural studies began to develop in the 1980s, and although they emerged from the world of academia, they were entwined with the practical process of redemocratization and based on intense observation of the social movements of the time, which makes their perspective different from that of the British and North American currents. The reflections and concepts of Antonio Gramsci influenced Latin American intellectuals, especially Nestor Garcia

Canclini and Jesús Martin-Barbero (Dorneles, 2011), and shaped a structure of political engagement. The area of cultural studies was formed quite recently in Brazil, with Heloisa Buarque de Holanda, Ana Carolina Escosteguy, and Thomaz Tadeu da Silva among its founders. Some scholars consider Antônio Candido, Roberto Schwarz, Silvio Santiago, and Renato Ortiz to be theorists whose writings could be classified under cultural studies (Prysthon, 2000; Canclini, 2006). The studies on cultural policies conducted between 2003 and 2011 integrate several areas, such as economy, geography, social service, and communication, among others. These studies present the impact of the cultural policy developed, examining the concepts of culture around which the different cultural programs and actions revolved, namely, culture as economy, culture as citizenship, and culture as symbolic production. The area of cultural studies in Brazil has developed under different approaches and with a multi- and interdisciplinary design, seeking to understand the relationships between culture, individual, and society. This has included looking more comprehensively at disputes around cultural capital, borders, hierarchies between cultural forms and practices, hybrid and intercultural aspects, media, and cultural consumption. From this perspective of cultural criticism, the studies propose an investigation of the cultural field, its daily practices, and cultural and social products and processes of all its production. Despite the extensive literature on the theme of "cultural policy," there are few works that actually define it. Overall, the approaches to this subject work with implied and presupposed ideas, but they are never systematized or explicit to the reader (Dorneles, 2011).

There are different understandings of the meaning of "cultural policy." Coelho (1997) advocates an anthropological view of the imaginary and claims that studies in this area expose a central motivation of the cultural impulse, a desire that can be resurfaced and expanded. For Coelho, it is necessary to assume that the object of cultural policy is almost always superfluous; he states that the highest expression of cultural policy is "cultural action," which must be understood as the availability of conditions for individuals and groups to create their own ways. Certeau (1997) understands cultural action as interventions that connect agents to specific objectives, as well as an operational segment where the means of achieving it are associated with the objectives to be defined. Cunha (2003) emphasizes that the term "cultural action," which emerged after World War II and was included in the efforts toward Europe's social and educational reconstruction, reached Brazil in the 1970s and that the term has often been used as a synonym for social or sociocultural motivation. Freire (2012) argues that the concept of cultural action can be linked to working-class education movements established in France. For the Brazilian educator, cultural action is political action, that is, collective action engaged in liberation (Freire, 2012); therefore, it is characterized by a liberating dialogue, which promotes knowledge and praxis, and the communion of subjects who participate in the transformation of reality (Freire, 1979).

Theorizing the field of cultural production as a space for struggle for the appropriation of symbolic capital, Bourdieu (2000) presents the struggle between various parties to define the concepts and paradigms associated with cultural actions and policies. Conservative or avantgarde trends are organized according to the positions held in relation to this capital.

Certeau (1997) conceptualizes "cultural policy as a more or less coherent set of objectives, means, and actions that aim to modify behaviors according to explicit criteria or principles" (p. 195). According to Cunha (2003), cultural policy is a "set of interventions of the public powers on the artistic-intellectual or generically symbolic activities of a society." Such interventions should be understood from a "legal framework of taxes and duties, incentives and protection to assets and activities, as well as, more concretely, of the cultural action of the state" (p. 15).

Coelho (1997) highlights that cultural policy is usually understood as a program of interventions conducted by the state, private institutions, or community groups, always with the objective of promoting and satisfying the development of symbolic representations. Thus, cultural policy should be understood as a set of initiatives aimed at fostering the production, distribution, and uses of culture and the preservation and dissemination of historical heritage. These initiatives can be developed by agents of groups and entities, both private and public. For Barbalho (2005), Coelho defines cultural policy as cultural management, stressing that cultural policy cannot be limited to an administrative task and/or to programs and sets of initiatives that act consensually but that it results from the relationship between cultural and political forces. Rubim (2012), citing Fernández,[2] emphasizes that the foundation period of cultural policies ranges from the 1930s to the 1960s. From this perspective, the political-cultural initiatives of the Second Spanish Republic in the 1930s and the English Arts Council in the 1940s can be regarded as inaugural efforts in this area. According to Cunha (2003), cultural policy as an intervention of the state emerged in the Soviet Union at the beginning of the 20th century, integrating economic, social, and educational plans, as well as playing

---

[2]Cited reference: Fernandez, X. B. (2007). Financia acerca del origen y genesis de las politicas culturales occidentales: arqueologías y derivas. O público e o privado. *Fortaleza, 9,* 111–147.

an ideological role. In modern times, the institutionalization of cultural policy is a common feature, and the creation of the Ministry of Cultural Affairs in France in 1959 was an international milestone. The French initiative to create a specific culture ministry was rooted in the aforementioned experiences (Rubim, 2012; Fernández, 2007; Calabre, 2008).

Revisiting the history of Brazil from the time of the empire to the military dictatorship of the 1960s and 1970s, it is possible to observe, among the paradigms of culture and public cultural policy, the perspectives of Eurocentrism, protection and valorization of the artist, and an understanding of culture as an expression of the classical arts. The Brazilian Ministry of Culture was created during the political liberalization of the 1980s. A national cultural policy was established based on tax incentives provided to large companies, and the market became the power defining cultural values and languages based on companies' private interests in creating associations for their brands. The expression used by the Brazilian Ministry of Culture in the mid-1990s—"culture is a good business"—signals the paradigm of cultural policy of that period (Dorneles, 2011). The agenda of citizenship and cultural diversity emerged at the federal level in the early 2000s. Before that, the efforts of the Brazilian left in public management at the municipal level had established the social right to culture, expanding democratization with respect to the production, dissemination, and access to culture through their actions and policies.

ON CITIZENSHIP AND CULTURAL DIVERSITY

Cultural citizenship and cultural diversity today represent concepts and practices of cultural actions and policies that expand social rights to include culture. Franz Boas, an American anthropologist of German descent, addressed the issues of cultural diversity at the beginning of the 20th century. By emphasizing the historical dimension of cultural phenomena and the cultural relativism behind the diversity of cultural systems, he breaks with theories of biological determinism and provides a counterpoint to the anthropological theories that prevailed until then, which defended the existence of a hierarchy between cultures rooted in ethnocentrism (Cuche, 2006).

According to Gruman (2008), addressing the issue of ethnocentric arrogance was one of the main objectives of the November 1945 constitution of the United Nations for Educational, Scientific, and Cultural Organization (UNESCO). Gruman highlights that the events of the then-recent World War II were worrisome, as is made explicit in the preamble to the document: "ignorance of each other's ways of life has been a common cause, throughout

the history of humanity, of suspicion and mistrust between the peoples of the world, causing wars," and "dissemination of culture and education of humanity for justice, liberty, and peace are indispensable to the dignity of human beings and constitute a sacred duty that all nations must fulfill within the spirit of mutual assistance" (UNESCO, 1945, p. 1, in Gruman, 2008, p. 174).

It is known that the mobilization around social rights, characteristic of the 20th century, was at the center of national debates after World War II, linked to the contemporary view of human rights and as a counterpoint to the horrors of the war. The Universal Declaration of Human Rights of 1948, with its new conception of universality and indivisibility, established being a person as the minimum requirement for the ownership of rights and held that human rights should be considered indivisible; in other words, civil and political rights should be combined with social, economic, and cultural rights (Fernandes, 2011).

Through regulations and the creation of opportunities and institutions, cultural issues begin to be the object of state policies after World War II. Although the relationship between culture and politics is older, it is worth emphasizing that they became interspersed with the advent of capitalism. In the Western world, guidelines for education and culture, among others, were first included in state constitutions with the Mexican constitution of 1917 and Weimar Constitution of 1918 in Germany. If in the first half of the 20th century reference to culture was vague and synthetic, in the second half, national constitutions expanded the idea of cultural rights as fundamental rights, with Article 27 of the Universal Declaration of Human Rights as a reference. In Brazil, the theme of culture first appeared in the constitutions of 1934 and 1988. In 1934, there were provisions to protect the sciences, arts, and culture in general in a chapter on education and culture. Article 215 of the 1988 constitution included cultural rights in the category of fundamental rights (Fernandes, 2011).

It is evident that the issue of cultural citizenship and/or cultural rights begins to be included in the agenda when minority groups fight for alternatives to survive the abandonment of the state or reduced assistance from the minimal state. These alternatives are expressed in collective and community actions that seek solutions of subjective, as well as economic, sustainability in their territories. Development actions toward innovative and collective identities also result in aesthetic, artistic, and cultural manifestations. From this perspective, they have become elements of resistance to the hegemonic culture centered on the view of "culture as good business" and that maintained the logic of financing and fostering the classical arts of the elite and spectacle. Such actions demonstrate the cultural process of a group, a *modus operandi*, a way of living "that appreciates exactly what is disqualified in the dominant culture" (Yúdice, 2006, p. 42).

It is interesting to observe that, in the theoretical field of cultural policies, there are few studies addressing the influence of social movements in the formulations of concepts and cultural policy agendas. As highlighted by Alvarez, Dagnino, and Escobar (2000), social movements, in addition to translating their agendas into public policies by expanding the frontier of institutional policy, have struggled significantly to redefine the sense of citizenship and conventional notions of political representation, participation, and democracy. Alvarez et al. state that in Latin America, the term "cultural policy" usually means the actions of the state or other institutions toward culture, which is considered a specific matter separate from the politics, quite often reduced to the production and consumption of cultural assets, such as art, cinema, theater, and so forth. Alvarez et al., from the field of cultural studies, use the concept of "cultural policy" to draw attention to a constitutive correlation between culture and politics and to the redefinition of politics that this view implies, noting that, as a set of meanings that integrate social practices, these cannot be adequately understood without understanding the power relations inherent to them. Therefore, it is impossible not to recognize the cultural character in the configurations of power relations; thus, the idea of "cultural policy" they refer to is associated to the process by which the cultural aspect becomes the political aspect. Among the topics of human rights and social justice included in the Brazilian civil society agenda and politics in the last decades of the 20th century, Gohn (2008) points out the "right to difference." This generated several social movements and gave rise to numerous nongovernmental organizations (NGOs) based on the demands and claims of so-called minorities—women, African Brazilians, and Indians, among others—that are in different historical contexts than the majority of the population. According to Gohn, the development and union of social movements with NGOs assist with uniting the terms "culture" and "rights" and with "constituting a new political culture in society, from the redefinition of values, symbols and meanings, in a game of interaction and reciprocity between what is instituted and instituting" (p. 41).

Contrary to assimilationist policies, American theorists focus on the multiculturalist view that proposes a pluralistic or relativistic egalitarian position, whereby different cultures have equal shares in the constitution of society and are expressions of a form of humanity (Yúdice, 2006). From this perspective, Renato Rosaldo "postulated that cultural citizenship implies that groups united by certain social, cultural and/or physical aspects should not be excluded from participation in public spheres of a particular political constitution based on those aspects or characteristics"

(Yúdice, 2006, p. 42). In dialogue with other authors, Yúdice encourages reflection on how, in a legal context based on litigation against exclusion and a cultural ethos, culture has served as the base or guarantee for "claiming rights in the public sphere" (Rosaldo, 1997, p. 36, cited in Yúdice, 2006), considering that culture is a space of identity where individuals can feel they belong to a group. Premised on difference, it functions as a *resource* (Flores & Benmayor, 1997, p. 5, cited by Yúdice, 2006; emphasis in the original[3]) for the formation of citizenship and guarantee of legitimacy, from the claim of difference. Culture becomes a resource for politics, because claims to cultural recognition are usually a means of undermining domination or wrongful deprivation. The result is that politics trump the content of culture (Yúdice, 2006).

At the international level, the question of the concept of cultural citizenship is permeated with the right to communication and cultural difference. Cultural difference is deeply marked by discussions on migration and ethnic processes. Miller (2011) makes interesting provocations on the theme of cultural citizenship and points out the perspectives of international studies in this field, which basically focus this theme on the processes related to immigration and cultural rights in the migrated territories. According to Miller, citizenship is cultural and, presenting political strategies in various North American and European countries where culture is used as an instrument of identity, he reaffirms territories of exclusion and belonging, depending on the economic and political interests of different states. In this context, he criticizes culturalist celebrants, arguing that cultural citizenship should not be understood only as the outcome of social movements but also as an adjustment to economic transformation; the "right's project of deregulation has played a role in creating and sustaining cultural citizenship" (p. 61). Miller focuses on seven groups of American and European researchers[4]

---

[3]Cited reference: Rosaldo, R. (1997). *Cultural citizenship, inequality, and multiculturalism.* In: William B. Flores y Rina Benmayor (comps.).
[4]The seven formations are cultural studies sociologist Tony Bennett and colleagues in Anglo-Australian cultural policy studies; anthropologist Renato Rosaldo and colleagues in the discipline of cultural studies/anthropology, with a field of influence in Chicano studies (United States); Canadian-based political theorist Will Kymlicka in the discipline of political theory, with a field of influence in the Baltic states; Bhikhu Parekh in the discipline of political theory; Amelie Orsenberg Rorty in the discipline of philosophy, with a field of influence in neoliberalism; Middle Eastern historian Bernard Lewis and Cold War political scientist Samuel Huntington in the discipline of history and international relations, with a field of influence in North American media and foreign policy; and Amy Chua in the law discipline, with a field of influence in US public culture.

and advocates of cultural citizenship and, considering their analyses, points out the contradictions of cultural policies that promote cultural citizenship based on different supports of liberal subjectivity. Thus, among other warnings, Miller (2011) points out that it is necessary to cope with the incommensurability of neoliberal prescriptions and statesmen to qualify cultural citizenship processes; one must reconcile the fact that the state is often the court of appeal for vernacular protests and assume the economic limits of liberal philosophy. It is important to be concerned with the stubbornly collectivist and hybrid nature of culture and with the fact that neoliberalism is not more metacultural than any other form of thought. The constitutive inequality and brutality of capitalism must be recognized.

CITIZENSHIP AND CULTURAL DIVERSITY IN PUBLIC POLICIES IN BRAZIL

It is common knowledge that social and intellectual movements contributed fundamentally during Brazil's transition from military dictatorship to democracy in the 1970s. The significant participation of these political actors in the drafting of the 1988 constitution, with the inclusion of new rights, potentiated new relationships between cultural life and the state. The reflections of these intellectuals during that period greatly extended the concept of culture, overcoming the classical meaning that referred only to "cultural work" (symbolic products socially valued and linked to the arts and humanities) and adopting an "anthropological sense of culture." This led to a new dimension of culture, highlighting its presence in everything, producing and fostering identities and meanings that shape social experience and configure social relations. The agendas of the social movements for popular participation in public management and human rights reframed the sense of citizenship by "associating it with emancipation and democracy" (Oliveira, 2010, p. 250). Thus, it can be said that with the political opening of Brazil, a new era of cultural policies was also inaugurated.

The perspective of cultural democracy presents challenges for new designs in the public management of culture. The concepts of culture decentralization and cultural citizenship become the guides for new forms of organizing and administrating culture, and a new institutionalization process is required in the cultural field. In Brazil, initiatives for cultural democratization in cultural policies were introduced in the cities of Porto Alegre and Sao Paulo in the early 1990s. The concepts of cultural citizenship, formulated by Marilena Chauí, the secretary of culture for the city of Sao Paulo (1989–1992), and culture decentralization, proposed by the administration of Porto Alegre during the same period, present similar guidelines for the development of a culture policy: the right to enjoy,

appropriate, and resignify existing cultural spaces; popular participation in cultural management and decision making; and the right to experimentation, innovation, and cultural and artistic formation, among others. From the aforementioned perspectives, neither the concept of culture decentralization nor of cultural citizenship holds culture to be responsible for directing or indoctrinating; on the contrary, they indicate that it is the responsibility of the state to encourage and provide conditions for the population to create and enjoy cultural invention. This involves breaking with investment monopolies on cultural initiatives centralized in the southeastern region and by famous artists in the media, as well as with geographical separation and sociocultural stigma, and fostering the expanded participation of civil society and entities in the public management of culture through different instruments such as conferences, councils, and forums (Dorneles, 2011). These experiences and the processes of culture democratization observed throughout that period inaugurated a new model of cultural management and influenced its perspective in Brazil in the 2000s, when cultural diversity and cultural citizenship were included in the national cultural policies. According to Chauí (1987), cultural citizenship means culture as the right of all citizens regardless of social class and without viewing them merely as consumers or taxpayers. It arises from the denial of three cultural policy concepts that have been in force in public bodies at different times: official culture, populist tradition, and the neoliberal position. The concept of official culture positions public power as a cultural subject that establishes the forms and contents of culture defined by the ruling group, reinforcing its ideology, and legitimating it through culture. Populist tradition is conceptualized as that in which public power plays a pedagogical role for the masses. By appropriating popular culture, the populist tradition transforms and returns culture as a model that can be recognized by the population, in addition to dividing it into elitist and popular, sanctifying the former and assigning a messianic tone to the latter. This tradition transforms the public agencies that use this populist model of cultural policy into agents of salvation, encouraging the population to recognize itself in the forms and contents that are provided to them by the state. The neoliberal perspective of cultural policy minimizes the role of the state in the field of culture, regarding it primarily as a source of historical heritage, and allowing cultural contents and standards to be determined by the capitalist cultural industry (Dorneles, 2011).

Chauí's assumptions gained acceptance in the cultural environment as a concept under construction, and "cultural citizenship" became a new term in the agendas of cultural policy. When studying the concept of "cultural citizenship," Cunha focuses on the fields of political and juridical sciences. Trying to conceptualize the noun "citizenship" prior to understanding the adjective "cultural," he points out that the exercise of cultural citizenship is not expressly mentioned in the specific legislation pertaining to this area, since it is already presupposed in the general discipline of citizenship or even in legal science.

Reflecting on cultural citizenship in the field of law, Cunha Filho (2010) highlights an overfill to "substantive citizenship" and, partially, the scope of the concept created from the experience and formulations of Chauí. In his opinion, Chauí's concept of cultural citizenship refers only to the rights and not to the duties of citizens. Unlike "formal citizenship," which refers only to membership in a nation-state, "substantive citizenship" implies that individuals are part of a sociopolitical body and that their rights and duties have been arranged both concretely and because they are members of this body (Edgar, Sedwick, & Cunha Filho, 2010, p. 183[5]). Thus, it can be affirmed that "substantive citizenship" is the realization of one's own citizenship. For Cunha Filho (2010, p. 186), the overfill to an environment favorable to the manifestation and development of "substantive citizenship" thus constitutes a set of guarantees. Reflections on cultural policies present a common defense of the importance of the juridification of so-called cultural citizenship. It can be argued that Cunha Filho (2010), as well as Yúdice (2006), based on different authors (Niec, 1996; Sreiner & Alston, 1996), agree that the definition of cultural rights is still ambiguous, and even if they present universal validity in different cultural contexts, they will not be applied in the same way as if they were legalized. Cunha Filho (2010) draws attention to the necessity to create specific legislation with the participation of all.

Reflections on the impact of globalization processes on the field of culture, which promote international debates and respectability policies among nations, address the issues of assimilation, hybridism, interculturalism, and so forth. In the postmodern world, the question of identity has become fundamental to the discussion about cultural processes, whereas the relations between global and local aspects mobilize managers and social movements of the cultural area in the implementation of the new. In the view of managers, these actions, which are based on democracy and diversity, promote more than access to cultural creation and production. In addition to aesthetic and artistic manifestations, issues of identity, territory, and

diversity are part of the cultural policy agendas. Agenda 21 for Culture (Barcelona, 2004) and the Convention on the Protection and Promotion of the Diversity of Cultural Expressions (UNESCO, 2005) are examples of forums and white papers on this new paradigm of cultural policies. In 2007, Brazil ratified the aforementioned UNESCO convention and became a signatory through decree no. 6.177.

The proposal of cultural policy in three dimensions[6]—culture as symbol, citizenship, and economy—demonstrated the concept that popularized the terms "cultural citizenship" and "cultural diversity" in Brazil. The inclusion of popular, indigenous, and gypsy cultures; the aesthetic and artistic expression of individuals under psychological distress and with disabilities; and the promotion of community-based cultural initiatives developed by civil society resulted in the concept of cultural policy in Brazil, with an emphasis on mechanisms of participation in the construction of these policies. The public calls adopted during that period generated new administrative impacts on management. This policy, in addition to adopting specific mapping and simplifications, enabled the identification of specific groups, such as public calls directed to popular, indigenous, and gypsy populations and individuals under psychological distress and with disabilities (Brasil, 2010). These public calls served both to map the existing initiatives and to bring the state closer to the symbolic expressions and cultural agents of these groups, previously unknown to the public policy of national culture.

The symbolic dimension of culture should include the "endless possibilities of creation expressed in social practices, ways of life, and worldviews" (Brasil, 2010, p. 8). Therefore, in addition to the arts and heritage policies, more heavily focused on the material perspective of architectural listings—although implementation of Article 16, Section II, Chapter III of the 1988 constitution on tangible and intangible heritage had already been timidly initiated—the perspective of the symbolic dimension promoted a shift to the cultural riches of African and indigenous origins, expanding and providing visibility to what was produced outside the spaces previously established as cultural. "Every Brazilian is the subject of their culture and history, and the policies of the Brazilian Ministry of Culture sought to recognize and value this symbolic capital, given the multiplicity of expressions" (Brasil, 2010, p. 8). Workshops and forums were set up with representatives from all regions and groups identified in the diversity policies, which aimed at the participatory construction of proposals for the

---

[5]Cited reference: Edgar, A., & Sedgwick, P. (Eds.). (2003). *Cultural theory: The key concepts* (Marcelo Rollemberg, Trans.). São Paulo: Contexto, p. 55.

[6]*Culture in three dimensions: The policies of the Brazilian Ministry of Culture from 2003 to 2010* (Brasil, 2010).

cultural policies and programs of the federal government. Article 215 of the 1988 constitution sheds light on the dimension of cultural citizenship: "The state shall guarantee the full exercise of cultural rights to all." Access to cultural production and enjoyment is therefore a right of all, and from this perspective, culture should be considered a basic need—a vital, constructive, and transformative element. Culture, which underlies our individual and collective affirmation, should be understood as an important element of quality of life, strengthening the self-esteem of individuals. Access to culture must be universal because it creates identity ties between individuals while differentiating them. The participation of civil society in the preparation and monitoring of cultural policies should be considered another important element of the civic dimension of culture. This coresponsibility of civil society in the formulation of cultural policies has been present in the conferences, in the creation of various forums and sectoral councils, and in the proposal of shared management programs (Brasil, 2010). Regarding the economic aspect of culture, its potential as a development vector is highlighted as an important source of labor and income, among other contributions (Brasil, 2010).

THE MARK OF THE "CULTURA VIVA - PONTOS DE CULTURA" PROGRAM

The *"Cultura Viva - Pontos de Cultura"* (Living Culture - Points of Culture) Program was established in Brazil in July 2004 as a broad action of cultural policy that, supported by participatory and decentralizing assumptions, invigorated the ideas and ideals that previously operated more locally. The initial proposal of the Living Culture Program was to support artistic and cultural initiatives of civil society in Brazilian peripheral neighborhoods. Through partnerships with institutions that had already been carrying out different cultural actions "in deep Brazil," the Ministry of Culture legitimized them as Points of Culture.[7] By 2010, more than 3,000 Points of Culture had agreements with the Ministry of Culture and state and municipal governments. According to official data, 8 million Brazilians had been directly and indirectly included in the program until 2009 (Brasil, 2009). The Living

Culture Program, which has become a technology for public cultural policy, has become a model replicated in several countries worldwide. A movement began in 2012 for the creation of the Latin American Network of Community Living Culture,[8] which involves universities, governments, and civil society institutions that work to recognize and foster community popular culture. The cultural policy proposal of the Living Culture Program became a reference for some countries in Europe and Africa, which studied its model for further implementation. Pope Francis has been meeting with the creators of the Brazilian program with the aim of producing a worldwide proposal for the Living Culture Program.

Based on the aforementioned observations and narratives, the Brazilian protagonism regarding the policies of citizenship and cultural diversity is affirmed. These policies are guided by international organizations with participation from different actors in the field of culture in the construction of public cultural policy through various instruments, which were fundamental for the articulation of these policies and for the mobilization and participation of civil society and other entities in its construction. The Brazilian experience in the process of cultural democratization fostered in this period (2003–2011) continued, albeit less intensely, until mid-2016, with the culmination of a political and institutional crisis (Pinto, 2017).

As discussed at the beginning of this chapter, cultural citizenship is under construction, and for it to advance, we must still strive so that legislation based on universal rights is effectively ensured at all levels of aesthetic and artistic languages and for all cultural groups and identities. The Living Culture legislation has been enacted, which transformed the program into public policy. However, with the inauguration of the current federal administration (2018–2022), Brazil is undergoing a process of weakening with respect to the guarantee of human rights in the country. The Ministry of Culture was extinguished by decree on the first day of the current federal administration, as well as other ministries and secretariats that cared for the rights of *quilombolas*, Indians, immigrants, and the LGBTQ+ population, among others. Thus, it is necessary to fight so that the policies achieved are not abandoned under the current administration, with the implementation of the National System of Culture (SNC), and, fundamentally, for the continuity of democratic participation in the construction of the public cultural policy.

---

[7]Points of Culture are institutions that develop initiatives for cultural actions, mostly promoted by civil society, working in the "opaque zones." The Living Culture Program was conceived as an organic network of cultural creation and management mediated by the Points of Culture—its main action. A Point of Culture "can be installed in a small house, a shed, a large cultural center, a school, or a museum" (Brasil, 2004).

[8]The First Latin American Congress of Community Living Culture was held in La Paz, Bolivia, in 2013.

POLICIES OF CITIZENSHIP AND CULTURAL DIVERSITY: AN OCCUPATIONAL THERAPY THEME

As has been discussed previously, there is a new national cultural policy agenda that deserves attention: identity, diversity, culture, and territory. It represents more than evolving artistic and aesthetic trends. In this process of monitoring and assisting with the implementation of Brazil's innovative cultural policies, there are many occupational therapists currently conducting actions in cultural policies within the scope of citizenship and cultural diversity.

In the state of Sao Paulo, there are occupational therapists carrying out activities at the Points of Culture, including managing them, as well as in the states of Rio Grande do Sul and Rio de Janeiro. In Rio de Janeiro, the Department of Occupational Therapy of the Federal University of Rio de Janeiro offers the Cultural Accessibility Specialization Course, which involves occupational therapy lecturers and undergraduate students in its work. In the agenda geared toward human occupation, identity, culture, and territory, occupational therapists are working with urban identities, collectives, LGBTQ+ youth networks, indigenous communities, *quilombolas*, and foreign immigrants in cities of the states of Sao Paulo, Espírito Santo, and Rio de Janeiro. There are also occupational therapy experiences in the field of mental health, art, and madness; these are historical concerns of occupational therapy that, when approached from the perspective of art education and the aesthetic development of languages, are linked with the cultural field.

Based on the foregoing, the theme "for occupational therapy in the management and actions of cultural policies" was created, which is addressed in works developed at the postdoctoral level in the Post-Graduate Program in Occupational Therapy of the Federal University of Sao Carlos (PPGTO/UFSCar). One of our objectives was to verify the possibility of establishing an area of academic study and practice for occupational therapists in cultural policies and actions. Combining university research and practical actions based on research action, four meetings entitled "Conversation Circles: Occupational Therapy and Culture" were held during the second half of 2014 in the southeastern region of Brazil. These were realized in partnership with occupational therapy departments of public universities in the states of Sao Paulo, Rio de Janeiro, Minas Gerais, and Espírito Santo, with the participation and collaboration of lecturers, professionals, and undergraduate students. From these conversation circles, it was possible to disseminate, map, and discuss propositions and interfaces of occupational therapy practices that dialogue with actions and policies of cultural diversity. It was also possible to gather data for sources of ongoing research, which proposes to present the design of curricula content for professional education in the field of culture to enhance the contribution of occupational therapists to actions of citizenship and cultural diversity.

Initially, based on the reflections and experiences of the invited lecturers, it was observed that the area of social occupational therapy (Barros et al., 2005) was responsible for the construction of practices similar to the activities that are currently identified in cultural policies as cultural actions in favor of citizenship and cultural diversity. Part of the practices presented—which were identified as actions in the health field guided by the discourse of interconnection, multi- or interdisciplinarity, and/or interinstitutionality, and which develop mapping, cultural planning, and democratization of culture through the promotion of aesthetic experience—could be identified as an occupational therapy approach based on the work of professionals as social articulators (Barros et al., 2005; Lopes & Malfitano, 2017). By developing activities that enhance the articulation and promotion of inventive and collective identities through different cultural actions in the life territories of individuals, social occupational therapy practice approaches the different actions of culture actors that guide citizenship and cultural diversity in their actions, favoring the principles of autonomy and protagonism and horizontal participation in the construction of common well-being and community life. These are the guiding principles of Brazil's largest cultural policy, the *Cultura Viva* Program.

It is not by chance that there are many occupational therapists currently developing practices and partnerships at the Points of Culture. The Points of Culture "school" was formed by the projects of the social movements that, organized in civil society institutions between 1980 and 1990, were initiated through the struggle for rights and democracy, different sociocultural projects of informal education, providing accessibility, mediation, and the promotion of aesthetic-artistic cultural production in Brazilian peripheries. With the purpose of breaking with cultural apartheid, civil society has taken on the responsibilities of the state in response to its absence, expressed in the neoliberal logic of the minimal state. Cultural actions were developed in different formats aiming to foster the democratization of knowledge and its production and to act against all forms of distribution and production of material and symbolic (cultural) goods up to that time (Dorneles, 2001, 2011).

Thus, it is worth highlighting that, currently, social occupational therapy is the "school" of occupational therapy that acts on the agendas of cultural policy. Belatedly recognized by the category as a specific field of practice by resolution no. 383, issued by the Brazilian Occupational Therapy Regulatory Council, social occupational therapy, which participated in the country's redemocratization processes through different intersectoral approaches, broke with tradition and expanded the profession beyond the health–disease binomial (Barros et al., 2005). Historical authenticity and the social and political context have been the structuring axes of social occupational therapy practice, and it is this perspective that has been potentiating the approach of this area of practice to the cultural field with its current paradigms. As previously discussed, the institutionalization processes of democratization and cultural citizenship in the Brazilian cultural policy agenda are recent; therefore, it is possible to understand why these experiences have not been previously identified as activities of occupational therapy in the field of culture. Similarly to other social actors, emancipatory occupational therapy actions in favor of citizenship and human rights, through esthetic-artistic-cultural activities, as well as those that foster the strengthening and dissemination of identities and mediate cultural boundaries, involve cultural practices and actions currently identified as a profile required for practice in the context of the effectiveness of cultural policies. Undoubtedly, this debate does not end here. If the mapping and education of cultural actors remain a challenge for cultural policies, it becomes necessary to expand the discussion on the participation and articulation of occupational therapy in the processes of democratization and inclusion in the agenda of cultural policies. Based on what participants in the meetings and conversations about occupational therapy and culture presented, it is important to incorporate the creation and institutionalization of disciplines addressing theoretical and practical contents involving the interface between social occupational therapy and culture into the education and profile of occupational therapists who will work with the previously mentioned populations of cultural diversity, as well as with the cultural actions and policies that mobilize and favor the promotion and institutionalization of cultural citizenship.

There is a need to discuss how to operationalize (also from a financial perspective) occupational therapy practice in cultural services, programs, and projects in a configuration that is not limited to the frameworks of clinical life. The border between social occupational therapy practice and occupational therapy acting from the perspective of cultural policy brings a new debate for the area. In the current political situation of Brazil, it is still necessary to consider how occupational therapists, engaged in the struggle for human and social rights, will face the dismantling of the emancipatory public policies achieved so far, in the scope of both their professional practice and vocational education.

REFERENCES

Alvares, S., Dagnino, E., & Escobar, A. (Eds.). (2000). *Cultura e Política nos Movimentos Sociais Latino- Americanos* [Culture, economics, and politics in Latin American social movements theory and research]. Humanitas. Ed. UFMG. Universidade Federal de Minas Gerais – UFMG. Belo Horizonte, Brasil.

Barbalho, A. (2005). Política Cultural [Cultural policy]. In L. Rubim (Ed.), *Organização e Produção Cultural – Edição Sala de Aula* [Cultural organization and production – Classroom edition]. EDUFBA. Universidade Federal da Bahia. Salvador, Brasil.

Barros, D. D., Ghirardi, M. I. G., & Lopes, R. E. (2005). Social occupational therapy: A socio-historical perspective. In F. Kronenberg, S. S. Algado, & N. Pollard (Eds.), *Occupational therapy without borders: Learning from the spirit of survivors* (pp. 140–151). London: Elsevier Science – Churchill Livingstone.

Bourdieu, P. (2000). *O Poder Simbólico* [Symbolic power]. Rio de Janeiro: Bertrand Brasil.

Brasil. (2009). *Avaliação Do Programa Cultura, Educação E Cidadania - Cultura Viva. Brasil em desenvolvimento: Estado, planejamento e políticas públicas* [Brazil under development: State, planning, and public policies]. Instituto de Pesquisa Econômica Aplicada. Brasília, DF: IPEA. (Brasil: o Estado de uma Nação [Brazil: The state of a nation].)

Brasil. (2010). A Cultura em três dimensões: as políticas do Ministério da Cultura de 2003 a 2010 [Culture in three dimensions: The policies of the Ministry of Culture from 2003 to 2010]. Ministério da Cultura. Brasília, DF. Brasil.

Calabre, L. (2008). Políticas culturais no governo militar: o Conselho Federal de Cultura [Cultural policies in military government: The Federal Council of Culture]. In *Identidades, Itaguaí*. Anais eletrônicos XIII Encontro de História Anpuh-Rio. Available at: http://encontro2008.rj.anpuh.org/resources/content/anais/1212692933_ARQUIVO_Anpuh2008.pdf. Retired on August 2020.

Canclini G. N. (2006). Estudos sobre Cultura: uma alternativa latino-americana aos cultural studies [Studies on culture: A Latin American alternative to cultural studies] [Interview]. *Revista FAMECOS, 13*(30), 7–15.

Chauí, M. (1987). *Conformismo e resistência: aspectos da cultura popular no Brasil* [Conformism and resistance: Aspects of popular culture in Brazil]. São Paulo: Ed. Brasiliense São Paulo.

Coelho, T. (1997). *Dicionário crítico de política cultural* [Critical dictionary of cultural policy]. São Paulo: Iluminuras.

Cunha, N. (2003). *Dicionário SESC: a linguagem da cultura* [The SESC dictionary: The language of culture]. São Paulo: Perspectiva.

Cunha Filho, F. H. (2010). Cidadania Cultural: um conceito em construção [Cultural citizenship: A concept under construction]. In L. Calabre (Ed.), *Cultural policies: Dialogues and trends* (pp. 177–201). Rio de Janeiro: Edições Casa de Rui Barbosa.

Cuche, D. (2006). *A noção de cultura nas ciências sociais* [The notion of culture in social sciences]. Bauru: EDUSC.

De Certeau, M. (1997). *Culture in the plural*. Minneapolis: University of Minnesota.

Dorneles, P. (2001). *Arte e Cidadania – Diálogos na experiência do Projeto de Descentralização da Cultura da Administração Popular em Porto Alegre* [Art and citizenship – Dialogues in the experience of the Culture Decentralization Project of the Popular Administration in Porto Alegre]. (Master's thesis in Geography). Universidade Federal de Santa Catarina (UFSC), PPGE.

Dorneles, P. (2011). *Identidades Inventivas: territorialidades na Rede Cultura Viva na Região Sul* [Inventive identities: Territorialities in the network of the "Culture Viva" Program in the south region of Brazil] (Dissertation in Geography). Porto Alegre: Universidade Federal do Rio Grande do Sul.

Fernandes, N. M. (2011). A cultura como direito: reflexões acerca da cidadania cultural [Culture as a right: Reflections on cultural citizenship]. *Semina: Ciências Sociais e Humanas, Londrina, 32*(2), 171–182.

Freire, P. (2012). *Pedagogy of the oppressed* (30th anniversary ed.) (3rd ed.). New York, NY: Bloomsbury Academic.

Freire, P. (1979). *Ação cultural para a liberdade e outros escritos* [Cultural action for freedom] (4th ed.). Rio de Janeiro: Paz e Terra.

Gohn, M. G. (2008). O *protagonismo da sociedade civil: movimentos sociais, ONGs e redes solidárias* [The protagonism of civil society: Social movements, NGOs and solidarity networks] (2nd ed.). São Paulo: Cortez.

Gruman, M. (2010). Unesco e as Políticas Culturais no Brasil [UNESCO and cultural policies in Brazil]. *Políticas Culturais em Revista, 2*(1), 174–186.

Lopes, R. E., & Malfitano, A. P. S. (2017). Social occupational therapy, citizenship, rights and policies: Connecting the voices of collectives and individuals. In D. Sakellariou & N. Pollard (Eds.), *Occupational therapies without borders: Integrating justice with practice* (pp. 245–256). Edinburgh: Elsevier.

Miller, T. (2011). Cidadania cultural [Cultural citizenship]. *Matrizes, 4*(2), 57–74.

Niec, H. (1996). Cultural rights: at the end of the world decade for cultural development. Preparatory paper for the power of culture. The intergovernmental Conference on Cultural Policies for Development, Stockholm (30 March – 2 April).

Oliveira, L. L. (2010). Cidadania e cultura: do povo à sociedade civil [Citizenship and culture: From the people to civil society]. In L. Calabre (Ed.), *Políticas Culturais: diálogos e tendências* [Cultural policies: Dialogues and trends]. Rio de Janeiro: Edições Casa de Rui Barbosa.

Pinto, C. R. J. (2017). A trajetória discursiva das manifestações de rua no Brasil (2013-2015). [The discursive trajectory of street demonstrations in Brazil (2013-2015)]. *Lua Nova, 100*, 119–153. doi:10.1590/ 0102-119153/100

Prysthon, A. (2000). Estudos culturais brasileiros nos anos 90 [Brazilian cultural studies in the 1990s]. V Congresso Internacional da Brazilian Studies Association (BRASA), Recife- Pernambuco.

Rosaldo, R. (1997). Cultural citizenship, inequality, and multiculturalism. (pp.27-38). In: Flores, W.V. & Benmayor, R., *Latino cultural citizenship: claiming identity, space, and politics*. Boston: Beacon Press. 27–38.

Rubim, A. (2012). Panorama das políticas culturais no mundo [Overview of cultural policies in the world]. In A. A. C. Rubim & R. Rocha (Eds.), *Políticas Culturais* [Cultural policies] (pp. 13–27). EDUFBA.

Sreiner, H., & Alston, P. (1996). *International human rights in context: Law, politics, morals* Oxford: Clarendon Press.

Yúdice, G. (2006). *A Convivência da Cultura: usos da cultura na era global* [The expediency of culture: Uses of culture in the global era] (Marie-Anne Kremer, Trans.). Belo Horizonte: Editora UFRG.

10

Traditional Peoples and Communities: Traditional Occupation as a Theme of Social Occupational Therapy

*Samira Lima da Costa, Maria Daniela Corrêa de Macedo,
and Sandra Benites*

> *"We grow into the world, as the world grows in us."*
> *(Ingold, 2012, p. 28)*

INTRODUCTION

The concept of tradition has been influenced by various theoretical viewpoints. It is understood that "tradition" evokes associations with permanence and conservation, of antiquity and immutability. In this vein, Benjamin (1999) signals the emergence of a concept of traditional culture that, for the media, is an "exotic adornment." From a critical perspective, Magnani (1997) points out that a preoccupation of scholars of traditional practices, the so-called folklorists, has been to "discover" and "preserve" ancient cultural practices. The author criticizes the opinion held by folklorists that every transformation is a mere representation of the original, pure form, so that any change entails the death of tradition. Following the same train of thought, Ingold and Kurttila (2000, p. 180) refute the concept of traditional knowledge that implies "the idea of biological and/or cultural heritage [being] 'passed' along from one generation to another." The authors point to the misconception of a traditional knowledge concept based on the idea of heritage through which it can be verified that certain groups are no longer traditional. More relevant than seeking to verify the supposed losses of authenticity, however, would be to analyze customs and values as they are presented today. Tradition refers to culture, and it is more similar to a process than to a static condition confined to a specific space and time. Social transformations are inherent in continuous development. Thus, it could be stated that defining tradition as something that remains unchanged over time would be to simultaneously conceptualize it and terminate it.

In this chapter, we will consider tradition from the perspective of collective signification, constructed in space and time and legitimized within the context of a group. Thus, we understand that in tradition, there is always something that changes and something that remains—and indeed, that which changes *maintains* that which remains—within a signification code for a particular group.

In this context—understanding occupation as the various everyday activities carried out by people individually and collectively—this chapter proposes to discuss tradition by means of a reading of traditional occupation as an object of interest in social occupational therapy. Traditional occupation is herein presented as an important element in the organization of the lives of social collectives known as traditional peoples and communities (TPCs), in their relationships with each other, work, and nature.

SOCIETY-NATURE RELATIONSHIP

Our discussion is informed by theoretical frameworks that present multiple views on the society–nature relationship given by contextual conditions that have been transformed politically and historically. The existence of conceptual conflicts reflects the battlefield of issues associated with the relationship between human beings and natural resources. In Brazil, these conflicts have culminated in legislation that ensures, on the one hand, the conservation of certain areas called environmental protection areas (EPAs) and, on the other hand, the participation and involvement—to varying degrees—of the populations of those areas in their use and management. However, the central objective is the same: economic growth and the defense of private rights.

Throughout the 20th century, Brazil's cities grew rapidly in a disorderly process, replacing relationships of coexistence with the expanded exploitation of natural resources and crowding people in proximity to profitable activities and the promises of urban life. At the same time, the country experienced the gradual growth of its environmentalist movement, with strong North American influences, which emphasized the experience of national parks as places to protect *nature* from *people*. These urban growth and environmental protection movements have often taken antagonistic paths, separating society from nature in a polarized and naturalized way (Costa, 2008). Western contemporary society is still based on disjunction between society and nature. According to Vaz (1999) and Loureiro and Costa (2003),

> this separation constitutes the paradox that would be the driving force of capitalism: people no longer know themselves or their environment and, therefore, must dominate these strange fields and keep them under their own control and exploitation. Capitalist logic rules the society-nature relationship from the perspective of environmental exploitation, repeating the relationship of exploitation of the bodies. We live in a production system in which social relations are mainly based on the concentration of wealth obtained through private appropriation of the work of others and natural heritage and, consequently, of power through the socioeconomic inequality established. . . . To this end, there is predatory and inconsequential appropriation of nature and the human body.
>
> (Loureiro & Costa, 2003, pp. 184–185)

From this perspective, one can understand the growth of cities and of the capitalist economic model as processes in which, gradually and systematically, social collectives have distanced themselves and reified their relationships with society, with their own bodies and those of others, and with natural resources. This movement assists in understanding society's growing alienation from nature, both from its own nature and from that corresponding to its immediate environment. "We become others in relation to ourselves, objects before the mirror. . . . Hence the idea that we *have* a body, and that we can possess and dispose of the bodies of other human beings" (Vaz, 1999, p. 91, emphasis added).

On the possible approximations between society and nature, Diegues (1998) identifies a preservationist relationship, which implies avoiding human contact with EPAs "for the good of humanity," and a conservationist relationship, which governs the relationship between human beings and

natural environments, assuming that contact is inevitable. Within the environmentalist movement, both views share the common objective of seeking to understand the separations and possible (re)approximations between society and nature. Loureiro (2004) goes further and proposes a third view, emancipatory or socioenvironmental, which is based on the logic that society culturally redefines the way of existing in nature by societal dynamics in the history of nature and that this relationship is essentially dialectic.

Another perspective, proposed by Descola (2000), questions how different societies/peoples express understanding about the relationship between culture and nature, considering that different concepts about the environment come from an anthropocentric framework, enabling "borders to be marked, identities to be assigned, and cultural mediations to be prepared" from the outside (Descola, 2000, p. 162).

In this process of attempting to understand and regulate society–nature relationships, the environmental movement faces certain people who may be regarded as either allies or opponents, depending on which view of the society–nature relationship is being advocated. They are people who do not experience this disjunction or, at least, do not experience it in a completely modern way (see Figure 10.1). These social collectives are currently known as TPCs. Indigenous peoples, such as Guarani, teach that the relationship with nature does not fit into the "human being–nature" classifications. Interaction with the land is not a matter of private use nor of the exploitation of nature by humans. People, trees, rivers, *Nhanderu* (a Guarani god), and the whole spirituality compose this territory, this *tekoa* (native village):

> For us, Guarani, this tekoa is yvyporã *(happiness)* that allows us to have a tekoporãrã *(good life),* live well. If we have no access to yvyporã *(good land),* we will lose our mbyaarandurã *(wisdom).*
>
> (Benites, 2015, p. 22)

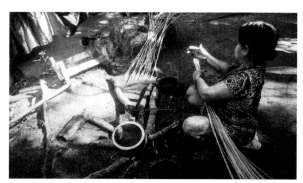

Fig. 10.1 *Mbya Jaka:* Guarani baskets. (Author: Jaxuca Rete, Mbya Guarani (Maria Helena). *Ara Howy* native village. Maricá, Rio de Janeiro, Brazil, 2017.)

For a long time, these groups have existed on the fringes of discussions around urban growth and environmental protection and have had a different relationship with their own bodies and those of others and with the land and natural resources. They are perhaps less alienated than wage laborers, concentrating the core of their society on the notion that people are tied to nature/spirituality in these relationships.

CONTEMPORARY PRODUCTION OF TRADITIONAL PEOPLES: THE *NEW* TRADITIONS

In Brazil, social construction of the category "traditional peoples" has been responding to demands associated with both national and international contexts. Therefore, a historical and critical understanding of the evolution and limitations of this term is needed.

Due to strong, widespread international movements for environmental protection spurred by alarmist studies about the end of humanity on Earth (Brundtland, 1987), Brazil has steadily and solidly expanded the creation of environmental conservation units (CUs), many of which were established in their present locations because of the impossibility of humans living within their borders. This project to preserve some environmental areas is ultimately an offshoot of continuous urban growth and investment in economic development, where protecting certain environmental areas serves to "alleviate" environmental responsibility.

As one of the axes of resistance to this preservationist, environmentalist movement that understands the society-nature relationship as the need to protect the latter from the influence of the former, Brazil has experienced, in recent decades, discussions on the expansion of the concept of peoples who live a self-sustaining extractive relationship with the natural environment. One of the discourses present in this resistance movement is one that affirms the "sustainable" relationship between TPCs and the environment, considering these peoples as part of the local ecosystem and maintainers of ecological equilibrium. In contrast, some authors have insisted on understanding tradition and TPCs as sociohistorical products, transformed by and transformers of the world. Ingold and Kurttila (2000, p. 25) propose that traditional knowledge be "seen as inseparable from actual practices of inhabiting the land," that is, "a view of traditional knowledge as that generated in local practices."

As early as 1949, Sérgio Buarque de Holanda emphasized the strength and power that communities have when they accept or reject other cultures:

For the historical analysis of the influences that can transform the ways of life of a society, it is necessary not to lose sight of the presence, within the social body

of factors, that assists with accepting or rejecting the instruction of habits, conducts, techniques, and institutions strange to its culture heritage. Far from representing inanimate and alluvial clusters, without defense against external suggestions or impositions, societies, including and especially among natural peoples, usually present selective forces that act for the benefit of their organic unity, preserving them as much as possible of everything that can transform this unity, or modifying the new acquisitions to the point they are integrated into the traditional structure.

(Holanda, 1949, emphasis added)

This field of theoretical and political debates and conflicts contributed to a process of problematizing and broadening the concept of TPCs in Brazil, culminating in the approval of the National Policy for the Sustainable Development of Traditional Peoples and Communities (PNPCT) in 2007. The content of this policy expands the concept of TPCs (until then limited to indigenous peoples and *quilombolas*), which initiated discussions timidly and slowly in the colonial period. The text of the PNPCT extends this concept to the communities that live a daily traditional and sustainable relationship with the land and natural resources (Brasil, 2007), like the artisanal fishing we can see in Figure 10.2, from Regencia Augusta beach, Espirito Santo, Brasil, 2012 (author: Laura Pereira Monteiro). Thus, since the approval of this policy, different groups, which have in common *an artisanal and sustainable extractive relationship with the natural environment*, are now considered to fall into this population category, namely, *caiçaras*, rubber tappers, indigenous Brazilians, shellfish gatherers, peasants, river dwellers, and so forth. This policy, far from being a satisfactory end point, is a strategic move in the ongoing power disputes around the

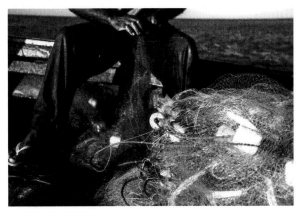

Fig. 10.2 Artisanal fishing. Regência Augusta Beach, Espírito Santo, Brazil, 2012. (Author: Luara Pereira Monteiro.)

issue of traditional peoples, complementing the expanding environmental protection policies and land exploitation policies that aim to stimulate unbridled economic development with no responsibility to future generations.

TPCs have become the focus of discussions and contradictions that now depend on the need to remove them from their habitats in the name of environmental protection or economic interest, emphasizing the importance of ensuring their rights. It was for that reason that discussions about *to be* or *not to be* a traditional person became of interest to these peoples and their advocates. In Brazil, TPCs have emerged as a category with the objective of defending their rights to remain in their original land. However, this concept is still subject to the influencing logic of sustainable development, which in some situations functions as a differentiator of these communities compared with contemporary urban society and values their existence, while at other times, it serves as a tool for maintaining the unchanged relationship with nature. This concept presents us with its own limitation because it is governed by the need to regulate relationships between human beings and CUs.

It is not a matter of putting the concept of TPC aside, therefore, but of understanding it in its limitations and pushing its boundaries, seeking to problematize, contextualize, and broaden discussions on the theme. "It is the recognition of the irrefutable value of a local life style maintained, assured, and verified in the practices and processes experienced by those who share it, including in the dialogue with broader society" (Prado, 2012, pp. 187–188).

The fact that TPCs exist politically and are recognized as a population category contributes to a series of struggles and conflicts of various orders. Nevertheless, it must be understood that in the daily life of the different peoples that are TPCs, there is not an individual homogenous identity or one social collective. The TPCs are multiple social collectives politically identified as one.

A certain "sense of community" can be identified within each of these TPC groups. The identity of a social collective is organized so that it can recognize itself. Far from representing a harmonious relationship, a collective identity is the result of disputes, conflicts, guerrillas, convergences, alliances, and divergences that do not de-characterize the community but, on the contrary, ensure its survival through its transformation potential. The TPCs constitute a *sense of community* in their lifestyle characterized by their traditional occupations.

TRADITIONAL OCCUPATION AND SOCIOENVIRONMENTAL CONFLICTS

Duarte (1999) researched groups of *caiçaras* (traditional fishermen) and found that the definition of a common work model, their commonality with what they extract from the natural environment, and the sense of subsistence in this occupation organize the individuals in a group. The author identified three plans for the practice of these traditional fishermen: "'association of interests' and the idea of a 'collective' of fishermen; 'non-differentiation' and the idea of a 'community' of fishermen; and 'stability' and the idea of a 'tradition' common to the fishermen" (Duarte, 1999, p. 36). Among these artisanal fishermen, there is a need to differentiate their *relationship with the sea* from the fragmented labor that characterizes both urban workers' activities and industrial fishing, which are centered on labor exploitation and on the accumulation of capital. In the case of the fishermen investigated by Duarte (1999), their definition as artisanal fishermen was based on the sum of their relationships as a *community of caiçaras*, their *relationship with the natural resources*, and their cohesion in a model of *campaigning* regarding work. But their *differentiation* from large fishing vessels merited their inclusion in the "traditional" category. Paraphrasing Bauman (2003), the internal organization erects borders and is recognized as traditional in the face of differences and conflicts with others.

In agreement with Costa (2012), traditional occupation will be herein identified in two different and complementary directions:

On the one hand, traditional occupation is understood as a significant practice and producer of patrimony (material and immaterial), characterized by labor as a mediator between human beings and nature; on the other hand, traditional occupation is understood as appropriation and collective use of land and natural resources, against the logic of occupation of territories for private use, hegemonic in the capitalist construction of social relations.

(Costa, 2012, p. 44)

Just as Duarte (1999) presents the characteristics of the relationship with the natural environment and of extraction for subsistence as important features of a traditional community of fishermen, the following is identified by Cândido (2001) in his research conducted with *caipiras* (peasants):

The traditional caipira *society has developed techniques that enable stabilization of the relationships between the group and the environment . . . through satisfactory knowledge about natural resources, systematic exploration, and establishment of a vital minimum diet – all related to a closed social life based on subsistence economy.*

(Cândido, 2001, p. 46)

This is the model of occupation of bodies and natural resources—and thus also of occupation of time and collective space—in which the capitalist logic is not a central issue, which we call traditional occupation. Similarly, when discussing the Guarani lifestyle (*Nhandereko*), Sandra Benites (2015) recognizes in her own people characteristics specific to their tradition, which define contact with nature as an inseparable part of the constitution of *being Guarani*:

> We, Guarani, learn by listening, observing, practicing, accompanying the elders, be they kyringue *(children), young adults, or our parents, grandparents, and uncles. The child has to listen, feel, observe, and this is done in practice, through experiencing, since childhood. They practice gradually, according to their age. This is how we learn, how we know. . . . Mbya arandu (Guarani knowledge), therefore, is transmitted in several places and at specific times. . . . This is how we learn to hunt, fish, make handcrafts, etc. . . . Our way of transmitting knowledge and teaching is something special for us. . . . For us Guarani, it is important to have in our* tekoa *(native village),* yxyry i *(running water),* yakāporā *(good, clean water), have our woods with a variety of trees, medicinal plants, and animals.*
>
> (Benites, 2015, pp. 22–27)

In this excerpt, it is possible to identify the inseparability of the Guarani people from their natural environment, which is characterized not only as a resource but also as a wise adviser and a necessary condition for the continuity of life, tradition, and knowledge. Detachment from or impaired maintenance of their activities associated with the natural environment can have consequences that some people identify as "illness." In this case, illness would be a consequence of a lack of the elements that compose traditional occupations in an indigenous community. The strength, spirituality, and wisdom of these peoples are associated with water, trees, plants, and nature (see Figure 10.3). Therefore, if there is any impact in the surroundings of the village—as in the case of villages that have no more forest or river—this will also influence the identity of those peoples. This is a serious problem that often occurs with indigenous peoples in Brazil today. The Guarani people call it *nhemyrō*: disenchantment, loss of life perspective. When the Guarani people lose reference to rites and identity, they recognize it as an illness. Thus, illness is not necessarily what they feel in their bodies but the effect of that impact on their psychological, cultural, and spiritual conditions as well. Indigenous wisdom and identity are constructed from the presence of the elders who, in contact with the ancestors and the sacred, guide the relationship with the natural elements in the daily activities of building houses, hunting, searching for plants in the woods to prepare medicine, and

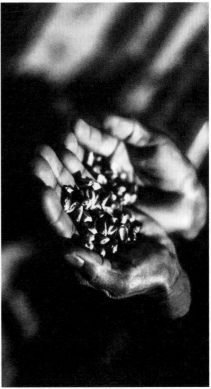

Fig. 10.3 *Auaxi Ete:* "True (sacred) corn," Guarani. (Author: Pará Mirim (Marcia da Silva). *Ara Howy* native village. Maricá, Rio de Janeiro, Brazil, 2017.)

so forth. The way they conduct their activities in a relationship with the elements of nature and with ancestral wisdom organizes the identity of the village. These are their traditional occupations that, in many cases, are characterized as ritual activities.

In 2007, the Brazilian government approved the PNPCT, aiming to determine the rights of TPCs to land occupation and extractive labor in a direct relationship with natural elements. This policy establishes the perspective of occupation as a determinant of tradition, both as a daily practice of constructing the world through the production of collective cultural heritage and as a practice of the use of land and natural resources.

It is worth recalling that the PNPCT and its concepts on occupation and tradition were supported by a historical series of documents that preceded and enabled it. As early as 1989, the International Labor Organization recognized the intimate relationship between the occupation of land and the traditional activities of these peoples, stating in Convention 169 that "measures should be taken to safeguard the right of the peoples interested in using the land . . . to which they have habitually had access to develop traditional and subsistence activities" (Organisation Internacionale Du Travail [OIT], 1989). In another article, the same convention states that "artisanal activities . . . and traditional and subsistence activities of the peoples concerned, such as hunting, fishing, trapping, and extraction, should be recognized as important factors for the maintenance of their culture and for their self-sufficiency and economic development" (OIT, 1989). This convention was belatedly regulated in Brazil by decree 5051/2004 (Brasil, 2004).

Nevertheless, depending on which interests participate in the games of power that occur in the relationships between traditional peoples and their territories, the meanings of the legislation are contradictory, sometimes showing a trend to cultural protection of the traditional peoples and other times favoring environmental protection of CUs. In many cases, neither of these trends is observed, and there is a movement toward a major goal: to secure economic development and the right to private property. Currently, processes that no longer polarize the protection of nature versus the protection of traditional culture are identified, but in many cases, these two protection perspectives are approached as a means of targeting another common enemy: unrestrained economic development.

In the discussions on this theme that occurred during the period of redemocratization in Brazil (reintegration of democratic institutions annulled by the military regime between 1964 and 1985 during the dictatorship), social participation in the form of public consultation was included in the processes of the approval and monitoring of the execution of large projects. However, in the 1990s, there was a progressive deconstruction/deceleration of many of the advancements made. The privatization and outsourcing processes experienced throughout the country during that decade also negatively influenced the recently initiated project of negotiation and social participation in issues related to social and environmental conflicts. Both the study of impacts and the social participation on these projects changed as a result of the new profile of national political management in the 1990s, which was based on neoliberal logic. Soares (2001) called these changes "neoliberal adjustments and social maladjustments." During the 2000s and until the mid-2010s, the social agenda was resumed, but the theme of economic growth remained in the spotlight. It was also at this historical moment that policies such as the PNPCT were approved—less as conquest, more as demarcation of a fighting arena. Discussions on TPCs have gradually taken up space in the governmental agendas of culture as an aspect of the defense of the right to cultural diversity or multiculturalism.

SOCIAL RIGHTS, TRADITION, AND THE PITFALLS OF MULTICULTURALISM

In the mid-20th century, the conception of equality as a category of the quality of relations between peoples and communities was replaced by the notion of equity. This change was due to the impossibility of achieving, in practice, the initial expectations of international organizations relating to the idea of "Equality among the Peoples" for the countries of the South (D'Ávila Neto, 1998; Costa, 2012).

> *The Economic Commission for Latin America and the Caribbean (CEPAL), faced with the failure of the policies for a better distribution of income adopted in Latin America, proposed "productive transformation with equity," where it intended to replace "equality" with "equity," whose concept is to be "equality with diversity."*
>
> (D'Ávila Neto, 1998, p. 2)

The proposal of equality with diversity gave rise to discussions on multiculturalism, which became a criticized concept and, at the same time, the theoretical support for protecting the positions of minority cultures, including TPCs. With respect to this new concept, Bauman comments:

> *Summoning up of "multiculturalism" as part of the enlightened classes, this contemporary incarnation of modern intellectuals, means:* Sorry, but we cannot rescue you from the confusion you got into. Yes, there is confusion about values, the sense of being human, the right ways of life in common; but it is up to you to find your own way and bear the consequences if you do not like the results.
>
> (Bauman, 2003, p. 112, emphasis in the original)

According to Bauman (2003), contemporary society would have created the concept of multiculturalism as a resource for affirming equality with diversity without compromising the elites and their hegemony. The adoption of the notion of multiculturalism in the 1990s occurred in parallel with state reforms in the context of globalization; with this, it resumes contradictions because "these reforms entailed, on the one hand, adjustment policies and retraction of social rights and, on the other hand, market relaxation and opening to transnational policies" (Yrigoyen Fajardo, 2009, p. 26).

We understand that, although some authors (such as Gonçalves & Silva, 1998) point to multiculturalism as a movement of opposition to cultural "centrisms," there is always the risk of being naive when considering differences by not questioning the problems inherent in the concept.

> *Multiculturalism defends cultural diversity, but without shaking the individualist basis of modern rationality,*

the same that produced the Western hegemonic culture. Thus, this current is insufficient to encompass the plural realities of Latin America and the Caribbean, where indigenous, Afro-descendant, European, Asian and mestizo cultures have long lived in permanent inter-ethnic and/or inter-racial conflict.

(Bragato, Barretto, & Silveira Filho, 2017, p. 35)

A pitfall then emerges: if TPCs as minority cultures can use the concept of tradition to assert themselves as a social category pervaded with rights, then "this notion can also be used for the maintenance of precarious living conditions, understood (not necessarily by the population in question) as 'local characteristics'" (Costa, 2012, p. 50).

There are many pitfalls, but the mistake seems to be repeated. For TPCs, appropriation of land by large enterprises, regulation of a "harmonic relationship" by the CUs, and determination of immutability as a record of tradition have in common the fact that they are external propositions that barely or do not at all include the effective participation of members of the diverse traditional Brazilian communities in their different and complex compositions. The possibility of effective social participation of TPCs in the definition of laws and rights occurs mainly through mechanisms of social control and community organization. This model of collective organization for the identification and defense of what it considers essential to its tradition is a modern construction forged on the notion of citizenship, which is not a traditional but rather a relatively recent notion in the history of humanity. Ancestral learning is excluded by this way of thinking. To participate in mechanisms defined by concepts such as "democracy," "citizenship," "sociofamilial nucleation," "human rights," and the like, many TPCs sometimes undergo violent processes of adjustment to legal models, social organizations, and imposed hegemonic epistemology. In this process, a violent exercise of continuous *coloniality of knowledge* is observed, which, according to Walsh (2008, p. 137), is "the positioning of Eurocentrism as the only perspective of knowledge, which governs the existence and viability of other epistemic rationalities and knowledge other than that of white European or Europeanized men."

Social participation, in this case, can constitute a tool that serves to defend the cultural characteristics, needs, and aspirations of TPCs, even if they organize outside the logic of citizenship.

SOCIAL OCCUPATIONAL THERAPY AND TRADITIONAL PEOPLES AND COMMUNITIES

In occupational therapy, discussion of the concept of occupation has not yet led to a consensus. This problem has been attributed in many cases to translations and internationalization of the profession: "as several authors point out, the term *occupation* has dubious meanings in English, and it cannot always be translated adequately into other linguistic contexts" (Magalhães, 2013, p. 256, emphasis in the original).

In many different ways, however, a commonality can be stated for the relevance of occupation—in its significant aspects—for the constitution of the individuals and their relationships with the world. In this way, based on the suggestion of Magalhães (2013), the concept of occupation proposed by the International Society of Occupational Science is used herein: "the various everyday activities of the individuals, in families and with communities, to occupy time and bring meaning and purpose to life. Occupations include things people need to, want to, and are expected to do" (International Society for Occupational Science, 2007, p. 1).

In a movement of appropriation of the socio-historical-political meanings that occupation can have for individuals and social collectives, and addressing not only the individuals and social collectives but also—and in some cases, mainly—their social rights, occupational therapists are inserting themselves and increasingly accompanying and contributing to social transformation movements in Latin America. In this process, from the 1970s onward and more strongly in the past two decades, Brazil has witnessed the growth and consolidation of occupational therapy with an essentially sociopolitical and cultural dimension. This is social occupational therapy, based on political sciences, sociology, and anthropology, presenting itself as a *project of applied social science*.

In agreement with Barros (2004, p. 92), we understand that "the processes of action in social occupational therapy become social spaces of cultural and relational negotiation, of production or facilitation of the person's participation in collective life, in the construction of life projects, and in the sense of belonging." Social occupational therapy consists of the relationship between individuals and social collectives and the world from the "complexity of social exchanges and of socio-historical contexts, investing in the participatory construction of projects that foster the guarantee of rights" (Costa, 2012, p. 44).

The perspective is that social occupational therapists assume the position of mediators of conflicts and agents of negotiations in cultural and socioenvironmental conflicts and in the guarantee of production, access, maintenance, and transformation of the relationships between the individuals and social collectives and their occupations, as an inalienable social right. The notion of conflict is inherent in collective life and "involves interaction between individuals, groups, social collectives, and classes. This interaction raises divergences, antagonisms, and contradictions of interests and perception" (Barros, 2004, p. 92). The occupational therapist is a guest, someone from the outside, a supporter, and a mediator who seeks to encourage understanding and defending the right to traditional occupations in accordance with what each traditional community indicates as their need.

The contexts of TPCs stand out as a focus of interest for social occupational therapy. The concept of traditional occupation was proposed in the context of occupational therapy by Wilcock (2006) when the author described indigenous peoples whose poor health could be associated with the loss or deprivation of "traditional occupations."

In this chapter, what defines traditional occupation is the relationships of a human being (1) with others, as a production of collective identity; (2) with work, as a significant practice (and not an alienating one); and (3) with nature, as a resource of collective significance (and not of private exploitation). These three elements (the relationships with others, work, and nature) imply a significant occupation in which the bodies are involved with what they produce (material and immaterial patrimony) in totality and with what they dialogue (land and natural resources) in their condition of alterity. Herein, society and nature compose games of power that resignify the capitalist senses of this relationship, sometimes escaping from them, sometimes negotiating with or marginalizing them. This does not mean that the relationships of TPC with labor, the bodies, and the natural resources are more or less violent than those established by capitalist society but only that they are different and defined by other worldviews.

The implications that exist between tradition and occupational therapy have raised the interest of some authors such as Zeldenryk and Yalmambirra (2006) and Smith (2011), who have investigated deprivation of access to significant occupations through which some groups experience forced processes of migration or separation from their communities. These authors share a designation of *traditional culture* as the social constructions from which these groups are separated by distancing themselves from their historical-geographical origins.

In Brazil, the *terreiro* people (populations mostly of Afro-Brazilian origin that are linked to religious communities of African matrices by kinship or initiatory ties) have been enabling the health, life, and culture of Afro-Brazilians through the continuous affirmation of their traditional occupations—planting, care, and spiritual practices—since the beginning of the slave trade from Africa. Similarly, the Guarani have continually cared for the health and continuity of the life and culture of their people through participation in their traditional occupations,

sustained by the direct relationship between individual, nature, and spirituality.

It is in the opy *(house of prayer) that sad and ill children recover* vy'a *(happiness). Also, if the children are too excited or whining, we do a ritual in the* opy *so that they calm down or stop crying so much. In fact, they are invited to participate in the* tekoa *(native village), according to their capacity. . . . They always work with older people, who are responsible for transmitting knowledge. The elders teach them how to do things, and the young people begin to practice these skills. It is by working that they listen to the stories of the lives of the elders, they hear advice on various subjects: marriage, family, learning how to treat women, drinking, what to do when having children.*

(Benites, 2015, p. 23)

Zeldenryk and Yalmambirra (2006, p. 43) investigated the history of indigenous children in Australia who were compulsorily removed from their native cultures and the consequences of this act, and they identified problems similar to those that the Guarani people call *Nhemyrõ* (disenchantment). These authors present three main aspects of these processes: deprivation of a culturally significant social environment—how indigenous children were denied access to their families and consequently prevented from learning their cultures and their associated roles and occupations; spiritual deprivation of one's land and story—how children were prevented from engaging in occupations relating to the stories of their people, their land, and their role within society; and deprivation of initiation processes—how children were denied their rightful place in initiation processes, ceremonies, and occupations, leading to the preclusion of the establishment of culturally significant roles within their community. These authors understand that the detachment of these children from their traditional cultures has led to deprivations of various orders, including those related to occupation.

Considering the bases of social occupational therapy, we include the perspective of traditional occupation as a right and a foundation for the construction of identity, culture, and alterity to understand the work of social occupational therapists with TPCs. As Costa (2012) noted, "we understand that the practice of social occupational therapy with TPC assumes that occupation, understood as a social right, is one that collectively means and produces social meaning" (p. 44).

This social meaning of traditional occupation has local characteristics and is different among different peoples because it is produced within the traditional communities in which it is constituted as a collective element. Traditional

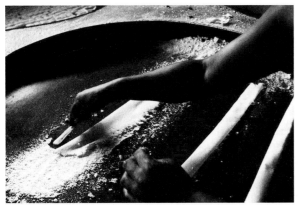

Fig. 10.4 *Beiju* at the "flourhouse." São Mateus, Quilombo Sapê do Norte, Espírito Santo, Brazil, 2016. (Author: Luara Pereira Monteiro.)

occupation is organized and transformed based on local knowledge as well, produced out of the relationship of the communities with the environment and with the products of this relationship (see Figure 10.4). "Knowledge is local because it is inherent in the activity of inhabiting the land, which in fact creates the locality. . . . People belong to the localities and environs in which they have grown up, just as much as the latter belong to them" (Ingold & Kurttila, 2000, p. 195).

The daily activities and occupation of the land produce the transformations in the territory and, at the same time, constitute this territory as a place of belonging. "By creating localities, the activities also make people belong to those localities" (Prado, 2012, p. 187). In the relationship between people and community and the space in transformation, traditional occupation—through the use of land and the production of material and immaterial patrimony—gains a collective meaning.

Social occupational therapists, in relation to TPCs, transit between the individual and the social collective, the singular and the generic, and occupation and territoriality. When approaching and establishing relationships of knowledge exchanges with TPCs, social occupational therapists need to suspend a certain limiting rationality imposed by the Eurocentric system, which relies on binary games (such as health vs. disease, individual vs. collective), to relate and intuit the presence of other elements that are not based on these binary games, such as spirituality, communitarianism, territoriality, and ancestry. It is then up to the social occupational therapist to understand TPCs as a political category when this formulation contributes to the advancement of their rights and to the understanding of the individuals involved in the situations presented, of the social collectives they identify with, and of the historical practices and contexts to which they belong.

FINAL CONSIDERATIONS

The perspectives of social occupational therapy have challenged us to consider the equation of social inequalities, the use of conflict mediation, the facilitation of emancipation processes, the guarantee of access to social rights, the possibility of transformations, and the sociocultural and ethnic valuation of rearrangements of the lives of TPC. This presents a challenge for social occupational therapists to learn from many of these peoples about more balanced ways of life with regard to relationships with others, the natural environment, and the spiritual dimension.

The situations that many of these traditional peoples cope with daily must be revealed to understand the ways in which they cope. This is necessary to observe the devastating effects of unequal socioenvironmental conflict, ranging from total loss of the land and natural environment with which an entire community or several communities maintained ancestral relationships to the production and naturalization of situations of misery. This inequality and the production of misery must be tackled, denounced, and overcome through intersectoral, international, and network efforts. It is necessary to identify potentialities, which each group understands as its own matters, in the relationship with nature and other social groups, valuing what they recognize as tradition.

Social occupational therapists, as they approach the issues of TPCs, generally imply the guarantee of social rights, public policies to achieve these rights, and their inclusion in participatory processes. Occupational therapists are involved in relationships both between people in community life and between them and the natural environment, in the processes of land transformation, of constitution of the community's place of belonging, and of production of material and immaterial patrimony through their actions. It is therefore important to understand and act in this complexity in ways that promote dialogue of the macro- and micro-spheres of life and the political existence of TPCs.

Overcoming situations of conflict and inequality with creativity will involve both public policies and the production of unique tools and strategies that are important socio-occupational resources in these processes.

REFERENCES

Barros, D. D. (2004). Terapia ocupacional social: o caminho se faz ao caminhar [Notes for a social occupational therapy: The way is done by the way we go]. *Revista de Terapia Ocupacional da Universidade de São Paulo, 15*(3), 90–97.

Bauman, Z. (2003). *Comunidade: a busca por segurança no mundo atual* [Community: Seeking safety in an insecure world]. Rio de Janeiro: Jorge Zahar Editora.

Benites, S. (2015). *Nhe'ẽ, rekoporãrã: nhemboeaoexakarẽ Fundamento da pessoa Guarani, nosso bem-estar futuro (educação tradicional): o olhar distorcido da escola* [Basis of the Guarani person, our future well-being (traditional education): The distorted look of the school]. Trabalho de Conclusão de Curso. Licenciatura Intercultural Indígena do Sul da Mata Atlântica da Universidade Federal de Santa Catarina (UFSC) Centro de Filosofia e Ciências Humanas (CFH), Departamento de História (DH). Florianópolis, Santa Catarina.

Benjamin, R. (1999). Culturas regionais: permanências e mudanças em tempo de globalização [Regional cultures: Permanences and changes in times of globalization]. In C. R. S. Bolaño (Ed.), *Globalização e regionalização das comunicações* [Globalization and regionalization of communications] (pp. 129–136). São Paulo: EDUC; Universidade Federal de Sergipe.

Bragato, F. F., Barretto, V. P., & Silveira Filho, A. S. (2017). A interculturalidade como possibilidade para a construção de uma visão de direitos humanos a partir das realidades plurais da América Latina [Interculturality as a possibility for the formation of a human rights view from the plural realities of Latin America]. *Revista da Faculdade de Direito UFPR*, *62*(1), 33–59.

Brasil. Organização Internacional do Trabalho. (2004). *Convenção n. 169 sobre povos indígenas e tribais e Resolução referente à ação da OIT*. Brasília: OIT.

Brundtland, G. H. (Ed.). (1987). *Nosso futuro comum* [Our common future]. Rio de Janeiro: FGV.

Brasil. (2007). Presidência da República. [Presidency of the Republic]. Decreto nº 6.040, de 7 de fevereiro de 2007. Institui a Política Nacional para o Desenvolvimento Sustentável de Povos e Comunidades Tradicionais [Decree No. 6,040, February 7, 2007, criate the National Policy for the Sustainable Development of Peoples and Communities Traditional]. *Diário Oficial da República Federativa do Brasil, Poder Executivo, Brasília*, DF, Seção 1.

Candido, A. (2001). *Os parceiros do Rio Bonito* [Partners of Bonito River] (9th ed.). São Paulo: 34/Duas Cidades.

Costa, S. L. (2008). *Os sentidos da comunidade: produção intergeracional de memória coletiva na Ilha das Caieiras* [The senses of the community: Intergenerational production of collective memory in the Island of Caieiras], *Vitória-ES*. Tese de Doutorado. PPPG Psicossociologia de Comunidades e Ecologia Social. Rio de Janeiro, Brazil. EICOS/IP/UFRJ, Rio de Janeiro, Brazil.

Costa, S. L. (2012). Terapia Ocupacional Social: dilemas e possibilidades da atuação junto a Povos e Comunidades Tradicionais [Social occupational therapy: Matters and action possibilities with traditional peoples and communities]. *Cadernos de Terapia Ocupacional da UFSCar, São Carlos, Brasil*, *20*(1), 43–54.

D'Ávila Neto, M. I. (1998). Os "novos" pobres e o contrato social: receitas de desenvolvimento, igualdade e solidariedade ou da solidariedade, seus mitos, laços e utopias [The "new" poor and the social contract: Development, equality and solidarity or solidarity recipes, their myths, ties and utopias]. *Arquivos Brasileiros de Psicologia*, *50*(4), 7–13.

Descola, P. (2000). Ecologia e Cosmologia [Ecology and cosmology]. In A. C. S. Diegues (Ed.), *Etnoconservação: Novos Rumos para a Conservação da Natureza* [Ethnoconservation: New directions for the conservation of nature] (pp. 149–163) São Paulo: HUCITEC-NUPAUB-USP.

Diegues, A. C. S. (1998). *O mito moderno da natureza intocada* [The modern myth of untouched nature]. São Paulo: HUCITEC.

Duarte, L. F. D. (1999). *As redes do suor: a reprodução social dos trabalhadores da pesca em Jurujuba* [Sweat nets: The social reproduction of fishing workers in Jurujuba]. Niterói, Brasil: EdUFF.

Gonçalves, L. A. O., & Silva, P. B. G. (1998). *O jogo das diferenças: o multiculturalismo e seus contextos* [Game of differences: Multiculturalism and its contexts]. Belo Horizonte: Autêntica.

Holanda, S. B. (1949). Índios e mamelucos na expansão paulista [Indians and Mamelukes in the expansion of São Paulo]. *Anais do Museu Paulista*, *13*, 176–290.

Ingold, T. (2012). Caminhando com dragões: em direção ao lado selvagem. [Walking with dragons: Towards the wild side]. In C. A. Steil & I. C. M. Carvalho (Eds.), *Cultura, percepção e ambiente: diálogos com Tim Ingold* [Culture, perception and environment: Dialogues with Tim Ingold] (Chapter 1, pp. 15–30). São Paulo: Terceiro Nome.

Ingold, T., & Kurtilla, T. (2000). Perceiving the environment in Finnish Lapland. *Body and Society*, *6*(3–4), 183–196.

International Society for Occupational Science. (2007). *The way forward plan for ISOS*. Canada. Retrieved March 25, 2013 from http://www.isoccsci.org

Loureiro, C. F. B. (2004). Educação ambiental transformadora [Transformative environmental education]. In P. P. Layrargues (Ed.), *Identidades da educação ambiental brasileira* [Identities of the Brazilian environmental education] (Chapter 5, pp. 65–84). Brasília: MMA.

Loureiro, C. F. B., & Costa, S. L. (2003). Educação Ambiental, Corpo e Sociedade: Tecendo Relações [Environmental education, body and society: Weaving relationships]. *Educação em Revista*, *38*(1), 173–192.

Magalhães, L. (2013). Ocupação e atividade: tendências e tensões conceituais na literatura anglófona da terapia ocupacional e da ciência ocupacional [Occupation and activity: Trends and conceptual tensions in the Anglophone literature of occupational therapy and occupational science]. *Cadernos de Terapia Ocupacional da UFSCar*, *21*(2), 255–263.

Magnani, J. G. C. (1997). *Festa no pedaço: cultura popular e lazer na cidade* [Party on the block: Popular culture and leisure in the city]. São Paulo: HUCITEC, UNESP.

Organisation Internationale Du Travail OIT - Indigenous and Tribal Peoples Convention (OIT C169). (1989). *Convention concerning indigenous and tribal peoples in independent countries. Geneva, 76th ILC session (27 Jun 1989)*. Art. 15.

Prado, R. M. (2012). Viagem pelo conceito de populações tradicionais, com aspas [Travel through the concept of traditional populations, with quotes]. In C. A. Steil & I. C. M. Carvalho (Eds.), *Cultura, percepção e ambiente: diálogos com Tim Ingold*

[Culture, perception and environment: Dialogues with Tim Ingold] (Chapter 10, pp. 173–190). São Paulo: Terceiro Nome.

Smith, Y. J. (2011). The Thai-Burma border - Issues of forced migration and the opportunity to provide OT Services. Research paper. Annual Research Conference of the Society for the Study of Occupation: USA. Retrieved January 11, 2015, from http://commons.pacificu.edu/sso_conf/2011/11abstracts/9/

Soares, L. T. R. (2001). *Ajuste neoliberal e desajuste social na América Latina* [Neoliberal adjustment and social maladjustment in Latin America]. Petrópolis, Brasil: Vozes.

Vaz, A. F. (1999). Treinar o corpo, dominar a natureza [To train the body, to subdue nature: Notes for a sports analysis from corporal training]. *Cadernos CEDES*, *48*(1), 89–108.

Walsh, C. (2008). Interculturalidad, plurinacionalidad y decolonialidad: lãs insurgencias político-epistémicas de refundar el Estado. *Tabula Rasa*, *9*(1), 131–152.

Wilcock, A. A. (2006). *An occupational perspective of health* (2nd ed.). Thorofare, NJ: Slack.

Yrigoyen Fajardo, R. (2009). Aos 20 anos do Convênio 169 da OIT: Balanço e desafios da implementação dos direitos dos Povos Indígenas na América Latina [Indigenous peoples in Latin America]. In R. Verdum (Ed.), *Povos Indígenas: Constituições e reformas Políticas na América Latina* [Indigenous peoples: Constitutions and political reforms in Latin America] (pp. 9–62). Brasília: Instituto de Estudos Socioeconômicos.

Zeldenryk, L., & Yalmambirra. (2006). Occupational deprivation: A consequence of policy assimilation. *Australian Occupational Therapy Journal*, *53*(1), 43–46.

11

School and Youth: Contributions of Social Occupational Therapy

Roseli Esquerdo Lopes, Carla Regina Silva, and Patrícia Leme de Oliveira Borba

INTRODUCTION

Occupational therapy includes multiple fields of practice, each related to different fields of knowledge. In Brazil, interventions by occupational therapists in the context of the social welfare system were initially developed in the mid-1970s (Barros, Lopes, & Galheigo, 2007; Barros, Ghirardi, & Lopes, 2005), prompting a discussion that remains a characteristic of social occupational therapy (Galheigo, 2003a). In the context of the struggle to end the military dictatorship and re-establish democratic freedoms (Gaspari, 2004), the social-political function of technical professionals, including occupational therapists, was brought into question. This led occupational therapists to take up roles in projects and institutions outside of the health service sector, focused on social care, education, and, mainly, remedial spaces (Barros, Ghirardi, & Lopes, 1999; Barros et al., 2005).

The following decade was marked by discussion of the fundamental concepts in occupational therapy, paying special attention to historical perspectives and philosophical or methodological issues. In parallel, a discourse formed arguing that the term "social" could apply to every practice of the occupational therapist, resulting in the dilution of the theoretical and practical framework that was being constructed by those who advocated for social occupational therapy (Barros, Lopes, & Galheigo, 2007a; Barros et al., 2005).

It is worth emphasizing the difference between "social occupational therapy" and "occupational therapy in the social field or context." Social occupational therapy is unique because it refers to practice in certain fields, dealing with certain problems/issues, and with specific populations with a focus on the social aspect. It is also defined by a theoretical and methodological framework developed for this specific type of practice. These framework

articulated its own cores of knowlegdes and outside the scope of clinical practice, including the so-called extended clinic.

In the late 1980s, the political and economic changes in Brazil brought new frameworks for occupational therapy practice. Importantly, in the early 1990s, incorporation of occupational therapists into social services occurred, especially health care and child and youth care, in the municipalities that adopted the implementation of the national constitution's precepts as a guideline (Lopes, 1999). It can be said that Brazil experienced, more than 40 years later, what most central countries of the world economy experienced in the postwar period: the struggle between social classes (workers and bourgeoisie) for access to public funding. Hence, these constitutional concepts, based on strategies and processes informed by social rights, were submitted to the scrutiny of Brazilian civil society, including its occupational therapists (Lopes, 2012).

Theoretical changes were also observed as interdisciplinary perspectives and the understanding of the diversity of occupational therapy practices that had been established in a particular social and political context were expanded. Simultaneously, there emerged the need to introduce a field of action whose main focus was to meet the demands of individuals and collectives with no access to cultural and social assets (Galheigo, 2003b; Lopes, 2004). Lima (2003) states that the ethical and political commitment of occupational therapists to transform spaces of exclusion has expanded the scope of the disciplinary logic and produced other paths for their practices, which have affirmed the right to difference and found positivity in the most singular and adverse situations.

The perspective of the authors who founded social occupational therapy is based on two main ideas: (1) the inseparability of the individual's needs and collective dimensions, recognizing that individuals are agents that produce and reproduce social practices and structures, and (2) the need to develop contextual and specific approaches for social occupational therapy because clinical and biomedical approaches are neither sufficient nor applicable (Malfitano, Lopes, Silva, & Silva, 2014).

The first decade of the 2000s was marked by the expansion of the fields, groups, and collectives on which professionals and their studies were focused in Brazil, including the social occupational therapy perspective. The assumptions of social occupational therapy (Barros et al., 2005) provided the foundation for the development of new practices that expanded the scope of the practice for occupational therapists in the sectors of social assistance, education, culture, social security, justice, and sociolegal services in Brazil. It should be remembered that the insertion of occupational therapists into the field of education gained momentum in the 1970s, when they were hired mainly by "special education" providers to support children with disabilities (Rocha, 2007).

However, within the framework of the transformations that occurred in the 2000s, other possibilities for occupational therapy's contribution to education have been identified, building on the issues associated with the inclusion of individuals with disabilities in school, showing a broader, more inclusive perspective. This new perspective of work for occupational therapists in the field of education has been developed by the Metuia-Federal University of São Carlos (UFSCar) Project (Barros, Lopes, Galheigo, & Galvani, 2007, Barros, Ghirardi, Lopes, & Galheigo, 2011). It has been considering the demands for autonomy and social participation that permeate the life of the "popular and urban youth" and has been making efforts with public school teachers and managers for the construction of a school environment that is more democratic, plural, and welcoming for the diversity of individuals that it needs to assist.

The public school network is understood as a privileged setting for occupational therapy practice. This is the school environment that, in Brazil as in other parts of the world, entered the 21st century demanding contributions from different professions, including occupational therapists, since one of its basic dilemmas had not yet been solved: how to be a mass school and respond with quality to collective and individual demands, as well as promoting education concerned with human emancipation, that is, with development of the intellectual and cultural autonomy of its students (Nosella, 2016).

In spite of all the historical and contemporary dilemmas associated with public education, it is necessary to affirm and reaffirm that the public school is an indispensable social component and a priority partner, because the vast majority of children and adolescents in Brazil and in the world are included within that system. The following considerations focus on the aim of public school to provide essential elements for the understanding of actions developed within this institutional structure based on social occupational therapy.

DEFENSE OF SCHOOL FOR ALL: THE DEFENSE OF THE PUBLIC SCHOOL

Each country establishes, based on its social-economic policy, the conditions by which its educational policies will be defined. In spite of its importance, the advances observed in the past decades, and the fact that education is considered a fundamental human right, school education is still not a global reality for all. Inclusion, equity, gender equality, and educational quality remain major challenges worldwide.

> *Despite the significant progress observed since 2000, it is estimated that 59 million children at primary school age and 65 million adolescents at first-level secondary school age—of whom girls are a majority—were still out of school in 2013. In addition, many of those attending school were not acquiring basic knowledge and skills. At least 250 million primary school age children—of whom over 50% attended school for at least four years—cannot read, write, or do mathematical operations sufficiently well to meet minimum standards.*
>
> (UNESCO, 2016)

Considering education as a human right and a public asset, it is the responsibility of the state to guarantee universal, equal, free, and compulsory access to quality, inclusive, and equitable learning (UNESCO, 2016). Public policies must therefore promote adequate strategies to achieve these goals, and thus public school is a central and indispensable part of the response to the right of education and an advantageous candidate for meeting and responding to such demands.

It was defined in Brazil's federal constitution and reaffirmed in the Child and Adolescent Statute (Brasil, 1990) that education must be provided by the state and the family with collaboration of society. Moreover, there is an official position in relation to its objectives indicating (1) full development of individuals, (2) their preparation for the exercise of citizenship, and (3) their qualification for work. Given these goals, school has become a public investment space conducting actions aimed at ensuring the rights of children and adolescents to personal, intellectual, and social knowledge and to educating through access, permanence, and learning opportunities.

According to the synthesis originally presented by Lopes, Borba, Trajber, Silva, and Cuel (2011), the Brazilian public school has undergone an intense transformation process. Although Brazil mandates compulsory education for children and youths, difficulties continue to arise in relation to students' permanence, progression, and completion at an appropriate age.

The right to democratic education, which is defined by equity and quality for all, remains a goal (Lopes, Silva, & Malfitano, 2006; Manacorda, 1989).

Ferreira Jr. and Bittar (2006) revealed three major problems in today's educational context: access, permanence, and effective learning. Of these, teachers have a direct influence on the latter two if they have been adequately trained and are reasonably remunerated. Nevertheless, the question of access has been the only one concretely tackled by successive governments, whose efforts have not been sufficient to transform the reality of Brazilian education. According to Gimeno Sacristán and Pérez Gómez (1998), only school can fulfill the function of critical and reflective re-elaboration of the dominant culture, and it should strive toward it, considering the fact that it has lost its hegemonic role in the transmission and distribution of information in contemporaneity.

In the 1990s, changes in the labor market drove demand for education to be expanded, as jobs required increasingly higher qualifications of potential employees. In this context, the National Education Guidelines and Framework Law of 1996 reformulated secondary school with the objective of increasing its availability and improving its quality (Marcílio, 2005). Despite being a fundamental sector in the public policies for youth, secondary school is faced every day with the conflict between its objectives and its real conditions of projecting the vast majority of Brazilian adolescents and youths toward a life of fulfillment, whether in the labor market or in preparation for higher education. A significant proportion of youths are excluded from school in Brazil in a process in which they experience the violence of this discrimination produced in the school context, with lack of access maintenance and education quality. This process of school exclusion is related to the enormous barrier of inequality in the construction of their life projects, barriers mostly imposed by socioeconomic conditions (Lopes & Silva, 2007).

According to Silva (2007), school is part of the search for the meaning of life through which a "self" is formed. However, individuals are subjected to control exercised by the institution, which standardizes, observes, and exposes them and reproduces social judgments and disqualifications. Considering that the role of school is to emancipate individuals, a paradox arises: on one hand, students should be enabled to understand the processes of submission and domination to which they are exposed (to foster emancipation and autonomy), leading them to resist and seek transformations; on the other hand, school does indeed maintain and legitimize social inequalities (Bourdieu & Saint-Martin, 2008).

"The challenge of being a great stage for collective projects" (Debortoli, 2002, p. 44) should be the responsibility of the school, seeking to transform itself to perform its function in the production and dissemination of cultural heritage and in the formation of autonomous individuals, avoiding the reproduction of established differences and coping with inherent diversity. According to the reflections of Paulo Freire (1996) on cultural heritage and by Bourdieu and Passeron (1977) on cultural capital, cultural heritage is understood as the set of assets, knowledge, beliefs, practices, behaviors, and "habitus" of humanity. School that does not conform as a machine of hierarchization, reproduction, and nurturing of a system of exclusion and injustice can offer the opportunity to break with the logic of domination, becoming a place of expression, subversion, and creation (Freire, 1996). Pedagogy as a cultural and intentional practice must use all its potential to actualize the formation of individuals and citizens in the most varied instances of contemporary life—school, work, family, social groups, and so forth—using two factors inherent to the pedagogical practice: intentionality and difference. School, particularly as a place intended for this practice, should be a space of meeting and valuing differences as referential multiplicity. By embracing differences, school can rethink and deconstruct the classic scourges of its history, such as evasion, grade repetition, and violence, traditionally viewed as "school failures" or as "individual failures" when in fact they are social, intentional, and educational (or pedagogical) failures.

The matter of the exercise of power in school would have to be assumed and made explicit so that it could be transformed. However, it is necessary to be clear about the dimension of this task and its difficulties, directly associated with what Bourdieu (1983a) calls "rites of institution," which means each and every rite that exercises an "effect of consecration," which assigns an individual a specific stigmatized identity (Bourdieu, 1983a). To enter and remain in school, all are subjected to rites that establish them as belonging or not belonging to the school system and to a specific school. It is important to highlight that a rite has an arbitrary character that is often concealed, hidden, under the naturalization of certain artificially promoted "differences." It is culturally reproduced by the hidden knowledges that are in operation in the school environment, shaping practices in school and consequently the identities of children and young people.

Instead of contributing to the emancipation of individuals, school establishes who will and who will not reach the end. One of the functions of the institution is often to permanently discourage the possibility of passage, resulting in transgression, desertion, and dismissal. In the schools frequented by the majority of young Brazilians (public schools), students are subjected to frightening violence (physical or symbolic). In these institutions, school evasion is interpreted as desertion by the students, an act of resignation, given the clear realization that the space is of little concern to them. It is also worth considering that the rites of institutions to which students are subjected have not even fulfilled their role of promoting "feeling a part," because there are always more insurmountable, if not excluding, rites in an inside-out process—that is, expelling those who had been "accepted as a part." In other words, schools, which should make people feel a part of them, do not in reality work on the integration principle; rather, they work based on the discipline principle, expelling those who fail to integrate. There is a cyclic logic that affects everyone—officials, teachers, oppressors, and oppressed—which constitutes a system that has not managed to achieve the social changes that are theoretically characterized as the central demands of education. According to Freire (1979), if pedagogy of autonomy is intended, experiences to motivate decisiveness and responsibility are needed, and they should be based on respect and freedom.

Constructing democracy in the school environment is not an easy task. Real participation could be ensured by availability of information, spaces of speech, basic infrastructure, collectivization of decisions, and the commitment (or "belonging") of each individual in relation to the process (Sorrentino, 2002). Despite the numerous problems and challenges identified in the current Brazilian educational system and the school institution, it is undeniable that formal education occupies a central place in social organization, mainly as one of the only legal means by which deprived populations can reach less unfavorable social positions. Thus, it is up to education as a whole, and to school in particular, to be a space of freedom of expression and creation, a priority place, from its basic infrastructure to the availability to opportunities for reflection and awareness, for the training of individuals to be capable of not only conducting their own lives but also participating, directly or indirectly, in the organization of the society in which they live. Thus, the interventions promoted and undertaken by the social occupational therapy of the Metuia-UFSCar Project aim to strengthen the school institution, with a view to offering approaches to meet its demands, as well as developing its resignification for youths and the expansion of the ways educational action is conceived.

Presenting and Discussing Some "Doings" and "Knowledge"

The work that the Metuia-UFSCar Project has been doing in public schools in the municipality of Sao Carlos, Sao Paulo state, Brazil, since 2005 has addressed these problems and contributed intervention proposals that seek to solve them. This project is composed of undergraduate students, mainly from the area of occupational therapy, but also from education, psychology, and audiovisual courses, as well as by graduate students at different levels, occupational therapists, researchers, and academic staff. In activities integrated with university teaching, research, and extension activities (partnership between university and schools), the project proposes the use of participatory methodologies with a view to resignifying the experience of schooling and being in school, from the creation of conditions for better apprehension of formal contents to the valuing of school as a space of sociability for youth.

Different perspectives on this practice will be presented with the aim of offering possible dimensions of the action of occupational therapists in the public school that seek inclusion and the democratization of education for youths, typically those who are economically deprived and belong to marginalized urban communities.

Workshops of Activities, Dynamics, and Projects: Violence "in" and "from" School

In 2006, workshops were started in five public schools for students in their last year of secondary school (called *Ensino Médio* in Brazil) in different regions of the city. These involved a survey and reflection on violence "in" and "from" school as their structuring axes. The "activity workshops" (Lopes et al., 2011) occurred on a weekly basis, grouped to the curriculum of three classes of each school, during the day and night periods, and on Saturdays in the case of one particular school.

At each school, the workshops considered the context of the school and its students; the link established with the different classes; the interest of adolescents in discussing and engaging in the dynamics; the duration of each workshop (50 minutes); and the pre-established themes that guided the discussions. The following themes were used: Who am I? (dynamics of presentation and understanding about who those adolescents and youngsters were and what they thought about school); violence (familial, urban, physical, verbal, moral, etc.); actors involved in situations of violence; possible causes of violence; the victims and the tormentors (and whether they could be understood as such); and proposals for a better school (Silva, 2007).

Proposals for the "activities" conducted varied as follows:

"Presentation": By means of writing words and/or sentences, students reported on activities they liked to do, as well as everyday and personal characteristics or elements shaping their identities, and included accompanying photos/images.

"Group discussion": Posters were produced with the following questions: What does school mean to you? What do you like most about school? What would you change in the school? How does school contribute to your perspective on the future?

"Production of a collective newspaper": With the theme of violence in the world and at school, the students developed reports, drawings, titles, and headlines for their newspapers.

"Role plays": Scenarios and dramatizations of situations previously experienced by the students regarding school violence were prepared and presented.

"Trial and Justice": The whole class staged the trial of a 16-year-old student who had been arrested with drugs inside the school, experiencing the different roles of the school organization and exposing their various points of view.

"Proposals for a better school": Opinions and suggestions on how to make school a space of participation were expressed and, as a result, a board was produced using mixed techniques of collage, drawings, and writing.

"Mime or drawings": Techniques were used to act out the causes of school violence that the students identified and had already witnessed.

"Documentary": For the elaboration of an audiovisual presentation, testimonies, interviews, simulations of television programs, and discussions were recorded, providing material on the urban and school violence experienced by the students in their daily lives.

"Exhibition": Assessments were carried out on the workshops and the themes were discussed at the end of the meetings. All the material produced by the youngsters was included in a synthesis exhibition held to facilitate appreciation of their work by the whole school community. These activities are described in more detail by Silva (2007).

In these workshops, it was possible to verify the refined strategies of the social inclusion and exclusion processes reproduced by the school, as well as the dynamics of the school agents regarding the processes of violence, their reproductions, and confrontations. Given the widespread nature and extent of violence today, school suffers with internal and external threats present in its daily life and faces the laborious task of reconciling repressive/punitive methods with the construction of democratic practices (Lopes, Silva, Rocha, & Oishi, 2009).

The young students revealed several situations of violence that had occurred in their schools and in their lives. Although most of the participating students did not consider their schools violent, they referred to the occurrence of situations of disrespect, humiliation, and verbal and physical aggression; such episodes of violence have been integrated into everyday school life and have been trivialized.

There is a need to move forward to construct spaces that ensure young people the right to speak and be heard, through direct participation, so that dialogue can be made effective. The "Metuia workshops," as the students called them, progressed in this direction (Figures 11.1 and 11.2).

Audiovisual Workshops and the Social Expression of Poor Youths

Considering the need to simultaneously include new methodological perspectives for working with youth and power and improve educational actions, a project was conducted with the objective of promoting possibilities for learning, relationships, and technical training. It was intended that the unveiling of the audiovisual productions could foster new ways of recognizing and formulating the material students were communicating, as well as supporting different reflections about the students' views of the world and of themselves, through works with self-image and other visual exercises. Audiovisual technology enables different ways of encoding information. However, the ways these instruments are consumed and/or decoded by young people need to be questioned. Audiovisual content as the product of a culture and the disposition of the syntactic elements that form the audiovisual discourse and of those responsible for such disposition must be considered by the individual who apprehends and interprets the information. For these objectives to be achieved, the technical intervention was associated with the creation of bonds with the young people, which allowed new possibilities of experiences, relationships, events, and everyday life, always working under the perspective of juveniles as agents, which understands youths as individuals with rights.

Audiovisual workshops were held in two weekly meetings in a school located on the outskirts of the city over 8 months. The themes of the meetings enabled the apprehension of priority contents in the preparation of an audiovisual product, using a theoretical-practical approach, and culminated in the completion of a short film entitled *Mutirão* (joint effort) (DVD 14) (Silva et al., 2008). The importance of creating an audiovisual product is to provide students with a space not only for technological training but also of collective experience and sociability, with moments appropriate for exploration of identity

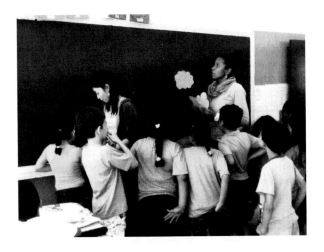

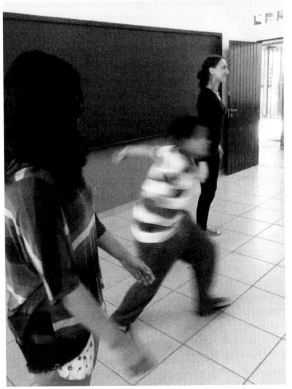

Fig. 11.1 and 11.2 Workshops of activities, dynamics, and projects inside the classroom.

and expression of subjectivities (Silva, Cardinalli, & Lopes, 2015).

It is worth emphasizing the need for interventions that move from an individualized view to a social and collective view to create strategies that foster relationships with the social environment, expanding actions that allow people to perform better in their living environment. These actions must occur not only to meet the needs of these individuals but also to produce subsidies for public policies whose influence is in the direction of promoting the universalization of citizenship rights, in the production of forms of creation and expansion of social support networks for the majority of young Brazilians (Lopes et al., 2008).

Reading and Writing Workshops

The reading and writing workshops were a demand of this school, with which a partnership had already been established in previous projects, because it identified students with literacy deficits and consequent evasion. Amaral, Silva, and Lopes (2008) fully present this experience and their reflections.

The proposal of the school board was to create "literacy classrooms" supported by teachers and pedagogical coordinators, who were replaced with the Metuia-UFSCar Project team after an agreement with the school board and teachers. The proposal was to conduct the reading and writing workshops based on teachers' indications of which students could benefit from them. The theoretical framework was supported by the work of Paulo Freire due to the educational precepts and the importance and recognition in his experience of the literacy of youths and adults. The political motivation that existed in the workshops, which encouraged not only reading and writing but also the students' interpretation of what was being absorbed and produced, was a characteristic of the chosen methodology (Freire, 1979). Working from the perspective of questioning rather than establishing a truth was the differential in these workshops.

The team was composed of two undergraduate students of the Pedagogy and Occupational Therapy courses of UFSCar, under the coordination of an occupational therapist. Teaching and learning with the students was always based on the performed actions, because the team members were not teachers or specialists in the area of reading and writing but professionals who intended to construct valid knowledge with these students and highlight its connection to the school environment.

Seven primary school students (fifth to ninth grades) and 11 students enrolled in the night course of Youth and Adult Education (EJA) participated in the workshops. Workshops were conducted in parallel with the regular classes but at alternate times so as not to compromise the classes of the same discipline. The activities prepared by the team always sought a correlation between the proposed reading and writing dynamics and their links to the everyday life, culture, and context of the students, involving themes that could be significant for them. Thus, frequently over the course of the workshops, motivation to participate was observed, in addition to students' perception about the need to use reading and writing, as well as the presence of self-esteem.

Fanzines and Expression of Youths

Another assertive proposal was the production of fanzines at school across 2 years, with four editions, each with 200 copies (Figure 11.3). The fanzine was named *Espaço Fala Aí* (Speak Out Space) in a voting session with the students. The full report of this experiment and the results of the research involving it can be found in Lopes, Borba, and Monzeli (2013).

Fanzines are recognized as vehicles free of censorship because "their authors disseminate what they want, since they are not concerned about large print runs or profit; therefore, they are free of the ties of the publishing market and the obligation to increase sales" (Magalhães, 1993, p. 10). These publications may be distributed in places that the mainstream press cannot reach, mainly due to geographical isolation (peripheries and favelas), high cost and/or printing characteristics, or even the elitist language of these media, and also because they present content different from that in the mainstream press, which allows cultural identification with other groups that have not been plurally and respectfully absorbed by the mass media. From this perspective, fanzines can become a vehicle of free expression for those who do not have freedom or space in the mainstream mass media. Most of the time, they are productions created by adolescents and youths who want to express themselves but do not have another space to do so (Carnicel, 2007).

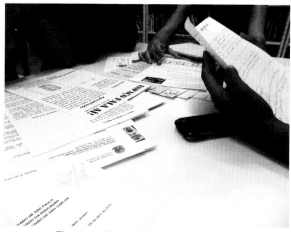

Fig. 11.3 Workshops of fanzine project.

The following processes composed the production of the fanzines: production of materials with the youths, publishing, printing, and distribution, aiming to enhance alternative forms of communication, free expression, and the creative process with the youths. The themes included citizenship and its related rights and duties in the context of the everyday reality of the youths, and issues associated with discussions on gender and the neighborhood where they lived. With this premise, the youngsters were asked to express/construct their opinions and positions based on each one's interest in different forms of expression, but there was also space for free creations, such as movie reviews, poetry, music lyrics, and drawings.

It was observed that the distribution of the fanzines in the school and the neighborhood engendered the personal satisfaction born of producing something, of being an author; this effectively highlights another important characteristic of the fanzine: the visibility of its creators. The youngsters said they liked both the process and the results, referring to personal satisfaction in producing and distributing something of their own, of seeing their creation materialized. This positively reframed the relationship established with the Metuia-UFSCar Project team and with the other youths, influencing the construction of other possibilities of material and other forms of constituting their own projects, arousing interests that had not been imagined, or simply curiosities that did not previously exist.

Among the results, it was verified that the processes involving the fanzine constituted a resource for the promotion of reflections associated with the experiences of these youths, for the expansion of their repertoires and possible individual and collective projects, and for discussion on the exclusion reality faced by many of them. It allowed expression of opinions that questioned institutions such as "family," "school," "police," and "drug trafficking." The possibilities of the circulation of the fanzine and its contents add to this resource, making it paradoxically interesting and "dangerous" from the standpoint of its creators because of the exposure it causes, requiring dialogue and articulation between youth, community, and social communication, fostering social technologies.

Propositions in Sociology Classes

A very productive partnership involving the creation of participative methodologies and the possibility of reflection on themes pertinent to the everyday life of the adolescents was created with the secondary school's sociology teacher. This teacher approached the Metuia-UFSCar Project team complaining that the content of her classes had a very theoretical, abstract character, and that she found it difficult for the students to comprehend it, a problem compounded by the fact that the classes were taught in the night course, in which most students work during the day and thus come to class tired or exhausted.

The proposed activities followed the discipline syllabus and the theme addressed by the teacher, respecting the density of the content, becoming simpler or more complex according to the grade and the participation/involvement of the students. The goal was to introduce the studied theme in a more active and participative way, utilizing activities and improved group dynamics, and enabling discussions and joint reflections, always trying to articulate them. The following two examples employed these dynamics.

In one class, the theme addressed was "men as social beings." The proposal was to leave the classroom and form a circle in the schoolyard in which each member of the team held a sign representing an institution (school, work, friends, family, religion, community). The "social being" stayed in the center, composed of/represented by the students, who held strings in their hands. Holding the strings, they walked to each institution, depending on the questions that were asked (Which place do you like the most? Which one do you think is more important? Where do you spend most of your time? Which one do you feel obligated to be in? Where do you invest your future?). With each question, they affixed their strings to the signs/institutions and, thus, a network (social network) was configured. A large entanglement with different densities was formed, and the greater concentration of strings reflected the "institution" of greater significance for that group. In the different groups with which this activity was conducted, "family" was quite central, as were "work" and "school."

In another class, the theme was "popular participation and political option." A podium, cameras, and microphones were taken to the school, and the class was divided into five groups. In each subgroup, after discussing and preparing proposals related to the theme, the students chose one of the members to represent them. This representative climbed the "podium" and expressed the proposal defined by the group. After that, the best representative was chosen collectively. As it was election time for the president and São Paulo state governor, this activity was directed toward a consideration of these positions.

Interactive Resources for the Break Time

Throughout all the time that it was inserted in school, the Metuia-UFSCar Project was able to participate very creatively in the break time—a very short period (20 minutes), but so productive (Figure 11.4). Twice a week in the evening, the members of the team were in the schoolyard proposing activities, called interactive resources, to inform, clarify, and motivate the young people about the themes of their realities. Two examples of these interactive resources

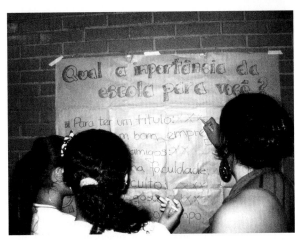

Fig. 11.4 Workshops of activities at break in the school.

are as follows: (1) A dynamic panel with proposals from the political programs of the candidates running for the positions of president, governor, deputy, and senator was shown to the students so that they could compare these proposals with the demands they had presented in the previous weeks (when approached by the team), each corresponding to a theme of social policies; these were discussed, and then proposals for improvements to be made by the governments were summarized on a card. (2) A panel with slang, customs, emblems of cultures, cuisine, and clothing, from various places in Brazil, was created; the students interacted in an attempt to associate these data with countries, Brazilian states, and other cultures.

Many relationships of trust with the youngsters were constituted during the breaks, because the constant presence of the team was more important than time spent. Being available for years in the same space, bringing color, receptiveness, and reflections, allowed the Metuia-UFSCar Project team to become recognized and known by the youngsters, some of whom were still children when the action started in 2005 (Pan, 2019). Boys and girls began to voice the demands of their lives that went beyond the school issues. Because of the inclusion of team members in that neighborhood, such as the project in the community center, it was possible to extrapolate from the institutional limit of the school, seeking to respond, also through other contributions, to the demands of the young people.

CONCLUDING REMARKS

In the context of public school, considering the education of adolescents and youths rather than specifically addressing the inclusion of children with disabilities, social occupational therapy seems strange. It is strange to both school and to occupational therapy itself. Although occupational therapy theoretically addresses its expansion into new fields, it is still recognized as a profession under the category of "health," making it seem resistant to the notion of being practiced in other contexts and areas of public policy. Because of this conflict, many questions have arisen regarding the occupational-therapeutic action and its field of knowledge. At times, occupational therapy has been presented as a field of knowledge that is pre-established rather than something under permanent construction and tension, both internal and external, in the confrontation between fields of power (Bourdieu, 1983b).

Interestingly, this conflict acted as a bonus; since the identity of occupational therapists in public school is not preconceived/preconceptualized, it allowed greater flexibility for how occupational therapy practices could be integrated into the school routine. Nevertheless, venturing into the territory of others calls for more care and respect. In this dialogic relationship, the presupposition of the action of social occupational therapy in its Freirean aspects is fundamental to the creation of action that can occur and that can interfere with the doings of this contradictory institution, the school, defending it so that it can be enjoyed by the youths of popular groups in a democratic, participatory, and inclusive way. Thus, all interventions carried out by the Metuia-UFSCar Project (only some of which could be reported in this chapter) are guided by dialogue with the students and the school staff. It was not always possible to establish this dialogue, especially with the school board, but we persisted and insisted, and after quite a few years, during which familiarity and connections were created, the Metuia-UFSCar Project and occupational therapy have come to be recognized by school boards as a group that collaborates in creating reflection and actions aligned with the needs and demands of popular and contemporary urban youth. Testimonials to this effect can be found in Malfitano et al. (2014).

An important demarcation that has become clearer over time is that with the action of occupational therapists, the repertoire involving the creation of activities, dynamics, and projects is very enriching, both to increase the experience of youths and for the everyday life of institutions. In fact, the resource arising from the "workshops of activities, dynamics, and projects" (Lopes, Malfitano, Silva, & Borba, 2014) allows closer contact with the youths, from which it becomes possible to deepen the reading of individual and collective needs, promote greater contact and coexistence between the participants, and provide experimentation regarding a pleasurable space of sociability and exchanges that can build on the physical space of the workshop and transcend into the wider school context. Another impact of the workshops has been the resignification, on the part of the students, of the importance of understanding the curricular contents of school, since the activities conducted usually foresee the mastery at different levels of "tools" such as reading, writing, mathematical skills, and historical elements, concretizing what is conventionally called work with cross-sectional themes.

However, these resources are useless if they are not connected to the debate and broader struggle for quality education for all. From the perspective of social occupational therapy, there can be no action limited to the interiors of institutions, or to "individual [although] territorial follow-ups" (Lopes et al., 2014). It is necessary to go beyond; there is need for the "articulation of resources in the social field" (Lopes et al., 2014) that includes an array of actions taken from the individual level to groups, collectives, and the levels of politics and management. There is also need for the "dynamization of the service network" (Lopes et al., 2014), articulating the different sectors and levels of intervention and facilitating the effectiveness and guidance of action strategies directed at the urban youths, and this cannot be done without the defense and effectiveness of free, quality public school for all in Brazil and in the world.

REFERENCES

Amaral, D. M., Silva, C. R., & Lopes, R. E. (2008). Sala de leitura e escrita com jovens e adultos em uma escola pública de periferia urbana na cidade de São Carlos (SP) [Reading and writing room with young people and adults in a public school of urban periphery in the city of São Carlos (SP)]. In T. Araújo Filho & M. J. M. Thiollent (Eds.), *Metodologia para projetos de extensão:apresentação e discussão* [Methodology for extension projects: Presentation and discussion] (pp. 336–348). São Carlos: Cubo Multimídia.

Barros, D. D., Ghirardi, M. I. G., & Lopes, R. E. (1999). Terapia ocupacional e sociedade [Occupational therapy and society]. *Revista de Terapia Ocupacional da Universidade de São Paulo, 10*(2–3), 69–74.

Barros, D. D., Ghirardi, M. I. G., & Lopes, R. E. (2005). Social occupational therapy: A socio-historical perspective. In F. Kronenberg, S. S. Algado, & N. Pollard (Eds.), *Occupational therapy without borders: Learning from the spirit of survivors* (pp. 140–151). London: Elsevier Science – Churchill Livingstone.

Barros, D. D., Lopes, R. E., & Galheigo, S. M. (2007). Terapia Ocupacional Social: Concepções e Perspectivas [Social occupational therapy: Conceptions and perspectives]. In A. Cavalcanti & C. Galvão (Eds.), *Terapia Ocupacional - Fundamentação & Prática* [Occupational therapy – Background and practice] (pp. 347–353). Rio de Janeiro: Guanabara Koogan S.A.

Barros, D. D., Lopes, R. E., Galheigo, S. M., & Galvani, D. (2007). El Proyecto Metuia en Brasil: ideas y acciones que nos unen

[Metuia's Project in Brazil: Ideas and actions that make us together] In F. Kronenberg, S. S. Algado, & N. Pollard (Eds.), *Terapia ocupacional sin fronteras: aprendiendo del espíritu de supervivientes* [Occupational therapy without borders: Learning from the spirit of survivors] (Vol. 1, pp. 392–403). Madri: Editorial Médica Panamericana S.A.

Barros, D. D., Ghirardi, M. I. G., Lopes, R. E., & Galheigo, S. M. (2011). Brazilian experiences in social occupational therapy. In F. Kronenberg, N. Pollard, & D. Sakellariou (Eds.), *Occupational therapy without borders: Towards an ecology of occupation-based practices* (Vol. 2, pp. 209–215). Edinburgh: Elsevier.

Bourdieu, P. (1983a). Algumas proprieties dos campos [Some proprieties of the scientific fields]. In P. Bourdieu (Ed.), *Questões de sociologia* [Questions of sociology]. Rio de Janeiro: Editora Marco Zero.

Bourdieu, P. (1983b). O campo científico [The scientific field]. In R. Ortiz (Ed.), *Pierre Bourdieu: sociologia* [Pierre Bourdieu: Sociology]. São Paulo: Ática.

Bourdieu, P., & Saint-Martin, M. (2008). As categorias do juízo professoral [The categories of the professorial judgment]. In P. Bourdieu (Ed.), *Escritos da educação* [Education writings] (10th ed.). Petrópolis: Voze.

Bourdieu, P., & Passeron, J. C. (1977). *Reproduction in education, society and culture*. London: SAGE Publications.

Brasil (1990). Lei Nº 8.069, de 13 de julho de 1990. Dispõe sobre o Estatuto da Criança e do Adolescente e dá outras providências [Law 8.069, from July 13th 1990, establishes the Children and Adolescentes Statute]. Retired on. July 2020, from: http://www.planalto.gov.br/ccivil_03/leis/l8069.htm

Carnicel, A. (2007). Fanzine. In M. Park, R. S. Fernandes, & A. Carnicel (Eds.), *Palavras-chave em educação não formal* [Key words in no formal education] (pp. 157–158). Campinas: Unicamp, CMU; Holambra: Setembro.

Debortoli, J. A. (2002). Adolescência(s): identidade e formação humana [Adolescent(s): Identities and human development]. In A. Carvalho, F. Salles, & M. Guimarães (Eds.), *Adolescência* [Adolescence] (pp. 31–47). Belo Horizonte: UFMG/PROEX.

Freire, P. (1979). *Educação e mudança* [Education and change]. Rio de Janeiro: Paz e Terra.

Freire, P. (1996). *Pedagogia da autonomia: saberes necessários à prática educativa* [Pedagogy of autonomy: Necessary knowledge to educational practice] (30th ed.). São Paulo: Paz e Terra.

Ferreira, J. R. A., & Bittar, M. (2006). *Proletarização e sindicalismo de professores na ditadura militar (1964–1985)* [Proletarianization and unionism of teachers in the military dictatorship (1964–1985)]. São Paulo: Terras do Sonhar/Edições Pulsar.

Galheigo, S. M. (2003a). O social: idas e vindas de um campo de ação em terapia ocupacional [The social: Paths of a field of action in occupational therapy]. In E. Pádua & M. M. Magalhães (Eds.), *Terapia ocupacional, teoria e prática* [Occupational therapy, theory and practice] (pp. 29–48). Campinas: Papirus.

Galheigo, S. M. (2003b). O cotidiano na terapia ocupacional: cultura, subjetividade e contexto histórico e social. [The Daylife by occupational therapy: Culture, subjectivity and

social-historic context]. *Revista de Terapia Ocupacional da Universidade de São Paulo, 14*(3), 104–109. doi:10.11606/issn.2238-6149.v14i3p104-109

Gaspari, E. (2004). *A ditadura encurralada* [The cornered dictatorship]. São Paulo: Companhia das Letras.

Gimeno Sacristán, J., & Pérez Gómez, A. (1998). As funções sociais da escola: da reprodução à reconstrução crítica do conhecimento e da experiência [The social functions of school: From reproduction to the critical reconstruction of knowledge and experience]. In J. Gimeno Sacristán & A. Pérez Gómez (Eds.), *Compreender e transformar o ensino* [Understanding and change the education] (4th ed., pp. 13–25). Porto Alegre: ArtMed.

Lima, E. M. F. A. (2003). Desejando a diferença: considerações acerca das relações entre os terapeutas ocupacionais e as populações tradicionalmente atendidas por estes profissionais [Desiring the difference: Considerations about the relationships between occupational therapists and the populations traditionally cared by these professionals]. *Revista de Terapia Ocupacional da Universidade de São Paulo, 14*(2), 64–71. doi:10.11606/issn.2238-6149.v14i2p64-71

Lopes, R. E. (1999). Cidadania, políticas públicas e terapia ocupacional, no contexto das ações de saúde mental e saúde da pessoa portadora de deficiência, no Município de São Paulo [Citizenship, public policies and occupational therapy, in the context of the actions of mental health and health of the person with disability, in the city of São Paulo]. 539f. 2 v. Tese de Doutorado em Educação. Faculdade de Educação da Universidade Estadual de Campinas, Campinas, SP. Retrieved from http://repositorio.unicamp.br/jspui/handle/REPOSIP/253885

Lopes, R. E. (2004). Terapia ocupacional em São Paulo: um percurso singular e geral [Occupational therapy in São Paulo: A general and unique path]. *Cadernos de Terapia Ocupacional da UFSCar, 12*(2), 75–88.

Lopes, R. E., Silva, C. R., & Malfitano, A. P. S. (2006). Adolescência e juventude de grupos populares urbanos no Brasil e as políticas públicas: apontamentos históricos [Adolescence and youth of urban popular groups in Brazil and public policies: Historical notes]. *Revista HISTEDBR Online, 23*, 114–130.

Lopes, R. E., Silva, C. R., Rocha, B. M., & Oishi, J. (2009) Violência, escola e jovens de grupos populares urbanos: o caso de estudantes de Ensino Médio de São Carlos/SP [Violence, school and youth of urban popular groups: The case of high school students of São Carlos/SP. *Revista HISTEDBR Online, 34*, 73–96. doi:10.20396/rho.v9i34.8639580

Lopes, R. E., Borba, P. L. O., Trajber, N. K. A., Silva, C. R., & Cuel, B. T. (2011). Oficinas de Atividades com Jovens da Escola Pública: Tecnologias Sociais entre Educação e Terapia Ocupacional [Activities workshops with public school youngsters: Social technologies between education and occupational therapy]. *Interface, 15*(36), 277–288. doi:10.1590/S1414-32832011000100021

Lopes, R. E. (2012). *Cidadania, Direitos e Terapia Ocupacional Social* [Citizenship, rights and occupational therapy] (p. 22). Conference that integrated the Erudition Proof of the Public Tender for the Position of Full Professor in the Occupational Therapy Area of the Department of Occupational Therapy of the Center of Biological Sciences and Health of the Federal University of São Carlos. Digitado.

Lopes, R. E., Borba, P. L. O., & Monzeli, G. A. (2013). Expressão livre de jovens por meio do Fanzine: recurso para a terapia ocupacional social [Free expression of young people through Fanzine: Resource for social occupational therapy]. *Saúde e Sociedade, 22*(3), 937–948. doi:10.1590/S0104-12902013000300027

Lopes, R. E., & Silva, C. R. (2007). O campo da educação e demandas para a terapia ocupacional no Brasil [The field of education and demands for occupational therapy in Brazil]. *Revista de Terapia Ocupacional da Universidade de São Paulo, 18*(3), 158–164. doi:10.11606/issn.2238-6149.v18i3p158-164

Lopes, R. E., Adorno, R. C. F., Malfitano, A. P. S., Takeiti, B. A., Silva, C. R., & Borba, P. L. O. (2008). Juventude pobre, violência e cidadania [Poor youth, violence and citizenship]. *Saúde e Sociedade, 17*(3), 63–76. doi:10.1590/S0104-12902008000300008

Lopes, R. E., Malfitano, A. P. S., Silva, C. R., & Borba, P. L.O. (2014). Recursos e tecnologias em Terapia Ocupacional Social: ações com jovens pobres na cidade [Resources and technologies in social occupational therapy: Actions with the poor youth in town]. *Cadernos de Terapia Ocupacional da UFSCar, São Carlos, 22*(3), 591–602. doi:10.4322/cto.2014.081

Magalhães, H. (1993). *O que é fanzine* [What's fanzine]. São Paulo: Brasiliense.

Malfitano, A. P. S., Lopes, R. E., Silva, C. D., & Silva, C. R. (2014). *Ações em terapia ocupacional social com a juventude popular urbana* [Actions in social occupational therapy with urban pour youth]. São Carlos - SP: Laboratório METUIA do Departamento de Terapia Ocupacional e Pró-Reitoria de Extensão da UFSCar (Produção Audiovisual – Vídeo Didático).

Manacorda, M. A. (1989). *História da educação: da antiguidade aos nossos dias* [History of education: From antiquity to our days]. São Paulo: Cortez.

Marcílio, M. L. (2005). *História da escola em São Paulo e no Brasil* [History of school in São Paulo and in Brazil]. São Paulo: Instituto Braudel/Imprensa Oficial.

Nosella, P. (2016). *A escola de Gramsci* [The school of Gramsci]. São Paulo: Cortez Editora.

Pan, L. C. (2020). Social occupational therapy in school: Experiences with a student association. In: Lopes, R. E. & Malfitano, A. P. S. *Social Occupational Therapy:* Theoretical and Practical Designs (pp.189–193). Amsterdam: Elsevier.

Rocha, E. F. (2007). A Terapia Ocupacional e as ações na educação: aprofundando interfaces [Occupational therapy and actions in education: deepening interfaces]. *Revista de Terapia Ocupacional da Universidade de São Paulo, 18*(3), 97–104. doi:10.11606/issn.2238-6149

Silva, C. R. (2007). Políticas públicas, educação, juventude e violência da escola: quais as dinâmicas entre os diversos atores envolvidos? [Publics policies, education, youth and violence in school: What are the dynamics between the various actors involved?]. 184f. *Dissertação de Mestrado.* Programa de Pós-Graduação em Educação da Universidade Federal de São Carlos, São Carlos, SP. Retrieved from https://repositorio.ufscar.br/bitstream/handle/ufscar/2423/DissCRS.pdf?sequence=1

Silva, C. R., Cardinalli, I., & Lopes, R. E. (2015). A utilização do blog e de recursos midiáticos na ampliação das formas de comunicação e participação social [The use of the blog and media resources in the expansion of forms of communication and social participation]. *Cadernos de Terapia Ocupacional da UFSCar, 23*(1), 131–142. doi:10.4322/0104-4931.ctoAO513

Silva, C. R., Lopes, R. E., Neto, A. A. F., de S., Marques, M., Kuhl, A. T., et al. (2008). *Mutirão* [Joint effort]. São Carlos - SP: Laboratório METUIA do Departamento de Terapia Ocupacional e Pró-Reitoria de Extensão da UFSCar (Produção Audiovisual – Vídeo Didático).

Sorrentino, M. (2002). Desenvolvimento sustentável e participação: algumas reflexões em voz alta [Sustainable development and participation: Some reflections out loud]. In C. F. B. Loureiro, P. P. Layrargues, & R. S. Castro (Eds.), *Educação ambiental: repensando o espaço da cidadania* [Environmental education: Rethinking the citizenship space] (pp. 15–21). São Paulo: Cortez.

UNESCO. (2016). Education 2030: Incheon declaration and framework for action: Towards inclusive and equitable quality education and lifelong learning for all. Retrieved January 19, 2018, from https://unesdoc.unesco.org/ark:/48223/pf0000243278

12

Social Occupational Therapy, Offenses, and School: Complex Plots in Fragile Relations

Patrícia Leme de Oliveira Borba, Beatriz Prado Pereira, and Roseli Esquerdo Lopes

INTRODUCTION

In this chapter, we describe aspects of the results of a doctoral dissertation (Borba, 2012) and undergraduate research studies (Lopes, Borba, Pereira, Dariolli, & Rodrigues, 2015) located in the themes of school, youth, and citizenship, with a focus on the relationship between school and offenses, conducted in a middle-sized municipality in the interior of the state of Sao Paulo, Brazil. All the research subprojects addressed the relationship between poor youths and their school trajectory, as reflected in interventions offered by institutions guided by the Child and Adolescent Statute (1990). This statute governs the protection of these individuals after they commit offenses.

In the excerpts selected for this text, we will present the history of three youths whose offenses unfolded from undisciplined acts that occurred within a public school. The three young people were supported by what we have agreed to call *individual territorial follow-ups* (Lopes, Malfitano, Silva, & Borba, 2014). This involved binding processes that occurred during the workshops of activities, projects, and dynamics (Lopes et al., 2014) conducted in social institutions—namely, a youth center and a public school. The actions were conducted by the Metuia Laboratory team of the Occupational Therapy Department at the Federal University of Sao Carlos (UFSCar), which is part of the Metuia Project[1] (Barros, Lopes, Galheigo, & Galvani, 2007). Since 2005, this team has conducted social interventions with youth in a specific neighborhood located on the outskirts of the aforementioned municipality. The team also actively engages in teaching and research activities at different levels (Lopes, Souza, & Borba, 2010).

The individual territorial follow-ups were influenced by specific theoretical and methodological frameworks, namely oral history (Meihy, 1997); ethnographic studies by Whyte (1993), Goffman (1961), Caria (2003), and Feltran (2008); and, especially, social occupational therapy (Barros, Ghirardi, & Lopes, 2005). Together this constituted a unique methodology of doing research based on the intervention relationship. Based on social occupational therapy, the territorial follow-ups are defined as a tool, characterized by a social technology that is guided by attentive listening to the needs of individuals and groups. It seeks to address essential issues in their lives, often determined by social inequality and lack of access to social services and assets (Lopes, Borba, & Cappellaro, 2011). These occupational-therapeutic follow-ups were one of the main methodological resources for this study. It allowed researchers the opportunity to understand the experiences of youth who had committed offenses and had to comply with socioeducational measures under assisted freedom, established by the Brazilian Child and Adolescent Statute. It was also possible to learn about their school and life paths, all of which became apparent during the field experience that was conducted by the Metuia/UFSCar Laboratory team.

In Brazil, when adolescents (12 to 18 years old) commit an offense, the authority may apply the following social-educational measures: I—warning; II—obligation to repair the damage; III—rendering of community services; IV—assisted freedom; V—insertion into a semiopen regime; or VI—confinement in an educational institution (Brasil, 1990). In the histories described in this chapter, we will discuss the social-educational measure of assisted freedom, which prioritizes the maintenance of social interaction. In this measure, a social assistance service is designated to follow up with the adolescent to promote an educational intervention focused on personal assistance through guidance, the maintenance of family and community ties, schooling, and insertion into the labor market and/or enrollment in vocational, formative courses (Morais & Malfitano, 2016).

The individuals' histories reveal their complex and conflicting relationships with the school and the legal assistance systems during particular times in their lives. Accessing, knowing, and eventually writing these histories occurred over a 6-year period of follow-up (2007 to 2012) and entailed many meetings, either mediated or not by activities and dialogue. It required not only a collective effort to integrate activities of university extension and research but also, most importantly, the opening up of these young people to share their lives, dreams, desires, and thoughts with us.

ABOUT THREE LIVES

Juninho, Nicolas, and Willian provide examples of three individual but also common and complementary juvenile trajectories. Over the years, it was possible to observe the transformation processes of their bodies, voices, hair, and gestures. At the end of the follow-ups, we were requested to call one of them by their adopted social name rather than by the official name by which we had previously known him (Lopes, Borba, & Cappellaro, 2011).

The combination of these three trajectories was motivated by processes that involve the mediation of conflicts within the public school and by the fact that these mediations involved the repressive intervention of the judicial network (police and juvenile justice system), which reached its peak with the account of the most tragic situation that their school had experienced until then. These three adolescents were the protagonists of this story, which had repercussions in their lives since they had a violent experience with the police, and this formed the root for their involvement in the juvenile justice system, leading to their compliance with the social-educational measure of assisted freedom. These histories are also combined because they subtly reveal a very specific universe; that is, they are directly associated with issues involving transsexuality and travestility and their repercussions within the school. These stories show how this social device promotes a series of difficulties around these adolescents, as well as how the school and its teachers and board, which are deeply rooted in certain moral values, resist establishing more pertinent and welcoming dialogues about gender and sexuality—a fact of life experienced by its entire student body.

Because of the proximity and personnel of the Metuia/UFSCar Laboratory team, the adolescents felt comfortable with sharing their experiences with the network of sexual exploitation, as well as the ambiguity between the exploitation itself and the presence of their desire to get involved in this network. This experience with the network meant they were able to access financial resources to buy consumer goods, help with the family bills, and especially live their travestility more intensely.

Numerically, there are few adolescent transvestites and transsexual youths in the context of the studied neighborhood; it can be inferred that they are exceptions. However, these histories raise concerns that call for attention to be focused on this issue beyond how it affects only this group. Rather, part of the concerns raised may be generalized to consider how all youths may be affected, especially with respect to how society, broadly, and schools, as a main public device for this age group, are challenged in coping with everything that involves the expression of sexuality. This difficulty is exacerbated when the need to respect travestility or transsexuality is called for. This has been evident in debates that have recently gained traction, such as the use of one's preferred social name or preferred restrooms.

We met these three adolescents at a school located on the city periphery, where they were attending night classes and had been "referred" to our social occupational therapy workshops. These workshops refer to a set of activities, projects, and dynamic activities that enable a powerful range of actions that can be classified, understood, and applied for different purposes, such as for dealing with different techniques and materials; using and producing materials and resources; transiting through different sectors (culture, art, sports, leisure, work, etc.); and preparing sessions that follow pre-established themes and objectives such as daily debates, life perspectives, exchanges and information about the world of labor, educational processes on rights and duties, and educational processes on the network of protection for children and adolescents in the city. It also involves a focus on the needs and possibilities of everyday life and the different senses and meanings the individuals in action can designate or apply according to their personal experiences. In this case, even if the proposals have previous indications or referrals, the interest is in the individual perception that the experience promotes in the participant of the action (Lopes et al., 2014). In the year when these individuals entered the workshops, the intervention focused on providing a space for students who showed relational and/or reading and writing difficulties. Although none of the three youths had difficulties in reading and writing, the central complaint on the part of the teachers was their behavior; they disturbed the whole school structure and they "drew attention" or, in other words, "disturbed" and "generated/caused conflicts."

Through their weekly participation in the workshops and their involvement in the activities carried out by the Metuia/UFSCar Laboratory team in the schoolyard at break time, we became references for these adolescents through the creation of interactive resources aiming to inform, clarify, and motivate the youths about the themes present in their realities (Lopes, Borba, Trajber, Silva, & Cuel, 2011), such as the matters of sexuality and gender. By translating these elements into a proposition of action and constant dialogue, many conversations were constructed, and thus, in different ways, their approaches and contacts with the team were intensified in that space and beyond it. The three youths had a discontinuous school trajectory, with successive failures and evasions that resulted in a significant school grade/age gap. They were and remained very good friends, a friendship that also existed outside of school premises. They were the sort of friends who were always arguing but were each other's confidants and who, in the course of their lives, were sometimes distant and sometimes close to each other, considering that their histories were not of success; in fact, we have witnessed the great resistance that these youths present and how they persevere in life. Let us therefore describe the event that generated the offense and their relationship with the social-educational measures.

Day of the Rebellion

To describe the day of the rebellion, we begin with this excerpt from Peregrino (2005), who focused on the expansion of the Brazilian public school in the state of Rio de Janeiro in her doctoral research:

> This one is like this: a school with no reading room, no laboratory, no cafeteria (except at lunch times, when the students who use this space have "no" classroom), no schoolyard, no sports, no library. School does not expand as a whole. It expands some of its "dimensions." The school of "expanded" access and reduced structure also sees its old "quality" references disappear. Through the data of the Brazilian National System of Evaluation of Basic Education, we have witnessed the gradual decrease in the performance of students in all grades (from elementary to high school), in all areas of knowledge. The "Platypus" produces its "offspring": the "expansion" of school access, without the concomitant expansion of minimum schooling conditions. It "creates," therefore, a school "full" of students, emptied of schooling conditions.
>
> (Peregrino, 2005, p. 359)

Peregrino (2005) evidenced a series of infrastructure problems impacting the late *universalization of basic education* in Brazil, creating a school full of students because of

the guaranteed access but deprived of its essence: production of schooling. The day of the rebellion, in fact, was a crisis announced by this emptying and the lack of infrastructure. The school was on the verge of imploding for some time. The situation, tragic in itself, arose from the growth crisis of a school without structural or organizational conditions. It was a crisis, a surge, a fright that marked the indelible trajectory of these three youths, and it was not mere coincidence that, from that year, they began a cycle of failures and evasions.

Juninho was the one who told us the story of the day of the rebellion in the greatest detail:

> Then I started getting involved with drugs. With friends, I helped in the school rebellion. . . . We broke all the school windows! Because of the school meals, because the women did it badly, they made a sort of oatmeal, they said it was peach cream . . . and it looked like baby poop. And then we started that food fight, remember? We got those fruits and began throwing them. I was going to throw the pigwash. When I saw the principal coming in, I threw it all over her. . . . That day at school was terror! Yeah, and because the cook said, "Why do you come to school, to eat or to study? You starving gang!" Then I got mad! I got mad 'cause she said, "Do you come to school to eat or to study, you starving gang." Then I was the first, I began knocking at all the doors, and I opened them and said: "Let's go, let's gather in the schoolyard," 'cause I was the mess boss! And I shouted, "I want everybody in the yard, let's go to the yard, go to the schoolyard!" I said there was a fight, then when everyone got there, there was no fight. . . . Then I said, "Listen, listen: she called us starving gang and many other names." I lied and made things bigger. . . . Then the food fight caught on, and everybody began throwing food, that peach cream. So disgusting! We started a fire inside a classroom, I passed with a lighter and put fire in those big trash cans. Wow, that day, the school looked like 'Carandiru'! [reference to Carandiru Penitentiary, an adult prison in the city of Sao Paulo where 111 inmates were massacred by the police in 1992; it was deactivated in 2002]. They didn't call the school guard; the police troop came . . . many police vans! Then they took everybody to the schoolyard and ordered us to take off our shirts and they chose a few and took us by van to the juvenile justice system, *but they drove on the highway! They went down "Aracy" [the neighborhood] and took the highway . . . and they threatened us! They didn't beat us, but they threatened us, they said they were going to kill us, were going to take us to the woods, and beat and leave us there. . . . When we arrived at*

the juvenile justice system, *they made everyone kneel facing the wall in a room . . . and the cop was there, looking at us!* I turned to him to ask for a cup of water, he got his billy club and hit me on the back! It was awful!

(Interview with Juninho, emphasis added)

And Willian simply said:

We tore the school down. We demolished it. Oh, I don't remember much. I just remember that they told us to sit down in a room, and if we said or did anything, they would beat us badly!

(Interview with Willian)

This story is in the memory of the school staff, and we had the opportunity to hear versions of it from the perspective of the school principal and the sociology teacher. Both reported the incident with great embarrassment and sadness, taking the blame for having called the police, as they did not anticipate the extent of the police truculence or the level of exposure of the students, children and adolescents. However, they justified that "the situation got out of hand," but they bitterly understood what it means to hand over to the police an out-of-control environment that is a priori educational, not a prison.

This situation evidences the violation of some rights prescribed in the Brazilian legislation, like the Child and Adolescent Statute (CAS). The first refers to Article 178:

Adolescents suspected of committing an offense cannot be taken or transported in a closed police vehicle, in conditions that threaten their dignity, or that put their physical or mental integrity at risk, under imputed liability.

(Brasil, 1990)

It also states:

Article 232: Submitting children or adolescents under one's authority, guard or vigilance to vexation or embarrassment: Penalty: 6-month to 2-year imprisonment.

(Brasil, 1990)

Unfortunately, if we still live in a country where law enforcement and its effectiveness are far from being a reality, the distance becomes much longer when the oppressor belongs to the state apparatus, which should ensure that these situations do not occur; thus, public security institutions escape what is mandated by the ECA. In addition, in Brazil, there is certain social authorization to treat those who are part of the masses—the poor—in a humiliating way.

Some excerpts from Juninho's narrative refer us to a repertoire of prison and rebellions in the rehabilitation units for adolescents. Invariably, people known by these boys pass through these places too; in this case, the three youths have not experienced it, but some of their cousins and friends have. It should also be emphasized that the police treated them in the same way that adolescents in the rehabilitation units are treated. What justifies all this violence and barbarism? This treatment of inmates in rehabilitation units is questionable and inconceivable, and a series of complaint reports on violations of human rights has already been made public (Conselho Federal de Psicologia; Ordem dos Advogados do Brasil [Psychology Federal Association; Brazilian Lawyers Association], 2006); nevertheless, the occurrence of such practices within a school publicly testifies to that school's collapse.

Juninho's narrative ranges from a certain excitement and pleasure, as if he were reliving the scene, to guilt merged with regret. Guilt and regret could be the result of how he perceives the situation today, with the influence of values that he has begun to profess (at the time of the interview, he was assiduously attending the Anointed Church, one of the neo-Pentecostal churches), moralizing the story and blaming himself for having done what he did, considering himself as a potential future father, and wondering what type of attitude he would have had if he were his son.

The situation that broke out in that school was the culmination of a crisis that had existed since 2006, when it became a full-time school despite lacking the minimum structural conditions. This proposal was implemented in 500 primary schools in the public school network in the state of Sao Paulo (Castro & Lopes, 2011). With this proposal, students at the end of primary school (children and adolescents aged 10 to 14) stayed in school daily for a period of 9 hours and attended curricular workshops: specifically, study and research guidance, activities of language, mathematics, the arts, sports and physical activities, and social integration (Castro & Lopes, 2011). The idealization and implementation of the proposal were faster than the conditions for its implementation, which led to inadequate spaces both for students to eat, for instance, and for the development of the so-called curricular workshops. This caused great discontent among the local school board, as well as the students and their families.

The precarious infrastructure of the school and the request for the military police to solve an internal conflict were added to accounts of the day of the rebellion. Calling the police to deal with behavioral matters was already a common practice in that school, and not only there, as has been studied by Cardoso, Gomes, and Santana (2013). This situation was worsened because the presence of a public security force in an educational space transformed an act of indiscipline, although serious, into an offense, as is expressed in the following two excerpts:

I was taken [to the social-educational legal system] because of a fight in the school. I fought with a boy in the schoolyard; at meal time, he came and cut the line in front of me. I told him, "No, you're not going to cut the line," and I pushed him out of the line. He tried to hit me; then I took his head and I slammed it on the table, right there, we were both taken to the juvenile justice system.

(*Interview with Willian*)

Gosh, I was taken before the judge seven times. I fought in school, cursed the teachers when they disrespected me, it was more like that, once the police got me on the corner, but I was never beaten by the teachers, or humiliated, it was more often fights between students like that, it's normal. They used to call the police school guard and they took us to school counseling when these things happened.

(*Interview with Nicolas*)

Reports such as Juninho's on the day of the rebellion reveal the normal practices used by the school board. In addition, it can be noticed that all situations started in a mismanaged conflict in the school space, an act of indiscipline that became, with the endorsement of the school board, an offense under the jurisdiction of the social-educational legal system. It is therefore relevant and necessary to understand the relationship between the school and adolescents who commit "acts of indiscipline," where the school treats them as offenses by requesting the action of the police school guard, the military police, the Guardianship Council, the childhood and youth court, social-educational measures, and so forth. In our experience in public schools, we have empirically realized that this type of request has been increasingly common for situations that, in the near past, were solved by the school staff. An act can be considered as indiscipline or offense, depending on the context in which it occurred, and different referrals should be used for each case. Not every act of indiscipline can be treated as an offense. Unfortunately, offenses are perfectly identifiable in the current legislation on the basis of the Adult Criminal Code. As for acts of indiscipline, they must be regulated according to the norms that govern the school, and the school regulations should play a relevant role in this matter. Schools must have internal regulations that include the rights and duties of students, teachers, the school board, and family members, and these should be known by the students, teachers, parents, and/or legal guardians so that they can be enforced or changed if necessary.

Proof of this is that at the first institutional court that judges juvenile offenses referred by schools, the technicians on call have difficulty finding "codes" that correspond to

the acts of indiscipline that occurred and so end up choosing criminal acts no. 33 or 34, because they are "general" acts. In this case, criminal act no. 33 refers to "suspicious inquiry," whereas no. 34 refers to "others." This occurs because offenses are based on the Adult Criminal Code (Brazil, 1940), and acts of indiscipline have no correspondence with that code; thus, general codes are assigned simply to characterize an offense and justify the existence of a criminal process (Borba, 2012; Borba, Lopes, & Malfitano, 2015). Considering discipline as behaviors governed by a set of rules, Ferreira (2010) defines two strands for the translation of indiscipline into offenses: the first is rebellion against these norms and the second is ignorance of their existence. Therefore, an act of indiscipline is presented as a breach of the norms established by the school and can be translated into disrespect to colleagues, teachers, or the school institution. Depending on the type of behavior, the student may be characterized as committing an act of indiscipline or an offense, each with specific consequences.

In contrast, the several uses and meanings of the word violence, alongside related terms such as indiscipline, allow significant changes of current meanings over the set of school actions. Acts previously classified as habitual products of student transgressions to disciplinary rules, hitherto tolerated by educators as inherent in their development, can now be summarily identified as violent.

(*Sposito, 1998, p. 3*)

Violent behavior and physical aggression can be treated as routine or simple transgressions of school rules. Thus, the practices relative to this issue in the school context are fundamental for the construction of definitions that normalize the conducts, whether violent or undisciplined, on the part of all parties involved: the school board, teachers, students, parents/legal guardians, and school officials (Sposito, 1998). It is also important to consider how some episodes that occur in school should be resolved within the educational system, based on the general regulations of this system and on those established by the school; mediation of the social-educational legal system should only be requested after all school resources have been exhausted; disciplinary cases should be the responsibility of the school (Ferreira, 2010). Finally, regarding the practice of offenses, the case must be investigated by the childhood and youth justice system, without the intention of having the police come into the school, which has invariably caused situations of humiliation and violence. According to Sposito (1998):

School violence has become the object of public action, especially from the standpoint of security and military police strategy, and less as an educational issue. It is not a matter of denying the validity of some of these initiatives, but misplacement in the way the problem is treated in evidence. (p. 13)

Resuming the experience of the three youths, they were taken to the juvenile justice system on the day of the rebellion, which resulted in the handing down of a social-educational measure: assisted freedom. The three adolescents, not coincidentally, failed their school grade in 2007 and 2008 and were compulsorily transferred to the night classes. All of them gave positive assessments of the experience of the assisted freedom:

Then I started to comply with the assisted freedom. . . . We talked, spent most of the weekdays there. There were workshops, we did various types of workshops, I liked it.

(Interview with Juninho)

I would go there, that's all! You would do the project, talk about your life, they stay in the school, participate in your life, it's like a mother somehow. They offer you courses, initiative, help you find a job, give you bus tickets so that you can go, then there's no reason not to go to the assisted freedom.

(Interview with Nicolas)

Ah, assisted freedom was just great, loved it. I used to go there and talked, eat, paint, draw, do handcraft, it was wonderful, I was there for four months. Ah, it was surely great . . . 'cause there was a different teacher each day, then it was nice.

(Interview with Willian)

The existence of a space where people listen to and welcome you, the possibility of circulating around the city, and the expansion of the experience repertoire through the workshops are elements that explain the positive aspect associated with assisted freedom. Unfortunately, the monitoring of the social-educational measure did not result in support for the permanence and progression of the adolescents in school. From the day of the rebellion and its consequences, the three individuals began a cycle of grade repetitions that culminated in their withdrawal from school. This reveals the fragility and contradictions of the so-called monitoring by those responsible for social-educational measure programs.

Studies such as those of Lopes, Sfair, and Bittar (2012); Borba et al. (2015); and Rocha, Bittar, and Lopes (2016) deepen the discussion on the dialogue between assisted freedom and school, which generates discontinuous, fragile, and inefficient monitoring of the school attendance of adolescents who comply with open-environment measures. Thus, these three lives and their dramas reflect a complex scenario in which they are immersed, equally, at different moments but did not remain in school. Even so, they expressed the desire to resume school and strongly believed, like all other young people of their generation (Peregrino, 2005), in the promise that a better life can be achieved through studying. In their own unique ways, the three of them express the same content:

My message is for those who want to listen and those you wish to show it to: Make the most of you! Take advantage of what I couldn't, because it's very necessary to study, to be well educated. I wish you to achieve everything that I couldn't, but I believe, I have faith that someday I will get there too! In leaps and bounds!

(Interview with Juninho)

If I don't finish high school, I won't get anything, it gives the opportunity to take courses. School, you go to school, and after some time you can get stuck in time, for a year or two, and then you realize everything you've gone through, what the teachers say and that I am, have always been, someone good, then how can I say I'll be bad, that someone that was bad can become good, right, you can reverse the situation and become good.

(Interview with Nicolas)

Gosh, it's great, school is falling down, you know that, falling down more and more. It's everything, isn't it, without education we're nothing, but I'll come back to school, but if there's trouble, I'll leave again, I won't take crap.

(Interview with Willian)

These excerpts show that school has lost (and keeps on losing) a great opportunity to "capture" boys and girls, since in some way it is internalized in them and in a whole generation, this desire to be and continue in this structure (Peregrino, 2005; Borba et al., 2015). But, on the other hand, these trajectories reinforce that school has drifted from the pulsating lives of these adolescents. Educational agents have enormous difficulties coming into contact with this pulsation, perhaps because it is too strong and intense, and perhaps because some of them are willing to hear but they do not truly listen: they approach but do not welcome, nor take responsibility, and lives break from a whole institutional structure because they first broke from its agents, demonstrating the centrality of human resources to the fulfillment of any institutional mission, evidencing that the reference is in the professionals that compose that (any) space. In this sense, it is necessary to think about how social occupational therapy in its space of professional action can contribute to ensuring the access and permanence of youths who commit acts of indiscipline and/or offenses in school.

CONTRIBUTIONS OF SOCIAL OCCUPATIONAL THERAPY TO SCHOOL

Since the 1970s, occupational therapists have been inserted in the education sector in Brazil, especially in the so-called special schools/classes, to address the demands of children with disabilities and their families (Rocha, 2007). However, we have noticed other possibilities of insertion for us, occupational therapists, who deal with school dimensions that extrapolate from those associated with disabilities. This new perspective of practice for occupational therapists in Brazil in the field of education is being generated mainly by the Metuia Network – Social Occupational Therapy Project in its centers at the UFSCar and the Federal University of Sao Paulo (UNIFESP) (Lopes & Silva, 2007, Lopes, Borba, Trajber, et al., 2011, Lopes et al., 2012, Lopes, Borba, & Monzeli, 2013; Silva & Borba, 2018). These occupational therapists, according to the problems arising from the social issue, as understood by Lopes (2016), especially issues related to the lives of the popular urban youth, have combined their efforts with those of the teachers and managers of certain public schools with the aim of constructing a school that wishes to be more democratic, plural, and welcoming for all the diversity of the population it needs to assist. For this group, of which we are a part, the public school is a privileged setting for occupational-therapeutic action; it is this institution that has reached the beginning of the 21st century demanding assistance from different professional areas, including occupational therapy (Lopes & Silva, 2007). In Brazil, one of the basic dilemmas of the public school has not been solved: how to be a school for all and respond with quality to the collective and individual demands, and also how to promote training that integrates a curriculum supportive of the professional development of its students in concert with the promotion of classical, humanistic culture (Buffa & Nosella, 1998). Despite all the historical and contemporary dilemmas that the Brazilian educational scenario expresses, it is necessary to affirm and reaffirm that the public school is a priority partner, because it is there that we, still, find the youth. That is why it is a fundamental strategy to promote and develop projects that can ensure better living conditions and experiences for the political and democratic participation of these young people (Lopes & Silva, 2007). We assume that if school is prepared to cope with the demands of adolescents involved in wrongdoing, it will be better prepared to address the demands of youth as a whole. This is based on

our understanding that the offense, because it is a limited situation that entails complexities that require review and questioning by every organization. Nonetheless, the reversal of this reasoning is equally true: once school and its agents are prepared to address the demands expressed by contemporary youth, they will also be better able to engage in dialogue with the narratives of youths involved in offenses.

It is in this context that the social occupational therapy we advocate understands the implications of its actions in the field of education and youth. The experiments developed by the Metuia Laboratory, in this perspective, have dealt with these problems and contributed intervention proposals that seek to solve them. Attention should be drawn to actions with a large number of adolescents and youth, with emphasis on *workshops of activities, dynamics, and projects; individual territorial follow-ups; articulation of resources in the social field; and dynamization of the services network* (Lopes et al., 2014), in this case, focusing on mediation and guidance together with teachers, the school board, and the social justice system. In addition, occupational therapists can also collaborate in better understanding the reality of students, with the improvement of resources to provide a new meaning to teaching in the 21st century, with the creation of collective strategies involving parents/legal guardians and the community in the process of teaching and learning, among other contributions. When the juvenile population is dealt with in terms of their offenses, the school faces other dilemmas and needs assistance in finding answers—for example: How can these adolescents be supported to remain in school in pursuit of the construction of a narrative that involves more lawful than illicit acts? How can we advise/train teachers, managers, and officials who dialogue with and understand the universe of youths that engage in illicit aspects of life? Unfortunately, with the development of our research, we have witnessed a school that ended up expelling the adolescents who committed offenses or had already "expelled" them long before the offense occurred (Borba et al., 2015). And this same school, due to mismanagement of its internal conflicts, ended up transforming acts of indiscipline into offenses, as can be verified by the narratives herein presented.

We have named a school, but it is necessary to remember that a school is composed of people and, therefore, it is important to highlight and reflect on the central role that professionals can play as positive references for the reception of demands that are imposed in the life and school trajectories of youths who have been marked by the occurrence of offenses. In this context, we consider the need both for professionals who are inside the school and who turn their attention to the territory/community and for professionals who are outside the school and assist it with dealing with its internal conflicts, as well as supporting the permanence of these adolescents in school with learning quality.

In considering the approach of occupational therapy professionals engaging in the field of education, we will explore the "outside of the school" that dialogues with its interior through the insertion of occupational therapists in the teams of social services (Almeida, Soares, Barros, & Galvani, 2012; Borba, Costa, Savani, Anastácio, & Ota, 2016; Morais & Malfitano, 2016). We would not be proposing the creation of a new service/professional but rather strengthening guidance that is already provided in the Unified Social Assistance System (SUAS) (Brasil, 2005), established in 2005, in the field of Brazilian social protection, with social assistance as a right of the citizens and a duty of the state. However, the implementation of this system has occurred at a slow pace regarding the hiring of occupational therapists to compose the aforementioned teams, given the disinvestment in the social public policies we have witnessed in Brazil in recent years and the intensification of disputes between professional fields. In spite of all the interdisciplinary scientific production observed, on the "shop floor," corporations close their doors when faced with the struggle for scarce resources.

Despite the times of scarcity, in a possible scenario, with the insertion of occupational therapists into social services and a school that dialogues with its own colleagues, the school board, instead of requesting the presence of the police school guard/military police, could rely on the support of these services when it identifies problem situations that are beyond their responsive ability. Identification of problem situations should not occur only when the conflict is already established but rather should occur gradually, through the ability of teachers to perceive the events of life that involve their students, verbalized (or silent) in the school daily routine through demands expressed in their behaviors and attitudes. Once the social services/school partnership has been established, depending on the level of rights violation, occupational therapists could be called upon for this mediation and conduct an individual territorial follow-up with this student based on the assumptions of social occupational therapy (Barros et al., 2005; Lopes, 2016). To follow up with students, we recommend being truly together with the other (Freire, 2012) in terms of time availability, in the spaces of life and in the spaces where the students circulate, with a view to assisting them to live new experiences, mediate family conflicts, expand their circulation spaces, and access new resources existing in the city in terms of culture, education, sports, and vocational training (Lopes et al., 2014).

However, to conduct this follow-up within a service that reports to the social assistance policy, it would be essential that occupational therapists make some ruptures and/or revisions. The first rupture and/or revision would be with the established logic of referral, which considers that recommending/referring/prescribing the individual to go somewhere is sufficient. This is due to the understanding that doing the process together is politically incorrect and denotes welfarism, because the assumption that everyone has the capacity to take action is shared, provided that they are motivated to do so. However, if they fail to do so, it is currently seen to be because they have not put enough effort into it, with the impossibility of complying being the exclusive responsibility of the individuals, not by interpreting the reality and conditions, social and subjective, that they are actually experiencing. The second rupture/revision is related to the logic of productivism and the bureaucratization of work in the area of social assistance. There are countless protocols, registrations, and reports to be filled out; the real need for these resources is doubtful, or perhaps their demand actually arises to create a distancing of the professionals from the harsh reality in which they are asked to intervene. However, the proposition of the follow-ups does not generate numbers as the registrations in the programs of income transfer do, and therein lies the challenge of how to demonstrate the result of a professional action that does not fit the logic of the punctual service. Finally, linked to this last aspect, a rupture/review would occur related to the logic of the time of assistance being limited to 1 hour, in keeping with the norms of clinical appointments. This rupture is necessary because being with another person in your life may take a whole afternoon one week and 15 minutes the next week. Time would have to be dimensioned according to the needs of the other, and not only to the work process organization of the professional—or rather, those demands have to be at the center of that organization.

We consider that, in a favorable scenario, the individual territorial follow-up should be conducted by occupational therapists, but it is also possible that it could be performed by professionals with complete basic education (high school) with a profile that fits the function of social workers, supervised by occupational therapists.

Collectively, we have learned from Juninho, Nicolas, and Willian the complex dimension of the realities in which lives are involved and, unfortunately, the fragile support that is provided to them for the redefinition of their trajectories. Nevertheless, theirs are lives in process, with unfinished follow-ups; thus, they are waiting for new perspectives, new and positive encounters and disagreements—ultimately, the continuity of life. For occupational therapy, the challenge remains to establish a dialogue and an understanding of these "new" fields of action, which are possible and viable and whose possibility of existence has been created at our insistence.

REFERENCES

Almeida, M. C., Soares, C. R. S., Barros, D. D., & Galvani, D. (2012). Processos e práticas de formalização da Terapia Ocupacional na Assistência Social: alguns marcos e desafios [Formalization processes and practices of occupational therapy in social assistance: Landmarks and challenges]. *Brazilian Journal of Occupational Therapy, 20*(1), 33–41. doi:10.4322/cto.2012.004

Barros, D. D., Ghirardi, M. I. G., & Lopes, R. E. (2005). Social occupational therapy: A socio-historical perspective. In F. Kronenberg, S. S. Algado, & N. Pollard (Eds.), *Occupational therapy without borders: Learning from the spirit of survivors* (Vol. 1, pp. 140–151). Londres: Elsevier Science – Churchill Livingstone.

Barros, D. D., Lopes, R. E., Galheigo, S. M., & Galvani, D. (2007). El Proyecto Metuia en Brasil: ideas y acciones que nos unen [The Metuia Project in Brazil: Ideas and actions that unite us]. In F. Kronenberg, S. S. Algado, & N. Pollard (Eds.), *Terapia ocupacional sin fronteras: aprendiendo del espíritu de supervivientes* [Occupational therapy without borders: Learning from the spirit of survivors] (Vol 1., pp. 392–403). Madri: Editorial Médica Panamericana, S. A.

Borba, P. L. O. (2012). *Juventude marcada: relações entre ato infracional e a Escola Pública em São Carlos – SP* [Youth marked: Relations between infraction and the Public School in São Carlos – SP]. 250f. (PhD thesis in Education). Universidade Federal de São Carlos, São Carlos. Retrieved February 2019, from https://repositorio.ufscar.br/handle/ufscar/2287

Borba, P. L. O., Costa, S. L., Savani, A. C. C., Anastácio, C. C., & Ota, N. H. (2016). Entre fluxos, pessoas e territórios: delineando a inserção do terapeuta ocupacional no Sistema Único de Assistência Social [Between flows, people and territories: Outlining the insert of occupational therapist in the Brazilian Social Assistance System]. *Brazilian Journal of Occupational Therapy, 25*(1), 203–214. doi:10.4322/0104-4931.ctoRE0758

Borba, P. L. O., Lopes, R. E. L., & Malfitano, A. P. S. (2015). Trajetórias escolares de adolescentes em conflito com a lei: subsídios para repensar políticas educacionais [School trajectories of adolescents with offenses: Subsidies to rethink educational policies]. *Revista Ensaio: Avaliação e Políticas Públicas em Educação, 23*(89), 937–963. doi:10.1590/S0104-40362015000400006

Brasil. (1990). *Estatuto da Criança e do Adolescente* [Brazilian's Statute of the Child and Adolescent]. Lei no 8069. São Paulo: Imprensa Oficial do Estado.

Brasil. (2005). Ministério do Desenvolvimento Social e Combate à Fome. Secretaria Nacional de Assistência Social. *Sistema Único de Assistência Social - SUAS. Norma Operacional Básica NOB/SUAS: Construindo as Bases para a Implantação do Sistema Único de Assistência Social* [Unique System of Social Assistance – Basic operational standard: Building the basis for the implementation of the single social assistance system]. Brasília: Ministério do Desenvolvimento Social e Combate à Fome.

Buffa, E., & Nosella, P. (1998). *A escola profissional de São Carlos* [Professional's School of São Carlos]. São Carlos, SP: EdUFSCar.

BRAZIL. Decreto-Lei 2.848, de 07 de dezembro de 1940 [Decree-Law 2848, of 07 of dezember of 1940]. Código Penal [Penal Code]. Diário Oficial da União, Rio de Janeiro, 31 dez. 1940.

Cardoso, J. C., Gomes, C. A., & Santana, E. U. (2013). Escola e polícia em três países: vinho novo em odres velhos ou a crise das instituições [School and police in three countries: New wine in old bottles or the crisis of institutions]. *Revista Ensaio: Avaliação e Políticas Públicas em Educação, 21*(81), 685–710. doi:10.1590/S0104-40362013000400004

Caria, T. (2003). A construção etnográfica do conhecimento em Ciências Sociais: reflexividade e fronteira [Ethnography construction of knowledge in social sciences: Reflexivity and frontier]. In T Caria (Eds.), *Experiência Etnográfica em Ciências Sociais* [Ethnography experiences in social sciences] (pp. 9–20). Porto: Afrontamento.

Castro, A., & Lopes, R. E. (2011). A escola de tempo integral: desafios e possibilidades [The full-time school: Challenges and possibilities]. *Ensaio (Fundação Cesgranrio. Impresso), 19*(71), 259–282. doi:10.1590/S0104-40362011000300003

Conselho Federal de Psicologia; Ordem dos Advogados do Brasil. (2006). *Direitos Humanos: um retrato das unidades de internação de adolescentes em conflito com a lei* [Human rights: A portrait of the units to restriction of freedom for adolescents with offenses] [Report]. Relatório de visita da comissão de inspeção, EdUFSCar.

Feltran, G. S. (2008). *Fronteiras de tensão: Um estudo sobre política e violência nas periferias de São Paulo* [Frontiers of tension: A study of politics and violence in the peripheries of São Paulo] (PhD thesis in Sociology). Universidade Estadual de Campinas (Unicamp), Campinas, São Paulo, Brasil. Retrieved February 2019, from http://bdtd.ibict.br/vufind/Record/CAMP_d25ccc41896a464ccd04c4098dc0d5e7

Ferreira, L. A. M. (2010). *O Estatuto da Criança e do Adolescente e o Professor: reflexos na sua formação e atuação* [The Statute of Child and Adolescent and the teacher: Reflections in education process and practice] (2nd ed.). São Paulo: Cortez.

Freire, P. (2012). *Pedagogy of the oppressed* (30th anniversary ed.) (3rd ed.). New York, NY: Bloomsbury Academic.

Goffman, E. (1961). *Asylums: Essays on the social situation of mental patients and other inmates.* New York, NY: Doubleday Anchor.

Lopes, R. E. (2016). Cidadania, Direitos e Terapia Ocupacional Social [Citizenship, rights and social occupational therapy]. In R. E. Lopes & A. P. Malfitano (Eds.), *Terapia Ocupacional Social: Desenhos Teóricos e Contornos Práticos* [Social occupational therapy: Theoretical designs and practice delimitations]. São Carlos, SP: EdUFSCar.

Lopes, R. E., Borba, P. L. O., & Cappellaro, M. (2011). Acompanhamento individual e articulação de recursos em terapia ocupacional social: compartilhando uma experiência [Individual support and resources articulation in social occupational therapy: Sharing an experience]. *O Mundo da Saúde, 35*(2), 233–238. doi:10.15343/0104-7809.20112233238

Lopes, R. E., Borba, P. L. O., & Monzeli, G. A. (2013). Expressão livre de jovens por meio do Fanzine: recurso para a terapia ocupacional social [Free expression of young people through Fanzine: Resource for social occupational therapy]. *Saúde e Sociedade, 22*(3), 937–948. doi:10.1590/S0104-12902013000300027

Lopes, R. E., Borba, P. L. O., Pereira, P. B., Dariolli, F., & Rodrigues, R. C. J. (2015). *Escola, Juventude e Cidadania: Relação entre a Escola e o Ato Infracional em São Carlos (SP)* [School, youth and citizenship: Relations with school and offenses in São Carlos (SP)] [Relatório de pesquisa – Research report]. 295p. METUIA/UFSCar; FAPESP; CNPq.

Lopes, R. E., Borba, P. L. O., Trajber, N. K. A., Silva, C. R., & Cuel, B. T. (2011). Oficinas de Atividades com Jovens da Escola Pública: Tecnologias Sociais entre Educação e Terapia Ocupacional [Activities workshops with public school youngsters: Social technologies between education and occupational therapy]. *Interface (Botucatu, Impresso), 15*(36), 277–288. doi:10.1590/S1414-32832011000100021

Lopes, R. E., Malfitano, A. P. S., Silva, C. R., & Borba, P. L. O. B. (2014). Recursos e tecnologias em Terapia Ocupacional Social: ações com jovens pobres na cidade [Resources and technologies in social occupational therapy: Actions with the poor youth in town]. *Brazilian Journal of Occupational Therapy, 22*(3), 591–602. doi:10.4322/cto.2014.081

Lopes, R. E., Sfair, S. C., & Bittar, M. (2012). Adolescentes em medidas socioeducativas em meio aberto e a escola [Teenagers and socio-educational measures at open environments and at school]. *Brazilian Journal of Occupational Therapy, 20*(2), 217–228. doi:10.4322/cto.2012.023

Lopes, R. E., & Silva, C. R. (2007). O campo da educação e demandas para a terapia ocupacional no Brasil [The field of education and demands for occupational therapy in Brazil]. *Revista de Terapia Ocupacional da Universidade de São Paulo, 18*(3), 158–164. doi:10.11606/issn.2238-6149.v18i3p158-164

Lopes, R. E., Souza, L. B., & Borba, P. L. O. (2010). *Memória e Ação Territorial: da história do Jardim Gonzaga às bases de intervenção em Terapia Ocupacional Social* [Memories and territorial actions: From the history of Jardim Honzaga to

the background of social occupational therapy] [Research report]. Iniciação Científica. Relatório de Pesquisa, Universidade Federal de São Carlos, Conselho Nacional de Desenvolvimento Científico e Tecnológico (CNPq).

Meihy, J. C. S. B. (1997). *História Oral* [Oral history]. São Paulo: Edusp.

Morais, A. C., & Malfitano, A. P. S. (2016). O terapeuta ocupacional como executor de medidas socioeducativas em meio aberto: discursos na construção de uma prática [Occupational therapist as socioeducational measures executor in open environment: Speech to practice construction]. *Brazilian Journal of Occupational Therapy, 24*(3), 531–542. doi:10.4322/0104-4931

Peregrino, M. (2005). Os jovens pobres e a escola [Poor youths and school]. *JOVENes, Revista de Estudios sobre Juventud, México, 9*(22), 356–368.

Rocha, E. F. (2007). A Terapia Ocupacional e as ações na educação: aprofundando interfaces [Occupational therapy and actions in education: Deepening interfaces]. *Revista de Terapia Ocupacional da Universidade de São Paulo, 18*(3), 97–104. doi:10.11606/issn.2238-6149

Rocha, M. F. J., Bittar, M., & Lopes, R. E. (2016). O Professor Mediador Escolar e Comunitário: uma Prática em Construção [The school and community mediator teacher: A practice in construction]. *Revista Eletrônica de Educação, 10*(3), 341–353. doi:10.14244/198271991523

Silva, C. G., & Borba, P. L. O. (2018). Encontros com a diferença na formação de profissionais de saúde: juventudes, sexualidades e gêneros na escola [Encounters with the difference at health education: Youth, sexualities, and genders at school]. *Saúde e Sociedade, 27*(4), 1134–1146. doi:10.1590/s0104-12902018170274

Sposito, M. P. (1998). *A instituição escolar e a violência* [The school institution and violence] [Cadernos de pesquisa]. São Paulo: Fundação Carlos Chagas/Cortez, n. 104. Retrieved February 2019, from http://publicacoes.fcc.org.br/ojs/index.php/cp/article/view/717

Whyte, W. F. (1993) *Street corner society: The social structure of an Italian slum* (4th ed.). Chicago: University of Chicago Press.

13

Social Occupational Therapy and the Eradication of Child Labor in Brazil: The Challenge of Articulating Social Protection and Autonomy

Carla Regina Silva Soares and Marta Carvalho de Almeida

With the support of international conventions, public policies that aim to tackle child labor have been developed in Brazil since the 1990s. Such actions involve different sectors of the economy, social movements, the government (i.e., executive, legislative, and judicial powers), and involvement at the national, state, and municipal management levels.

Among these actions, those associated with the ongoing nationwide Child Labor Eradication Program (PETI) are especially notable. In 2005, this program was included in the Brazilian social assistance public policy, which is implemented through the Unified Social Assistance System (SUAS) (Brasil, Ministério do Desenvolvimento Social e Combate à Fome [MDS], 2010). The program involves occupational therapists (Almeida, Soares, Barros, & Galvani, 2012) who contribute to the design and implementation of strategies aimed at promoting social protection for children and adolescents who are experiencing or have experienced child labor as well as those who seek autonomy and family emancipation. The occupational therapists involved in this program assist families and communities in creating and supporting a dignified life for children and adolescents that protects their rights. The purpose of this chapter is to present the work of occupational therapists in PETI.

HISTORY OF CHILD LABOR IN BRAZIL

Child labor is at the heart of Brazil's historical socioeconomic development (Moura, 2013; Vieira, 2009). From the 16th to the 19th centuries, children of indigenous and African origin were subjected to slavery or labor in rural and urban areas under the same conditions as adults. In the late 19th century and throughout the 20th century, the process of industrialization caused large numbers of children to be incorporated into manufacturing and service activities. For a long time, the social narrative that work educates and contributes to the moral development of children masked evidence that child labor is motivated by economic priorities: that children represent cheap, adaptable, trainable labor with a low capacity for political organization and are thus very useful to the exploitation of surplus value. This imagination provided strong support for a social practice that began long ago and was aggravated by the Industrial Revolution. As early as 1867, Marx pointed out that the reduced physical effort required for work and reductions in wages were factors that encouraged workers to include their whole family in the labor market, including their children (Kassouf, 2007).

The exploitation of child labor results from contradictions inherent to the process of capitalist accumulation. Its reproduction is ensured through prejudices against working-class people, which cite their supposed "inability" to educate children according to appropriate moral values (Carvalho, 2008). From this perspective, work can be presented as a suitable alternative to educate properly socialized adults. However, while child labor is considered appropriate for the "education" of the poor population, wealthier people increasingly postpone joining the labor market until after graduation, postgraduate education, internships abroad, or various other educational experiences that provide access to higher-paying occupations. The social class bias evident in the different ways of conceiving the rights of children and youths reveals prejudices underlying the discourse around child labor in Brazilian society (Repórter Brasil, 2013). But social bias is not the only factor; this discourse has long hidden employers' interests in reducing the costs of products or services to increase their profit margins through the work of children and adolescents. It has also hidden the abusive relationships that permeate the world of child labor, especially at home. More recent changes in the world of work have also concealed the fact that "exploitation of child labor is not dissociated from the global strategies of precariousness of workers' living conditions and reduction of labor cost" (Brasil, MDS, 2010, p. 22). The legitimacy of precocious work still prevails in discourses around different social groups. According to Sarti (1999), work is linked to the need to create a positive social identity (i.e., "worker") because it represents a moral value associated with the notion of dignity. For the upper classes, in addition to keeping salary levels low, the employment of poor children brings a sense of security "to the extent that it is a modality of social control over the 'dangerous classes'" (Di Giovanni, 2004).

As of the mid-1980s, Brazilian society's commitment to the protection of children and adolescents became the basis for fighting child labor. International pressure and Brazilian social movements in defense of children's rights gave rise to denunciations and awareness of the perverse character of child labor, characterizing it as a violation of human rights. In agreement with international documents such as the Declaration of the Rights of the Child of 1959, the Constitution of the Federative Republic of Brazil of 1988 (Brasil, 1988) established a "legal doctrine of integral protection," which advocates for the egalitarian and safe development of all Brazilian children and adolescents (Carvalho, 2008). Article 227 of this document states that this population should be guaranteed

the right to life, health, food, education, leisure, professionalization, culture, dignity, respect, freedom, and family and community life, and the safeguard from all forms of negligence, discrimination, exploitation, violence, cruelty, and oppression.

(Brasil, 1988, p. 37)

Addressing this population at the national level, the Child and Adolescent Statute (CAS) was enacted in 1990. This document established the rights of children and adolescents in Brazil as a priority for social protection and places the obligation on family, society, and the state to actualize them. The CAS aims to protect the rights of children and adolescents[1] and promotes the notion that childhood should be valued and that children and adolescents are human beings in development (Marcilio, 1998).

As this paradigm for social protection was implemented, Brazilian society's perception regarding child labor—that work was a positive force in the education of poor or underprivileged children—became increasingly challenged in the 1990s (Comissão Nacional de Erradicação do Trabalho Infantil [CONAETI], 2011). This perception was also challenged by the International Labour Organization (ILO), which, since 1973, has emphasized the harmful effects of child labor and characterized it as any type of work performed by children and adolescents that disagrees with the minimum age established by the law for entering the labor market, regardless of whether the work is paid or unpaid, regular or sporadic (ILO/Brasil, 2013). This societal perception was also contrary to the Constitution of the Federative Republic of Brazil of 1988, which established that work is totally prohibited until the age of 14 and is only acceptable between 14 and 16 years for young apprentices, who must be employed by an apprenticeship contract. As stated in decree no. 6.481 of 2008, which discriminates against the "worst forms of child labor" according to Article 4 of the ILO Convention 182 (Brasil, 1988), adolescents between the ages of 16 and 18 may work if their employment adheres to specific conditions such as not being nocturnal, being unhealthy, being performed in environments harmful to development, or hindering school attendance.

Although child labor is still present in Brazil and its existence is associated with notions of utility and benefit, societal movements have emerged to challenge it by promoting campaigns to raise awareness of its harmful consequences, holding events and discussions aimed at deepening knowledge, and creating political pressure for the introduction of laws and actions to tackle the issue.

CHILD LABOR: SCOPE, NATURE, AND HARM

According to estimates in 2016, approximately 152 million children and adolescents perform child labor worldwide, representing almost 1 in 10 children. Among this group, 73 million children and adolescents are engaged in activities considered to be the "worst forms of child labor," labor that involves painful, hazardous, or unhealthy activities that directly jeopardize safety, health, and moral development (ILO, 2017). Worldwide estimates using a comparative interval of 16 years show a decrease of 94 million children and adolescents performing child labor between 2000 and 2016 (ILO, 2017). Although there was a reduction of 16 million child laborers between 2012 and 2016, it was a slower decline than between 2008 and 2012, which showed the greatest rate of decline for that 16-year period. During the same time frame, the most significant reduction occurred among children aged 5 to 11. This age range

---

[1]According to Child and Adolescent Statute, the term "children" applies to citizens under 12 years old and "adolescents" to those aged 12 to 18 years old.

also accounted for the largest proportion of child laborers (44%). There was a greater reduction in the number of working girls (40%) than working boys (25%) (ILO, 2013).

Global data demonstrates that among all children and adolescents performing child labor, 43% are in the poorest countries (ILO, 2017). However, the child labor rate in other countries is still significant: 38% are in lower-middle-income countries, 17.3% are in upper-middle-income countries, and 1.3% are in high-income (1.3%) countries. According to the ILO (2017), 70.9% of child laborers work in agriculture, 17.2% work in services, and 11.9% are in industry.

In line with global perspectives, Brazil has shown a progressive decrease in its rates of child labor over the past two decades, despite experiencing a slower rate of decline as of 2005 (Repórter Brasil, 2013) and an increase in the number of working children and adolescents aged 5 to 14 in all macro-regions of the country between 2013 and 2015 (Instituto Brasileiro de Geografia e Estatística [IBGE], 2016). The Brazilian National Household Sample Survey (PNAD)[2] measured the incidence of child labor for the first time in 1992 and found that 19.6% of children and adolescents aged 5 to 17 worked. This percentage was reduced to 12.7% in 2001 and 10.2% in 2008. For the 5 to 15 age bracket, the rate dropped from 10.8% in 1998 to 5.6% in 2009 (CONAETI, 2011).

Despite the reduction in percentage, the absolute numbers of child labor in Brazil demonstrate that the problem remains important: 2.3 million children and adolescents in the 5 to 17 age bracket were working in 2016, which corresponds to 5.96% of the Brazilian child and adolescent population. Of these, 104,000 were aged 5 to 9, 347,000 were 10 to 13, and the majority, 1.8 million, were aged 14 to 17 (CONAETI, 2018). These statistics do not account for rates of child labor in domestic work, sexual exploitation, or the illegal drug trade. Santos (2017) also highlights that children working on the streets have been inadequately sampled, arguing that the PNAD methodology addresses work situations declared by residents of a household, which may conceal cases of child labor due to fear or lack of awareness among respondents.

Furthermore, studies indicate the existence of a "bastion" of child labor, resistant to change in the context of unpaid family work, agricultural activity, and informal urban activities (CONAETI, 2011). Moreover, according to a report by the Repórter Brasil (2013) nongovernmental organization (NGO), a major challenge for eradicating child labor in Brazil remains in addressing its worst forms in homes, landfills, sexual exploitation, family farming, the illegal drug trade, and urban informal commerce. According to the report, policies face great difficulty in tackling these forms of work because they are especially complex. Further, from 2000 to 2010, the problem increased by 1.5% among children aged 10 to 13, who belong to a very vulnerable age group and for whom all types of work are prohibited. The report states that if Brazil maintains this trend, it will not be able to meet its goal to eradicate all child labor by 2020 as set before the international community. For the period of 2019 to 2022 in Brazil, the Third National Program for the Prevention and Eradication of Child Labor and Protection of the Adolescent Worker included an updated research methodology that differentiated "paid work" from "other forms of work," including work that is "own-use production." The results included children and adolescents in both categories, which, according to the report, can explain the increase of child labor between 2015 and 2016 in the 5 to 9 (from 79,000 to 104,000) and 10 to 13 (from 333,000 to 347,000) age brackets. This demonstrates that the decrease in total child labor—from 2.7 million in 2016 to 2.3 million in 2017—was concentrated in the 14 to 17 age bracket (CONAETI, 2018).

The program highlighted some important characteristics of the child and adolescent working population and defined a set of central problems and actions with respect to the way child labor is being addressed. It showed that most (67%) child labor is performed by males (although females are more common in specific occupations such as housework) who are predominantly brown and black (66.2%). In Brazil, the highest child labor rate among 5- to 13-year-olds occurred in the Northeast region (33%), whereas the lowest rate was observed in the Central-West region (7.2%). As for workers aged 14 to 17 (1.8 million), 83.3% did not have a legal employment contract at the time of the survey (CONAETI, 2018). Among all workers aged 10 to 17, it was found that the average income was lower than the national minimum wage (R$ 724 ≅ USD 192) in 2014. Those working in domestic service received the lowest wages, on average equivalent to 33.6% of the legal minimum wage. In agriculture, fisheries, forestry, livestock, and aquaculture, working children received an average of 59.9% of the minimum wage. Incomes in rural areas were lower than those in urban areas. Unlike in the rest of the world, the program revealed that the child labor rate in Brazil is higher in nonagricultural activities (76.3%), with most agricultural activities (23.7%) concentrated in the Northeast and North regions (CONAETI, 2018).

It is worth considering that, despite its prohibitive legislation, the ILO emphasizes the importance of differentiating child labor from cultural traditions found in different

---

[2]The PNAD is an annual demographic and socioeconomic survey conducted by the Brazilian Institute of Statistics and Geography (IBGE).

parts of the world, which add meaning and value to children's work. In some regions, part of the cultural transmission and socialization process occurs through work under the supervision of parents. These cases should not be mistaken for those in which children and adolescents are forced to work to ensure their livelihoods and/or those of their families, with consequent harm to their development (ILO, 2011). In contrast, it is also worth noting that some forms of child labor are more socially tolerated or are so inherent to everyday life that they are not perceived as a violation of rights. In Brazil, sports and artistic activities, which are regulated by specific standards, are among these forms of child labor (Medeiros Neto & Marques, 2013), as is housework (CONAETI, 2018).

The harm associated with child labor occurs at many levels. Since the hours at work reduce opportunities for children and youths to perform an array of activities, one impact that is particularly problematic is the effect on access to education and activities that are integral to development. For example, barriers or limitations on the right to play interfere with essential aspects of the development of affection and affectivity (MDS, 2010). These barriers exacerbate concerns for the physical and mental health of these young workers (ILO, 2013). Many studies have shown that children who work are more likely to be out of school than children who do not. In Brazil, the 2016 PNAD revealed that the 14 to 17 age group has the highest rate of absenteeism from school and that although 84% of children and adolescents aged 5 to 17 years who worked were also in school, a high illiteracy rate was observed in the population aged 10 to 17 (CONAETI, 2018). Previous studies have shown that time spent at work impairs both school performance and social participation and interaction, which are equally important for the development of children and adolescents (CONAETI, 2011).

According to Kassouf and Santos (2010), the negative effects of child labor on individual income have also been studied using the PNAD data. These studies have reported that child labor correlates with a reduction in future income and that this reduction can be mostly attributed to the loss of education caused by child labor. Limited schooling and poor school performance restrict employment opportunities to low-skilled and low-paid jobs. Research also shows that the younger children are when they begin working, the lower their earnings are in adulthood.

With respect to the health impairments of children and adolescents engaged in child labor, studies report a high rate of injuries or illnesses resulting from work activities (CONAETI, 2011). Among 5- to 17-year-olds, the perceived negative effects of work were physical exhaustion, mental strain, and premature aging. In addition to the damages evinced by research, other negative effects of child labor should be highlighted. In Brazil, one of the arguments in favor of child labor is that it is better for children to be working than on the streets, unoccupied and vulnerable to drug use and crime. However, this assertion is easily refuted by considering how various forms of child labor in Brazil "push" children and adolescents into organized crime, illegal drug trade, human trafficking, sexual exploitation, and contexts where they are subjected to humiliation and violence of all kinds (Repórter Brasil, 2013). In this respect, the ILO (2011) also drew attention to the emotional harm experienced by children and adolescents engaged in child labor, referring to possible difficulties in establishing affective bonds due to exploitation and ill treatment. There is also concern about the harm caused by illicit work, such as child prostitution and the illegal drug trade. This type of work imposes limits on the lives of children and adolescents and often restricts their circulation as they are monitored and experience daily tension while fearing for their lives. Many of them sleep on the streets, roofs, or slabs to watch over the places where illicit activity occurs (MDS, 2010).

In Brazil, one of the most important factors contributing to child labor is serious socioeconomic inequality, which forces many poor families to rely on income from child labor as an essential source of survival. As previously mentioned, another important contributor to normalizing child labor is the popular social narrative that poor children and adolescents benefit from work (MDS, 2010).

Further, "the lack of universalization of the public assistance policies on the rights of children, adolescents, and their families" also contributes to the incidence of child labor in Brazil (MDS, 2010, p. 21). Despite advances in the implementation of public policies to eliminate child labor, the Third National Program for the Prevention and Eradication of Child Labor and Protection of the Adolescent Worker emphasized that political and social agendas need to prioritize this issue by improving protections for children and adolescents, fostering social mobilization, and increasing investment in education policies for this population (CONAETI, 2018).

TACKLING THE PROBLEM IN BRAZIL AND THE CHILD LABOR ERADICATION PROGRAM (PETI)

The previous overview sought to demonstrate that the eradication of child labor requires profound political, economic, cultural, and social transformation because it is a complex phenomenon that reflects and is perpetuated by the inequalities inherent to the capitalist mode of production. According to Araújo (2010), the relations of capitalist production engender exploitation of the child labor force for the perpetuation and expansion of capital. These relations preserve and reproduce workforce conditions, thereby promoting ineffective actions that attempt to regulate and mitigate the effects of child labor but fail to target and revolutionize the relationships that bring it about. From the perspective of social policy, the eradication of child labor requires multiple sectors from the state and society to develop a combination of strategies for prevention and punishment, to create real possibilities for education and professionalization, and to implement future projects for children and adolescents. Although limited, Brazil has implemented comparable measures, such as the National Program for the Prevention and Eradication of Child Labor and Protection of Adolescent Workers. Specifically, the International Program on the Elimination of Child Labor (IPEC/ILO) and the Child Labor Eradication Program (PETI) were implemented in 1992 and 1996, respectively. Currently, the latter is defined as an intergovernmental and intersectoral program, which joins the three levels of government and NGOs to protect all children and adolescents under 16 years of age from any form of work (except for work as an apprentice) (MDS, 2018). Families with children and adolescents up to the age of 16 who are eligible to participate in the program receive a financial benefit to replace the income generated by child labor, and in return, these families must enroll their children in school and prove a minimum monthly attendance rate of 85%. Pregnant women and infants should adhere to prenatal care, assist workshops on breastfeeding and child health, accept vaccinations, and attend follow-ups on the development of their children up to the age of 7—all offered by the free public health system. In addition, the PETI directs children who have withdrawn from work and their families to participate in activities by social assistance services in addition to the school classes.

Data from the 2010 census showed that 80% of child labor in Brazil was concentrated in 1,913 municipalities, which represents approximately 34% of Brazilian municipalities. This information was used to reformulate the PETI in 2013. Since then, 1,032 municipalities with a high incidence of child labor were prioritized as targets for an action plan to tackle the less visible forms of child labor—domestic child labor, family farming, and work related to the informal sector. These municipalities were offered greater availability of specific resources for the development of strategic actions within the PETI. According to current guidelines, children and adolescents withdrawn from work should have priority in accessing the Service of Coexistence and Strengthening of Bonds (SCFV), provided by the SUAS. This service offers opportunities for shared living and socialization while stimulating personal

---

BOX 13.1   Proactiveness

Fábio worked as a salesperson at his neighborhood street market twice a week. He was 13 years old when the Specialized Service of Social Approach (SEAS) team first encountered him during an active search in public spaces. Over the course of 2 weeks, the team carefully and gradually approached him. After establishing a bond of trust with the team, Fábio and his family agreed to receive a technical visit from the SEAS staff at their residence. In dialogue with his mother (Solange) during the visit, the team confirmed that Fábio had been working regularly. The team also learned about the family's composition and general information regarding their social and economic context. The family was identified as being socially vulnerable. The SEAS staff advised Solange to access the Social Assistance Reference Center (CRAS) of their neighborhood and notified the center of the family's situation.

---

development through play, sports, and artistic activities occurring during the school year in addition to their school classes. Participation in these activities and school attendance are required for families to continue in the program. Participating families receive follow-ups from other social assistance services to mitigate other social risks and to strengthen family and community bonds. In Social Assistance Reference Centers (CRAS), one of the aforementioned services, families with children and adolescents engaged in child labor can access activities that promote professional qualifications and productive inclusion to enhance their work opportunities (Brasil, Secretaria Nacional de Assistência Social [SNAS], 2014). The occurrence of child labor must be identified by territorial assessments by the Social Assistance Surveillance sector of SUAS and through active searching by technical social assistance teams from the Specialized Service of Social Approach (SEAS) (see Box 13.1).

Although Brazil is committed to the development of strategies to eliminate child labor, there are challenges that must be overcome, such as the increasing number of working children in the 5 to 9 age bracket and the failure to eliminate the "worst forms of child labor" by 2016—a goal established at the Second Global Conference on Child Labor. Further, only a small proportion of children and adolescents in child labor benefit from the actions of the PETI (Santos, 2017). To address this complex problem, it is necessary to broaden the range of public policies that target child labor at multiple levels and to augment public consciousness regarding the contemporary social mechanisms that contribute to child labor in Brazil. Most importantly, social inequalities must be reduced if this problem is to be eradicated.

SOCIAL OCCUPATIONAL THERAPY AND CHILD LABOR

As has been shown, child labor is a serious social problem in Brazil and has multiple negative effects on the lives of children, youths, families, and communities, causing observable losses during the time the work is performed and long after it ceases. Among these losses, there are several problems associated with everyday activities that are the focus of occupational therapy (see Box 13.2). In this context, several losses incurred through child labor can cause a cascade of successive additional losses. Occupational therapists who work in programs addressing child labor use social occupational therapy as the theoretical-methodological framework for their professional practice.

Table 13.1 provides an overview of the problems frequently experienced by children, youths (see Box 13.3), families, and communities involved in child labor. These will vary depending on the different contexts in which child labor occurs.

In general, occupational therapists seek to reduce the contextual factors that encourage child labor and aim to repair the aforementioned losses, which remain long after children and adolescents withdraw from work. Keeping this population away from labor is a complex challenge in Brazil due to the social context, the conditions of vulnerability, and the social risk to families and culture, which assign a positive value to child labor.

Occupational therapists consider the different environments in which children or youths who have withdrawn from work carry out their everyday activities to identify changes that are necessary to promote activities and relationships that establish/strengthen a space for children and adolescents to experience security and the motivation to achieve their full development. Schools, social assistance units, health units, cultural and sports projects, and other forms of social organization should be coherently coordinated to offer appropriate opportunities to these children and adolescents (Lopes, Malfitano, Silva, & Borba, 2014). All actors and organizations are responsible for addressing the damages caused by child labor (see Box 13.4). Therefore, it is important to understand the existing Brazilian network of policies and services that protect and defend the rights of children and adolescents, including government actions and civil initiatives. It is necessary for occupational therapists to work with the institutions, organizations, and individuals that compose this network to expand their territorial work to develop and implement strategies that bring the best community resources and experiences to this population (Lopes, Barros, Malfitano, Galvani, & Galluzzi, 2001; Borba, Costa, Savani, Anastácio, & Ota, 2017) (see Box 13.5). Families should actively participate in protecting the rights of children since they play a central

---

BOX 13.2 Social Approach

When Solange connected with services, the Social Assistance Reference Center (CRAS) team, which included an occupational therapist, sought to better understand the social conditions of her family such as its history, internal relationships, ties with the community, and family life dynamics. They soon learned that the family, which consisted of a mother and three adolescents, was undergoing a difficult time due to the parents' separation, which resulted in decreased income and changes in everyday life among other challenges. Solange was sad and worried. She had not worked for pay since her first daughter was born (at the time of accessing services, her daughter was 17 years old with an 8-month-old baby) and relied on Fábio's earnings to supplement the family income, which had decreased after the divorce despite payments she received from her former husband.

According to Solange, changes in the family affected the everyday lives of each family member. Her two sons, Fábio and his younger brother, aged 12, spent a lot of time away from home and often argued for no reason. Disagreements between Solange and her daughter were also more common and usually erupted over sharing household chores. Solange wanted her daughter, who had dropped out of school when she became pregnant, to assume more responsibilities in the house, including caring for her brothers and her baby. Fábio, who had previously interacted extensively with all family members, spent more time alone and in silence.

Solange was overwhelmed, and she felt unable to solve her problems. The father had been absent in supporting his family's welfare beyond the required payments, and in this context, Fábio's work was a relief to Solange, since she believed he would be safe from bad company and idleness. She was proud of Fábio's enthusiasm for work and concluded that he was well prepared to assume the responsibilities of adulthood. Her sole source of support was her sister-in-law, the wife of her deceased brother. According to Solange, they helped each other financially and emotionally.

TABLE 13.1   Impacts/Losses Involved in the Experience of Child Labor

Individual	Impacts/Losses
Child/youth	• Lack of activities and experiences recommended for the full development of children and adolescents. This refers to the absence of opportunities to develop an adequate occupational repertoire both qualitatively and quantitatively. Restriction of playful activities is especially harmful. • Absence or lack of activities that enable action–reflection–action focusing to focus on individual and collective life • Difficulty regularly attending classes and/or participating in school activities • Participation in activities that pose health risks • Participation in activities involving physical and/or psychological violence • Participation in activities with demands that exceed a person's physical, cognitive, and psychosocial capacities • Lack of opportunities for choice and self-determination regarding work and everyday activities. Such limitations tend to persist in adult life. • Absence or lack of experiences of support, protection, respect, and care from adults • Impediment of collective activity to ensure the rights of children and youths and to provide a dignified life for the community
Family	• Decrease in the number and quality of family activities • Absence or lack of activities that enable action–reflection–action focusing on family and collective life • Absence or lack of activities that foster interpersonal relationships wherein adults are positioned as protectors, caregivers, and providers of the needs of children and youths • Absence or lack of playful experiences or experiences with low levels of mutual participation in family activities • Absence or lack of cooperative/collaborative activities around family interests or interests common to its members • Absence or lack of activities that facilitate the development of a collective identity as a family unit • Absence or lack of activities that enable the expression and appreciation of the different skills or ways of being among members of the family and that contribute to the life and well-being of the family • Absence or lack of collective actions aimed at ensuring the rights of the family and its members, as well as a dignified life for the community
Community	• Absence or lack of activities requiring social exchanges that promote self-identification with the community as a collective that recognizes, guides, and demands the rights of its children and youths, as well as a dignified life for the community • Absence or restriction of participation in activities that promote the circulation of symbolic goods associated with childhood and adolescence • Absence or lack of activities that enable action-reflection-action with a focus on collective life. This strongly encourages the idea of considering child labor normal. • Absence or lack of collective actions aimed at a dignified life for the community

role in children's life. Occupational therapists have worked to make this network increasingly powerful so that it can protect the rights of children and youths and ensure that protections become established in their communities (see Box 13.6). Accordingly, a fundamental aspect of this work involves developing a critical and comprehensive understanding of social reality, which includes analyzing the territory where one works from a socioanthropological perspective (Barros, Ghirardi, & Lopes, 2005). This approach privileges the Child–family–community unit and respects its inclusion in the social reality that defines it throughout processes of assessment and intervention design.

BOX 13.3 Losses

On days when the street market occurred, Fábio got up at 4 a.m. to help unload boxes of fruits and vegetables that would be sold in the stand where he worked. He walked to the street market and arrived there before dawn. Even though he was quite thin and weak, he carried heavy boxes on these days. He worked alongside adults, older and stronger, performing the same functions, but received less pay for his work. At the end of the work shift, around midday, he was always too tired to go to school in the afternoon. His frequent absences had a negative effect on his performance at school and led Fábio to believe that he was not good at studying. He began to skip classes on days when he was not working and began to consider quitting school. Fábio said he liked working at the street market, which he had been doing for 6 months, because his mother let him keep some of the money.

BOX 13.4 Connections

As soon as this situation was confirmed as child labor, the family was included in the Child Labor Eradication Program (PETI) and began to receive monthly financial support. Adhering to the requirements for being enrolled in PETI, Fábio stopped working and resumed regular school attendance. The family received services at the Social Assistance Reference Center (CRAS) from various professions with different approaches. One intervention strategy enrolled Fábio in activities at the Sports and Leisure Center for children and adolescents located near his residence. An occupational therapist was responsible for following up on Fabio's process in PETI. The therapist's role was to suggest and assist with any changes necessary to improve Fabio's everyday experience at the center, to support his attendance at school, and to enhance his participation with his family and community.

To tailor their work to the particularities of a specific social field, occupational therapists have been guided by general guidelines, objectives, and intervention strategies that dialogue directly with the nature of the service, program, or project with which they are collaborating (Malfitano, 2005). Occupational therapists have been working to promote respect for the rights of children and adolescents through their professional expertise in using the power of human activity to generate welfare, products and materials, and symbolic practices significant for the individuals who perform them and for the collective in which they live (Castro, Lima, & Brunello, 2001). By exercising

BOX 13.5 Opportunities

The Sports and Leisure Center also provides the Service of Coexistence and Strengthening of Bonds (SCFV). Every working day, during the school period, in addition to his classes, Fábio participates in play, sports, and artistic and cultural activities appropriate for his age, sharing time with other young people of the same age group. Through this participation, he has found new opportunities for development that value and stimulate his autonomy. Through social and educational activities, Fábio learned about and reflected on the rights of children and youths in Brazil including the various situations that violate those rights. The theme of child labor, its consequences, and the need to tackle the problem were addressed in one of those activities.

Fábio's family has participated in these events to promote shared living among themselves and with the families of other children and adolescents who attend the center. Generally, these events are held on festive occasions, which are related to the local culture. Opportunities for joint action between parents and children are offered in recreational or playful activities.

BOX 13.6 Child–Family–Community

Solange participates in a group that meets for an hour and a half weekly and is coordinated by an occupational therapist. Most of the participants are mothers or grandmothers of children and adolescents who have had their rights violated. Group activities are varied (from watching a movie to making handcrafts) and are often determined by the group itself through consideration of the occupations, interests, and needs of participants. Through these groups, several opportunities are created: (1) discussion and reflection on the rights of children and adolescents and their importance for the construction of an equitable and more egalitarian society; (2) sharing of experiences among participants with an appreciation of each person's knowledge; (3) discussion about the difficulties faced by participants in their roles of protecting children and youths in their families; (4) support for decisions and life projects aimed at establishing family autonomy; and (5) referrals to professionals, services, and community resources that can broaden their social support network.

In these group activities, Solange expressed a desire to resume work.

their rights, children and adolescents can experience a wide range of activities that offer opportunities for full human development in individual and collective spheres.

To this end, the following operational guidelines are proposed:

- Foster the participation of children, youths, families, groups, and communities that are or have been involved in child labor in meaningful activities to offer opportunities for them to recognize themselves as individuals with rights. Participation in activities may be individual or in groups, and activities should be diversified to offer possibilities for experimentation, creation, personal development, personal expression, sharing of histories, and development of community and cultural identities, and for the acquisition or improvement of skills considered important by participants.
- Using activities and relationships established in the process of doing, provide opportunities for the exercise and valuing of autonomy, choice, being a protagonist in their life, and emancipation.
- Provide shared experiences based on mutual respect and valuing of individual and/or collective powers and knowledge to create and/or expand relational spaces in which these values are validated and practiced. Dialogue should support such experiences, as well as other concepts guiding the methodologies of social occupational therapy (Barros, 2004).
- Provide encouragement and support for ongoing lifelong projects, whose meanings emerge from human relationships and the intersection of the objective dimensions of an experienced problem and its subjective interpretation (Barros, 2004). Life projects associated with the exercise of rights, the protection and defense of interests, and the provision of needs for children and youths should be encouraged.

Finally, it is worth noting that efforts to enhance resources and activate the powers of children, youths, families, and communities to reflect and act on the problem of child labor should not be based on the logic of individualism and its emphasis on individual responsibility; otherwise, those efforts would become marred by politicization. Combatting child labor and deconstructing the social narratives that support it can only be achieved with parallel efforts to combat poverty and domination and the social narratives that reinforce them.

REFERENCES

Almeida, M. C., Soares, C. R. S., Barros, D. D., & Galvani, D. (2012). Processos e práticas de formalização da Terapia Ocupacional na Assistência Social: alguns marcos e desafios [Formalization processes and practices of occupational therapy in social assistance: Landmarks and challenges]. *Brazilian Journal of Occupational Therapy, 20*(1), 33–41. doi:10.4322/cto.2012.004

Araújo, C. M. G. (2010). *A exploração da força de trabalho infantil na fumicultura no município de Angelina* [Exploitation of child labor in tobacco forming of the city of Angelina (SC)] (Dissertação de Mestrado). Florianópolis, SC, Brasil: Sociologia, Universidade Federal de Santa Catarina. Retrieved from repositorio.ufsc.br/bitstream/handle/123456789/103270/280290.pdf?sequence=1

Barros, D. D. (2004). Terapia ocupacional social: o caminho se faz ao caminhar [Notes for a social occupational therapy: The way is done by the way we go]. *Revista de Terapia Ocupacional da Universidade de São Paulo, 15*(3), 90–97. doi:10.11606/issn.2238-6149.v15i3p90-97

Barros, D. D., Ghirardi, M. I. G., & Lopes, R. E. (2005). Social occupational therapy: A socio-historical perspective. In F. Kronenberg, S. Simó Algado, & N. Pollard (Eds.), *Occupational therapy without borders: Learning from the spirit of survivors* (pp. 140–151). Edinburgh: Elsevier/Churchill Livingstone.

Borba, P. L. O., Costa, S. L, Savani, A. C. C., Anastácio, C. C., & Ota, N. H. (2017). Entre fluxos, pessoas e territórios: delineando a inserção do terapeuta ocupacional no Sistema Único de Assistência Social [Between flows, people and territories: Outlining the insert of occupational therapist in the Brazilian Social Assistance System]. *Brazilian Journal of Occupational Therapy, 25*(1), 203–214. doi:10.4322/0104-4931.ctoRE0758

Brasil. (1988). Constituição da Republica Federativa do Brasil de 1988. [Constitution of the Brazilian Federative Republic]. Brasília, Governo Federal.

Brasil, Ministério do Desenvolvimento Social e Combate à Fome (MDS). (2010). *Orientações Técnicas: gestão do programa de erradicação do trabalho infantil no SUAS* [Technical guidelines: Management of the child labor eradication program in SUAS]. Brasília: Author.

Brasil, Ministério do Desenvolvimento Social e Combate à Fome (MDS). (2018). *Caderno de Orientações Técnicas para Aperfeiçoamento da Gestão do Programa de Erradicação do Trabalho Infantil (PETI)* [Technical Guidance Booklet for the improvement of the management of the Child Labor Eradication Program (PETI)]. Brasília: Author.

Brasil, Secretaria Nacional de Assistência Social (SNAS). (2014). *Perguntas e respostas: O Redesenho do Programa de Erradicação do Trabalho Infantil* [Questions and answers: The redesign of the Child Labor Eradication Program]. Brasília: Author.

Carvalho, I. M. M. (2008). O trabalho infantil no Brasil contemporâneo [The child labor in Brazil contemporary]. *Caderno CRH, 21*(54), 551–569. doi:10.1590/S0103-49792008000300010

Castro, E. D., Lima, E. M. F. A., & Brunello, M. I. B. (2001). Atividades humanas e terapia ocupacional [Human activities and occupational therapy]. In M. M. R. De Carlo & C. C. Bartolotti (Eds.), *Terapia Ocupacional no Brasil* [Occupational therapy in Brazil]. São Paulo: Plexus.

Comissão Nacional de Erradicação do Trabalho Infantil (CONAETI). (2011). *Plano Nacional de Prevenção e Erradicação do Trabalho Infantil e Proteção do Adolescente Trabalhador* [*National plan for the prevention and eradication of child labor and protection of the adolescent worker*] (2nd ed.). Brasília: Author.

Comissão Nacional de Erradicação do Trabalho Infantil (CONAETI). (2018). *III Plano Nacional de Prevenção e Erradicação do Trabalho Infantil e Proteção do Adolescente Trabalhador (2019–2022).* [III National plan for the prevention and eradication of child labor and protection of the adolescent worker (2019–2022)]. Brasília: Author.

Di Giovanni, G. (2004). *Aspectos qualitativos do trabalho infantil no Brasil* [Qualitative aspects of child labor in Brazil]. Brasília: ILO/Brasil.

Instituto Brasileiro de Geografia e Estatística (IBGE). (2016). *Pesquisa Nacional por Amostra de Domicílio (PNAD): Síntese do levantamento 2015* [National Household Sample Survey (PNAD): Summary of the 2015 survey]. Rio de Janeiro: Author.

International Labour Organization (ILO). (2011). *ECOAR O Fim do Trabalho Infantil – Educação, Comunicação e Arte na Defesa dos Direitos da Criança e do Adolescente: versão resumida* [Supporting Children's Rights through Education, Arts and Media – Short version]. Brasília: Author.

International Labour Organization (ILO). (2013). *Medir o progresso na Luta contra o Trabalho Infantil: Estimativas e tendências mundiais 2000–2012* [Marking progress against child labor - Global estimates and trends 2000–2012]. Geneva: Author. Retrieved from https://www.ilo.org/wcmsp5/groups/public/—-ed_norm/—-ipec/documents/publication/wcms_221799.pdf

International Labour Organization (ILO). (2017). *Global estimates of child labour: Results and trends, 2012–2016.* Geneva: Author. Retrieved from https://www.ilo.org/wcmsp5/groups/public/—-dgreports/—-dcomm/documents/publication/wcms_575499.pdf

International Labour Organization (ILO/Brasil). (2013). Documento Orientador da III Conferência Global sobre Trabalho Infantil [Guiding document of the III Global Conference on Child Labor]. In *III Global Conference of Child Labour.* Brasília: Author.

Kassouf, A. L. (2007). O que conhecemos sobre o trabalho infantil? [What do we know about child labor?] *Nova Economia, 17*(2), 323–350. doi:10.1590/S0103-63512007000200005

Kassouf, A. L., & Santos, M. J. (2010). Consequências do trabalho infantil no rendimento futuro do trabalho dos brasileiros: diferenças regionais e de gênero [Consequence of child labor on the future income of Brazilians work: Regional and gender differences]. In *38º Encontro Nacional de Economia ANPEC,* Salvador. Retrieved from http://www.anpec.org.br/encontro2010/inscricao/arquivos/000-7bfe42d90954e5040f9bdae429f51e3c.pdf

Lopes, R. E., Barros, D. D., Malfitano, A. P. S., Galvani, D., & Galluzzi, A. M. (2001). Terapia Ocupacional no território: as crianças e os adolescentes da Unidade do Brás – Movimento de Luta por Moradia Urbana [Occupational therapy in the territory: The children and adolescents of the Brás Unit – Urban Housing Movement]. *Cadernos Brasileiros de Terapia Ocupacional, 9*(1), 30–49. Retrieved from http://www.cadernosdeterapiaocupacional.ufscar.br/index.php/cadernos/article/view/233

Lopes, R. E., Malfitano, A. P. S., Silva, C. R., & Borba, P. L. O. (2014). Recursos e tecnologias em Terapia Ocupacional Social: ações com jovens pobres na cidade [Resources and technologies in social occupational therapy: Actions with the poor youth in town]. *Brazilian Journal of Occupational Therapy, 22*(3), 591–602. doi:10.4322/cto.2014.081

Malfitano, A. P. S. (2005). Campos e núcleos de intervenção na terapia ocupacional social [Intervention fields and cores in social occupational therapy]. *Revista de Terapia Ocupacional da Universidade de São Paulo, 16*(1), 1–8. doi:10.11606/issn.2238-6149.v16i1p1-8

Marcilio, M. L. (1998). A lenta construção dos direitos da criança brasileira. Século XX [The slow construction of the rights of the Brazilian child – 20th century]. *Revista USP, 37,* 46–57. Retrieved from http://www.direitoshumanos.usp.br/index.php/Obras-recentemente-publicadas/a-lenta-construcao-dos-direitos-da-crianca-brasileira-seculo-xx-1998.html

Medeiros Neto, X. T., & Marques, R. D. (2013). *Manual de Atuação do Ministério Público na Prevenção e Erradicação do Trabalho Infantil* [Manual of public prosecution in the prevention and eradication of child labor]. Brasília: Conselho Nacional do Ministério Público.

Moura, E. B. B. (2013). Crianças operárias na recém-industrializada São Paulo [Children operated in the newly industrialized São Paulo]. In M. Del Priore (Ed.), *História das crianças no Brasil* [*History of children in Brazil*] (pp. 259–288). São Paulo: Contexto.

Repórter Brasil. (2013). *Brasil livre de trabalho infantil: Contribuições para o debate sobre a eliminação das piores formas do trabalho de crianças e adolescentes* [Brazil free of child labor: Contributions to the debate on eliminating the worst forms of child and adolescent labor]. São Paulo: Author.

Santos, E. (2017). *Trabalho infantil nas ruas, pobreza e discriminação: crianças invisíveis nos faróis da cidade de São Paulo* [Child labor in the streets, poverty and discrimination: Invisible children in traffic signal in São Paulo] (Dissertação de Mestrado). São Paulo, SP, Brazil: Instituto de Estudos Brasileiros, Universidade de São Paulo.

Sarti, C. A. (1999). Família e jovens: no horizonte das ações [Family and youth: On the horizon of actions]. *Revista Brasileira de Educação, 11,* 99–109. Retrieved from http://anped.tempsite.ws/novo_portal/rbe/rbedigital/RBDE11/RBDE11_10_ESPACO_ABERTO_-_CYNTHIA_A_SARTI.pdf

Vieira, M. G. (2009). *Trabalho infantil no Brasil: questões culturais e políticas públicas* [Child labor in Brazil: Cultural issues and public policies] (Dissertação de Mestrado). Brasília, DF, Brazil: Instituto de Ciências Sociais, Universidade de Brasília.

14

Informing Social Occupational Therapy: Unpacking the "Social" Using Critical Social Theory

Debbie Laliberte Rudman

Social occupational therapy, grounded within the particular social, historical, and political context of Brazil and with a rich history of development since the 1970s, is well positioned to make significant contributions to a larger contemporary turn towards addressing social issues within occupational therapy and occupational science (Malfitano, de Souza, Townsend, & Lopes, 2019; Malfitano, Lopes, Magalhães, & Townsend, 2014). In particular, social occupational therapy has illustrated the importance of underpinning social practices committed to inclusion, social rights, and social participation with critical social theoretical perspectives, including concepts from Gramsci, Castel, and Freire (Lopes & Malfitano, 2017).

Within this chapter, I argue that to responsibly and effectively attend to the "social" within social occupational therapy, as well as within the broader field of occupation-based social transformation, it is essential to continue to shift away from individualistic frames that have often underpinned occupational therapy practices and occupational science scholarship, particularly in the minority world (Laliberte Rudman, 2013). This shift is essential so that social transformation efforts avoid individualizing social problems, reinscribing power relations associated with oppression and colonialism, and reproducing occupational inequities (Galheigo, 2011; Farias & Laliberte Rudman, 2019; Gerlach, Teachman, Laliberte Rudman, Aldrich, & Huot, 2018). In turn, critical social theories provide lenses and concepts that can enable in-depth analysis of the social, as well as occupation itself, in ways that attend to power relations, forms of discrimination, and the range of political, economic, gendered, and other contextual conditions that shape and perpetuate occupational inequities (Farias, Laliberte Rudman, & Magalhães, 2016; Hammell & Iwama, 2012; Malfitano et al., 2019; Townsend, 2017). Such analysis can underpin the further

development and enactment of ethical, culturally humble, and critically informed approaches to occupation-based social transformation that reimagine and reconfigure discourses, social structures, systems, and practices so as to expand occupational possibilities, particularly for individuals and collectives facing social marginalization and oppression.

OCCUPATION-BASED SOCIAL TRANSFORMATION: CALLS AND CHALLENGES

There have been growing calls over the past two decades within occupational therapy and occupational science publications for the further development and enactment of social transformative practices (Galheigo, 2011; Galvaan & Peters, 2017; Laliberte Rudman et al., 2019). For example, van Bruggen (2017) challenged occupational therapy "to develop a transformative discipline, in which occupation is contributing to social changes" (p. 418), while Farias and Laliberte Rudman (2016) argued that "an emancipatory agenda is emerging within occupational science, building on the work of scholars who have advocated for a more critical, reflexive and socially responsive discipline" (p. 33).

Within this chapter, I use the term "occupation-based social transformation" to encompass a range of practices that aim to inform and enact transformations of discourses, social structures, social systems, and social practices in ways that work against occupational inequities (Farias et al., 2019; Laliberte Rudman et al., 2019). In addition to social occupational therapy, various terms and models have been used to name and promote occupation-based practices aimed at transformation at the social level, such as transformative practice or scholarship (Laliberte

Rudman, 2014), political practice (Pollard, Sakellariou, & Kronenberg, 2008), occupational reconstruction (Frank, 2013), critical occupational therapy practice (Guajardo & Mondaca, 2017; Hammell & Iwama, 2012), and occupation-based community development (Galvaan & Peters, 2017; Richards & Galvaan, 2018). Although each form has unique aspects, related to historical features, context, and theoretical foundations, they share an intent to mobilize occupation in social change efforts that shift beyond a focus on individuals and their occupational needs to address social forces and conditions shaping and perpetuating occupational inequities (Galvaan & Peters, 2017; Guajardo & Mondaca, 2017; Malfitano et al., 2014). As well, such practices are often positioned as addressing sociopolitical conditions to uphold the rights of all people, regardless of age, ability, social class, gender identity, or other axes of diversity, to participate in the range of occupations they need and want to do to flourish as individuals, collectives, and societies (Galheigo, 2011; World Federation of Occupational Therapists, 2006). Integrating cultural humility and a justice of difference, there is recognition of the need to commit to participatory practices of "working with," rather than working "for" or "on," persons and collectives facing occupational inequities, and to create space for the articulation of perspectives that are often marginalized or silenced (Hammell & Iwama, 2012; Richards & Galvaan, 2018). Moreover, there is an underpinning belief in the transformative potential of occupation (Frank & Zemke, 2008; Laliberte Rudman et al., 2019).

The development of forms of occupational therapy practice addressing social issues in South America is politically and historically situated within particular conditions, such as colonization and dictatorial forms of government, that shaped and perpetuated occupational, social, economic, health, and other disparities (Galheigo, 2011; Malfitano et al., 2014; Malfitano & Lopes, 2018). Within the contemporary global spread of neoliberalism, associated with growing occupational and other disparities within and across nations, the turn toward the social is increasingly framed as a necessity and a moral responsibility rather than just an expansion of practice areas (Frank & Zemke, 2008; Galheigo, 2011; Kirsh, 2015; Lopes & Malfitano, 2017). This necessity is encapsulated by Guajardo and Mondaca (2017):

> Everything that is related to people, their well-being, quality of life, justice and participation in an unequal, structurally segregated and violent world is an issue for occupational therapy. The profession has to say something about these issues and be part of transformative actions aimed at changing them. Indifference is not an option. (p. 105)

At the same time, concerns have been raised regarding hesitancies to fully move forward in enacting occupation-based social transformation, insufficient uptake of research and practice approaches that focus on social issues, and a rupture between theoretical commitments to address social issues and actual practice (Kirsh, 2015; Hammell & Iwama, 2012; Magalhães, 2012). For example, both a critical interpretive synthesis of research articles addressing occupational injustice and a scoping review of occupational therapy articles attending to occupational justice concepts concluded that scholarship and practice have often focused on individualized solution frames and practice approaches, even when attending to injustices shaped through social forces (Benjamin-Thomas & Laliberte Rudman, 2018; Malfitano et al., 2019). Another key set of concerns relates to the risks of moving forward with occupation-based social transformation in ways that reinscribe situations of oppression through the imposition of ways of thinking about and addressing occupation that are dominantly underpinned by Western perspectives (Hammell, 2015; Galheigo, 2011; Magalhães, Farias, Rivas-Quarneti, Alvarez, & Malfitano, 2019).

Given these growing calls as well as concerns, it is crucial to both identify the challenges to moving forward with occupation-based social transformation and build theoretical underpinnings and knowledge that will enable occupational therapists and scientists to do so in socially responsive, ethically appropriate, and culturally relevant ways (Farias & Laliberte Rudman, 2019; Galheigo, 2011). Dissertation work carried out by Lisette Farias provides insights into key barriers working against the realization of the ideals of occupation-based social transformative practices (Farias & Laliberte Rudman, 2019; Farias et al., 2019). Based on a critical dialogical study done in collaboration with five occupational therapists and scientists who are leaders in developing various forms of occupation-based social transformation, three interrelated challenges were identified as bounding possibilities for enacting such practices. These challenges included two dominant tendencies existing within occupational therapy and broader society. The first tendency involved the individualization of occupation, social issues, and responsibilities. This tendency encompassed ways that social issues, such as substance abuse and unemployment, are often framed as individual problems and responsibilities to be resolved through remediation and action at the individual level. The participants described how individualization worked against efforts to move analysis of issues to the social level and bounded possibilities for enacting practices that addressed the root causes of social issues. The second tendency involved the prioritization of health as a focus for intervention, along with the dominant use of a biomedical lens. The participants expressed how this tendency presented a challenge to addressing occupational inequities that could not be framed as within the health field. This narrowing of what was understood as the legitimate terrain for occupational therapy was further amplified by biomedical understandings of health focused on bodily functions and individual-level deficiencies. The third challenge identified was the pressure to maintain professional power, status, and accountability. This pressure was described as working against efforts to share power, shift away from expert-driven approaches, integrate local knowledges, and fully embrace participatory approaches (Farias & Laliberte Rudman, 2019).

Taken together, these three key barriers reinforce the assertions of other scholars that moving forward in enacting occupation-based social transformation requires radically rethinking many basic assumptions and practice approaches that characterize dominant approaches to occupational therapy employed within health care arenas, particularly in the Western world (Galheigo, 2011; Kirsh, 2015; Richards & Galvaan, 2018; Malfitano & Lopes, 2018). In particular, forces of individualism, shaped and reinforced through neoliberalism and biomedical frames, are key to counter and resist (Frank & Zemke, 2009; Hammell & Iwama, 2012; Gerlach et al., 2017; Laliberte Rudman, 2014; Malfitano & Lopes, 2018).

THE IMPERATIVE OF COUNTERING INDIVIDUALISM

Individualism is a term associated with many meanings; for example, it has been described as a philosophical perspective, a political ideology, and a methodological and epistemological perspective. At a general overarching level, individualism can be framed as a socially constructed constellation of ideas that have heavily influenced how "Western" society and its various systems, such as those related to the economy, welfare, health, and knowledge production, have been shaped over time in ways that emphasize the rights, responsibilities, and freedoms of individuals (Lukes, 2006). When applied to the context of framing social problems, individualism results in an "individualizing of the social" that "involves viewing various social issues and phenomena, including occupation, as primarily residing in and being shaped through individuals" (Gerlach et al., 2017, p. 36). To effectively attend to social issues through occupation-based social transformation, it is key to counter individualism so as to acknowledge, analyze, and address the "root" social, political, economic, and other factors shaping and perpetuating such issues and their implications for occupation (Galheigo, 2011; Hammell & Iwama, 2012; Laliberte Rudman, 2013; Lopes & Malfitano, 2017).

The imperative of countering individualism is particularly significant given that the rise of neoliberal political rationality has further intensified the "individualizing of the social," leading to increasing social disparities (Ferge, 1997; Laliberte Rudman, 2013; Polzer & Power, 2016). Within social policies, discourses, and systems, many social issues, such as unemployment, poverty, gender inequity, social exclusion in later life, or homelessness, have been increasingly reframed as individual failures or deficiencies. In parallel, the responsibilities for the resolution of such issues have increasingly been shifted onto individuals, aligning with a neoliberal retreat of the state (Brady, 2014; Ilcan, 2009; Polzer & Power, 2016). As well, neoliberal individualistic problem and solution frames obscure the sociopolitical production of social problems and their inequitable distribution along lines of age, race, gender, ability status, class, and other axes of diversity. When the contribution of broader social factors is acknowledged, these are often framed as the "ways things are" or immutable. Once social issues are framed as individual problems occurring within immutable structures, solutions often focus on how individuals can cope with, manage, or overcome inequities. In turn, as increasing demands are placed on individual citizens to find personal causes and solutions to collective or social problems, the vulnerability of marginalized groups is enhanced, and health, occupational, economic, and other forms of social inequities are intensified (Coburn, 2000; Ilcan, 2009; Laliberte Rudman, 2013; Mooney, 2012). Thus, for example, ageism may be acknowledged as a form of discrimination embedded within policies, systems, and everyday relations, but "positive aging" discourses exhort aging individuals to combat ageism and take up the responsibility to age well through lifestyle, consumer, and other "choices." At the same time, the inequitable distribution of the resources required to make such "choices" becomes obscured, while social resources to support health, well-being, and occupational participation are simultaneously reduced (Laliberte Rudman, 2017).

Many authors, from diverse geographical locations, have raised concerns that occupational therapy and occupational science, as developed in the West or minority world, are also imbued with individualism (Hammell & Iwama, 2012; Galheigo, 2011; Guajardo & Mondaca, 2017; Hocking, 2012; Kronenberg & Pollard, 2006). It has been asserted that humans have primarily being conceptualized and studied as self-made, self-directed occupational beings (Guajardo & Mondaca, 2017; Hocking, 2012; Laliberte Rudman, 2013). In addition, individualism has influenced understandings of occupation and related constructs, such as choice, identity, adaptation, and motivation, embedded in dominant models of occupational therapy practice. This has meant that occupation, and these related constructs, are primarily understood, studied, and addressed as generated by individuals who are independent of or separate from environments (Hammell, 2015; Laliberte Rudman, 2013). Such understandings then shape, and reinforce, practice approaches that emphasize enabling occupation through remediating or developing individuals' skills, knowledge, behaviors, or bodily and mental capacities, as well as enhancing their abilities to cope with and adapt to the conditions of their lives (Gerlach et al., 2017; Hammell & Iwama, 2012). Individualistic practice approaches are further reinforced through the uptake of biomedical and postpositivist perspectives that frame illness, health, and disability as individual experiences and neglect the social and structural determinants of health and the sociopolitical production of disability (Farias et al., 2019; Gerlach et al., 2018; Guajardo & Mondaca, 2017).

Although not negating that this individualistic orientation as taken up in occupational therapy and science has generated valuable knowledge and individual-level practices that make important contributions to people's occupations and well-being, the dominance of individualism is a key constraint in moving forward in occupation-based social transformation. Its constraining force arises because the uptake of individualism in the profession and discipline leads to (1) conceptualizing and addressing challenges related to occupation as individual problems and experiences, rather than as collective or social problems; (2) insufficiently attending to the ways that occupation and occupational beings are socially and politically constituted; and (3) neglecting the sociopolitical conditions that create and sustain inequities for individuals and collectives (Hocking, 2012; Gerlach et al., 2018; Laliberte Rudman, 2013, 2014). As articulated by Hammell (2015), "the dominance of an individualistic ideology which posits individuals as responsible for their own achievements distracts our profession from challenging and changing those structural inequalities—economic, religious, socio-cultural and political—that constrain occupational opportunities and occupational rights, not only of individuals, but of entire communities" (p. 719).

Beyond being a poor fit with occupation-based social transformation, the use of individualistic perspectives and practices to address social issues may result in "the perpetuation, rather than the resolution, of occupational inequities" (Gerlach et al., 2018, p. 35). Within the broader neoliberal "individualizing of the social," this means that occupational therapy and occupational science may inadvertently be complicit in dominant power relations that shape and perpetuate occupational and other forms of inequities for particular collectives, such as aging persons with chronic disabilities, youth living in poverty, or immigrants facing restrictive integration policies (Galheigo,

2011; Laliberte Rudman, 2014). Put simply, if our approaches to analyzing and addressing occupational inequities also place "increasing demands on individuals to find personal causes and solutions to socially produced problems pertaining to occupation" (Laliberte Rudman, 2013, p. 302), we risk being complicit with the perpetuation of occupational inequities for collectives who are marginalized within contemporary power relations (Guajardo & Mondaca, 2017; Hammell & Iwama, 2012). If the term "social" in occupation-based social transformation "implies that human emancipation depends on the transformation of the social world and not just the individual inner self" (Farias et al., 2016, p. 239), it becomes imperative to be counter to individualism. One way forward in doing so involves taking up critical social theory to develop understandings of occupation and enact practices that attend to the sociopolitical production of occupational inequities (Gerlach et al., 2018; Hammell & Iwama, 2012).

QUESTIONING AND TRANSFORMING THE SOCIAL: CRITICAL SOCIAL THEORY

Critical social theories offer a key way forward in enhancing occupation-based social transformation. Such theories can support a shift in scholarly and practice attention toward ways in which occupation and occupational inequities are shaped within social, cultural, political, institutional, historical, and economic contexts, shifting away from viewing occupations as personal choices or as completely within the control of individuals. Such in-depth analysis will locate problems at the social level and, in turn, inform solutions that address social discourses, structures, systems, and practices perpetuating occupational inequities (Hammell & Iwama, 2012; Galheigo, 2011; Laliberte Rudman, 2013, 2014; Njelesani, Gibson, Nixon, Cameron, & Polatajko, 2013; Richards & Galvaan, 2018). In addition to questioning and countering individualistic analyses, critical social theories also provide a means to resist ethnocentric tendencies through enacting continuous critical reflexivity regarding guiding assumptions and positionality, as well as deploying participatory practices that embrace diverse ways of knowing and doing (Farias, Laliberte Rudman, Magalhães, & Gastaldo, 2017; Galvaan & Peters, 2017; Hammell & Iwawa, 2012).

The term "critical" has a multiplicity of meanings. Within the context of critical social theories, it encompasses a particular philosophical or paradigmatic stance that underpins a diversity of theoretical perspectives that address issues of social justice, diversity, equity, and transformation (Njelesani et al., 2013). As examples, critical social theories encompass theoretical perspectives such as critical race theories, postcolonial theories, critical feminist theories, queer theories, and critical disability perspectives, and theorists such as Foucault, Friere, and Bakhtin (Gibson, 2016; Hammell & Iwawa, 2015). Taking up critical social theories to rethink and reimagine conceptualizations of occupation, analyses of occupation-based inequities, and socially transformative practices extends beyond expanding current theories to encompass "re-examining the ontological bases, assumptions, values and ethics" (Farias & Laliberte Rudman, 2016, p. 34) underpinning occupation-focused scholarship and practices.

In relation to understanding the social, critical social theories adopt a position of tentative or historical realism. This position assumes that what is taken to be "real" within a particular societal context is always a product of ongoing power relations, constructed through sociopolitical forces that privilege certain collectives, ways of being, and ways of doing while simultaneously marginalizing and oppressing other collectives, ways of being, and ways of doing (Cannella & Lincoln, 2009, 2011; Farias & Laliberte Rudman, 2013; Njelesani et al., 2013). Thus, "truth" and knowledge are always viewed as value laden and partial, and there is a recognition that "what counts as legitimate knowledge arises from historical, political, and social conditions" (Gibson, 2016, p. 3). In turn, as social reality is always constructed, it has the potential to be transformed through deconstructing how inequities have come to be constructed and sustained within particular contextual conditions and social power relations and imagining and working toward enacting other ways of being and doing (Cannella & Lincoln, 2009).

From this ontological frame, occupations are conceptualized as situated, relational, and political. Occupation is viewed as inseparable from social, political, economic, historical, cultural, gendered, and other contextual forces, and occupational inequities are assumed to be shaped within social power relations. Thus, occupation itself is conceptualized as political, used as a means to govern others in explicit and implicit ways. In turn, occupation can also be taken up as a means to resist and reconfigure power relations, such as those related to racism, ageism, classism, sexism, and other forms of discrimination (Guajardo & Mondaca, 2017; Hammell & Iwama, 2012; Pollard et al., 2009).

The common epistemological starting point and commitment of critical social theories involves questioning what has come to be taken for granted as "true" about the way the world is, particularly when dominant discourses, structures, systems, and practices produce and perpetuate inequities (Gibson, 2016). Critically informed analysis and reasoning refuse to accept how a problem has come to be constructed within dominant discourses and policies, particularly when constructions individualize social issues

(Farias et al., 2017). Such analysis and reasoning involve questioning and deconstructing the dominant, taken-for-granted ways societal elements are structured; the ideas that shape and support such elements; and the practices that flow from dominant structures and ideas (Hammell & Iwama, 2012; Laliberte Rudman, 2013, 2014). There is also a focus on how various forms of power operate to shape everyday human possibilities for being and doing (Gibson, 2016; Njelesani et al., 2013). Within many critical theories, for example, there is a focus on power in relation to the construction of language and knowledge, as it is proposed that the construction of reality occurs through language in ways that shape how particular phenomena, such as mental illness or poverty, and particular types of people, such as migrants or persons experiencing unemployment, come to be understood and addressed at micro to macro levels (Foucault, 1982; Mumby, 2004). Overall, foundational questions guiding critically informed analyses of the social include attending to what types of subjects and ways of doing are helped, privileged, and legitimated by current societal arrangements and what types of subjects and ways of doing are harmed, oppressed, and disqualified (Cannella & Lincoln, 2009, 2011; Nixon, Yeung, Shaw, Kuper, & Gibson, 2017).

Taking up a critical epistemological stance within occupational therapy and science can promote a constant vigilance and questioning of the "way things are" within society, as well as within the profession and discipline, particularly when current structures, systems, and practices shape and perpetuate occupational inequities (Laliberte Rudman, 2013, 2014). Critically informed analysis and reasoning can support in-depth understandings of the sociopolitical production of occupational inequities, thus providing a road map for occupation-based social transformation (Townsend, 2017). An array of critically informed concepts has been developed within recent occupational therapy and science scholarship, such as occupational possibilities (Laliberte Rudman, 2010), occupational consciousness (Ramugondo, 2015), resource-seeking occupations (Aldrich, Laliberte Rudman, & Dickie, 2017), resistive occupations (Pyatak & Muccitelli, 2011), and nonsanctioned occupations (Kiepek, Beagan, Laliberte Rudman, & Phelan, 2018). Such concepts locate challenges to occupation within social, political, economic, gendered, ableist, and other contextual features. These concepts, in turn, have been used to critically analyze the boundaries and unintended consequences of current approaches in occupational therapy practice, as well as occupational inequities experienced by collectives within broader societal contexts (Njelesani et al., 2013).

Indeed, critical social theories have been increasingly incorporated into studies of occupation, with such studies illustrating how this incorporation enhances understanding of occupation as social, relational, and political and can inform occupation-based social transformation (Farias & Laliberte Rudman, 2016, 2019). As one example, Njelesani, Teachman, Durocher, Hamdani, and Phelan (2015) drew upon the concept of occupational possibilities and a critical occupational approach to "identify and problematize assumptions regarding the value of approximating normal occupational possibilities" (p. 252) as enacted in three different practice contexts. Their analysis raises concerns regarding how practice aligned with approximating normative occupations and normative ways of doing occupation may inadvertently limit the range of occupational possibilities addressed within practice, unintentionally shaping situations of social exclusion and marginalization and reproducing taken-for-granted social expectations for occupation. To more fully enact client-centered practice and support diverse occupational possibilities, these authors outline directions for incorporating critical reflexivity and advocacy into practice to counter societal normative expectations and "envision possibilities for occupation that would be missed altogether in the pursuit of normal" (p. 7). The work of Cloete and Ramugondo (2015), which addressed excessive drinking practices among pregnant women in a region of South Africa, provides a critically informed example addressing a broader social issue. Expanding beyond understandings of such drinking practices as an individual coping strategy within oppressive social conditions, these authors employ a critically informed occupational lens to frame such drinking practices as "imposed occupations." This concept of imposed occupations draws attention to how occupations, often those that are deemed to be nonsanctioned, can be structurally imposed upon collectives, over time, through historical, cultural, and sociopolitical factors. Enhanced understanding of such structural entrenchment aids in understanding the persistence of such occupations, even when they have detrimental individual and social implications. As well, this concept highlights that addressing "imposed occupations" needs to extend beyond individual-level interventions to transform the social, political, economic, and other factors that have shaped their structural entrenchment.

CONCLUSION

Moving in socially transformative directions is increasingly framed as a moral responsibility of occupational therapists and scientists, within a global context in which various forms of inequities, including occupational inequities, are increasing (Guajardo & Mondaca, 2017; Laliberte Rudman, 2018). Building on the foundations established by social occupational therapy, continuing to move forward in

developing and enacting occupation-based social transformation requires further integration of critical social theories to work against individualizing tendencies and attend to power relations. Critical social theories can be productively taken up in ways that promote in-depth analysis of the production of social problems and occupational inequities. Such theories can also inform the development of solutions that address how social elements—at discursive, structural, systemic, and practice levels—can be transformed to expand occupational possibilities for collectives who are marginalized within contemporary power relations and contextual conditions.

Overall, critical social theories are aligned with a commitment to social transformation (Farias et al., 2017); as stated by Nixon and colleagues (2017), "critical approaches are emancipatory in their aims, whereby new ways of seeing give rise to novel and more progressive actions to promote equity" (p. 250). Alternative spaces for knowing and doing can be opened up through problematizing what has come to be commonly accepted as "truth" regarding a social issue and its solution frames (Gibson, 2016) and through exposing contradictions, tensions, and inequities that exist within what has come to be dominantly viewed as "natural" or "the way the world is" (Laliberte Rudman, 2014; Njelesani et al., 2013). Within this space, dialogical and participatory approaches to imagining and enacting alternative discourses, structures, systems, and practices with collectives who are marginalized, silenced, and oppressed within current societal arrangements offer a way forward in transformative efforts (Guajardo & Mondaca, 2017; Hammell & Iwama, 2012; Sandwick et al., 2018). As described by Guajardo and Mondaca (2017), such critically informed occupational therapy practice would aim to transform social relations and everyday practices in ways that work against occupational inequities and would respect and dialogue with diverse worldviews "to imagine and build other possible worlds, other subjects, other ways of life" (p. 107).

REFERENCES

Aldrich, R. M., Laliberte Rudman, D., & Dickie, V. A. (2017). Resource seeking as occupation: A critical and empirical exploration. *American Journal of Occupational Therapy, 71*(3), 1–9.

Benjamin-Thomas, T. E., & Laliberte Rudman, D. (2018). A critical interpretive syntheses: Use of the occupational justice framework in research. *Australian Occupational Therapy Journal, 65*, 2–14.

Brady, M. (2014). Ethnographies of neoliberal governmentalities: From the neoliberal apparatus to neoliberalism and governmental assemblages. *Foucault Studies, 18*, 11–33.

Cannella, G. S., & Lincoln, Y. S. (2009). Deploying qualitative methods for critical social purposes. In N. K. Denzin & M. D. Giardina (Eds.), *Qualitative inquiry and social justice* (pp. 53–72). Los Angeles, CA: West Coast.

Cannella, G. S., & Lincoln, Y. S. (2011). Ethics, research regulations and critical social science. In N. K. Denzin & Y. S. Lincoln (Eds.), *The Sage handbook of qualitative research* (4th ed., pp. 81–90). Los Angeles, CA: Sage.

Cloete, L. G., & Ramugondo, E. L. (2015). "I drink": Mothers' alcohol consumption as both individualised and imposed occupation. *South African Journal of Occupational Therapy*, 45(1), 34–40.

Coburn, D. (2000). Income inequality, social cohesion and the health status of populations: The role of neo-liberalism. *Social Science & Medicine*, 51(1), 135–146.

Farias, L., & Laliberte Rudman, D. L. (2016). A critical interpretive synthesis of the uptake of critical perspectives in occupational science. *Journal of Occupational Science*, 23(1), 33–50.

Farias, L., & Laliberte Rudman, D. L. (2019). Challenges in enacting occupation-based social transformative practices: A critical dialogical study. *Canadian Journal of Occupational Therapy*. doi:0008417419828798

Farias, L. V., Laliberte Rudman, D. L., & Magalhães, L. (2016). Illustrating the importance of critical epistemology to realize the promise of occupational justice. *OTJR: Occupation, Participation and Health*, 36(4), 234–243

Farias, L., Laliberte Rudman, D. L., Magalhães, L., & Gastaldo, D. (2017). Reclaiming the potential of transformative scholarship to enable social justice. *International Journal of Qualitative Methods*, 36(4), 234–243.

Farias, L., Laliberte Rudman, D. L., Pollard, N., Schiller, S., Malfitano, A. P. S., Thomas, K., et al. (2019). Critical dialogical approach: A methodological direction for occupation-based social transformation. *Scandinavian Journal of Occupational Therapy*, 26(4), 235–245.

Ferge, Z. (1997). The changed welfare paradigm: The individualization of the social. *Social Policy & Administration*, 31(1), 20–44.

Foucault, M. (1982). The subject and power. *Critical Inquiry*, 8(4), 777–795.

Frank, G. (2013). Twenty-first century pragmatism and social justice: Problematic situations and occupational reconstructions in post-civil war Guatemala. In M. P. Cutchin & V. A. Dickie (Eds.), *Transactional perspectives on occupation* (pp. 229–243). New York, NY: Springer.

Frank, G., & Zemke, R. (2008). Occupational therapy foundations for political engagement and social transformation. In N. Pollard, D. Sakellariou, & F. Kronenberg (Eds.), *A political practice of occupational therapy* (pp. 111–136). New York, NY: Churchill Livingstone.

Galheigo, S. M. (2011). What needs to be done? Occupational therapy responsibilities and challenges regarding human rights. *Australian Occupational Therapy Journal*, 58, 60–66.

Galvaan, R., & Peters, L. (2017). Occupation-based community development: Confronting the politics of occupation. In D. Sakellariou & N. Pollard (Eds.), *Occupational therapy without borders: Integrating justice and practice* (2nd ed., pp. 283–291). Edinburgh, UK: Elsevier.

Gerlach, A. J., Teachman, G., Laliberte Rudman, D. L., Aldrich, R. M., & Huot, S. (2018). Expanding beyond individualism: Engaging critical perspectives on occupation. *Scandinavian Journal of Occupational Therapy*, 25(1), 35–43.

Gibson, B. E. (2016). Commentary: Critical rehabilitation research – Why it matters for all research. *rehabINK*, 1(2), 1–6.

Guajardo, A., & Mondaca, M. (2017). Human rights, occupational therapy and the centrality of social practices. In D. Sakellariou & N. Pollard (Eds.), *Occupational therapy without borders: Integrating justice and practice* (2nd ed., pp. 101–108). Edinburgh, UK: Elsevier.

Hammell, K. W. (2015). Respecting global wisdom: Enhancing the cultural relevance of occupational therapy's theoretical base. *British Journal of Occupational Therapy*, 78(11), 718–721.

Hammell, K. W., & Iwama, M. K. (2012). Well-being and occupational rights: An imperative for critical occupational therapy. *Scandinavian Journal of Occupational Therapy*, 19(5), 385–394.

Hocking, C. (2012). Occupations through the looking glass: Reflecting on occupational scientists' ontological assumptions. In G. E. Whiteford & C. Hocking (Eds.), *Occupational science: Society, inclusion and participation* (pp. 54–68). Oxford, UK: Wiley-Blackwell.

Ilcan, S. (2009). Privatizing responsibility: Public sector reform under neoliberal government. *Foucault Studies*, 18, 11–33.

Kiepek, N. C., Beagan, B., Laliberte Rudman, D., & Phelan, S. (2019). Silences around occupations framed as unhealthy, illegal and deviant. *Journal of Occupational Science*, 26(3), 341–353.

Kirsh, B. H. (2015). Transforming values into action: Advocacy as a professional imperative. *Canadian Journal of Occupational Therapy*, 82(4), 212–223.

Kronenberg, F., & Pollard, N. (2006). Political dimensions of occupation and the roles of occupational therapy. *American Journal of Occupational Therapy*, 60, 617–626.

Laliberte Rudman, D. (2013). Enacting the critical potential of occupational science: Problematizing the "'individualizing of occupation.'" *Journal of Occupational Science*, 20(4), 298–313.

Laliberte Rudman, D. (2014). Embracing and enacting an "'occupational imagination'": Occupational science as transformative. *Journal of Occupational Science*, 21(4), 373–388.

Laliberte Rudman, D. (2017). The duty to age well: Critical reflections on occupational possibilities shaped through discursive and policy responses to population aging. In N. Pollard & D. Sakellariou (Eds.), *Occupational therapy without borders: Integrating justice with practice* (2nd ed., pp. 319–327). Edinburgh, UK: Elsevier.

Laliberte Rudman, D. L. (2018). Occupational therapy and occupational science: Building critical and transformative alliances. *Cadernos Brasileiros de Terapia Ocupacional*, 26(1), 241–249.

Laliberte Rudman, D. L., Pollard, N., Craig, C., Kantartzis, S., Piskur, B., Simó Algado, S., et al. (2019). Contributing to social transformation through occupation: Experiences from a think tank. *Journal of Occupational Science*, 26(2), 316–322.

Lopes, R. E., & Malfitano, A. P. S. (2017). Social occupational therapy, citizenship, rights, and policies: Connecting the voices of individuals and collectives. In D. Sakellariou & N. Pollard (Eds.), *Occupational therapy without borders: Integrating justice and practice* (2nd ed., pp. 245–254). Edinburgh, UK: Elsevier.

Lukes, S. (2006). *Individualism.* Wivenhoe Park, UK: ECPR Press.

Magalhães, L. (2012). What would Paulo Freire think of occupational science? In G. E. Whiteford & C. Hocking (Eds.), *Occupational science: Society, inclusion, participation* (pp. 8–19). West Sussex, UK: Wiley-Blackwell.

Magalhães, L., Farias, L., Rivas-Quarneti, N., Alvarez, L., & Malfitano, A. P. S. (2019). The development of occupational science outside the Anglophone sphere: Enacting global collaboration. *Journal of Occupational Science, 26*(2), 181–192.

Malfitano, A. P., de Souza, R. G. D. M., Townsend, E., & Lopes, R. E. (2019). Do occupational justice concepts inform occupational therapists' practice? A scoping review. *Canadian Journal of Occupational Therapy, 86,* 299–312. doi:10.1177/0008417419833409

Malfitano, A. P., & Lopes, R. E. (2018). Social occupational therapy: Committing to social change. *New Zealand Journal of Occupational Therapy, 65,* 20–26.

Malfitano, A. P., Lopes, R. E., Magalhães, L., & Townsend, E. A. (2014). Social occupational therapy: Conversations about a Brazilian experience. *Canadian Journal of Occupational Therapy, 81*(5), 298–307.

Mooney, G. (2012). Neoliberalism is bad for our health. *International Journal of Health Services, 42*(3), 383–401.

Mumby, D. K. (2004). Discourse, power and ideology: Unpacking the critical approach. In D. Grant, C. Hardy, C. Oswick, & L. Putnam (Eds.), *The Sage handbook of organizational discourse studies* (pp. 237–258). Los Angeles, CA: Sage.

Nixon, S., Yeung, E., Shaw, J. A., Kuper, A., & Gibson, B. E. (2017). Seven-step framework for critical analysis and its application in the field of physical therapy. *Physical Therapy, 97*(2), 249–257.

Njelesani, J., Gibson, B. E., Nixon, S., Cameron, D., & Polatajko, H. J. (2013). Towards a critical occupational approach to research. *International Journal of Qualitative Methods, 12*(1), 207–220.

Njelesani, J., Teachman, G., Durocher, E., Hamdani, Y., & Phelan, S. K. (2015). Thinking critically about client-centred practice and occupational possibilities across the life span. *Scandinavian Journal of Occupational Therapy, 22*(4), 252–259.

Pollard, N., Sakellariou, D., & Kronenberg, F. (2008). Introduction. In N. Pollard, D. Sakellariou, & F. Kronenberg (Eds.), *A political practice of occupational therapy.* London, UK: Churchill-Livingstone.

Polzer, J., & Power, E. (2016). The governance of health in neoliberal societies. In J. Polzer & E. Power (Eds.), *Neoliberal governance and health: Duties, risks and responsibilities* (pp. 3–42). Kingston, Canada: McGill-Queen's University Press.

Pyatak, E., & Muccitelli, L. (2011). Rap music as resistive occupation: constructions of Black American identity and culture for performers and their audiences. *Journal of Occupational Science, 18*(1), 48–61.

Ramugondo, E. L. (2015). Occupational consciousness. *Journal of Occupational Science, 22*(4), 488–501.

Richards, L., & Galvaan, R. (2018). Developing a socially transformative focus in occupational therapy: Insights from South African practice. *South African Journal of Occupational Therapy, 48*(1), 3–8.

Sandwick, T., Fine, M., Greene, A. C., Stoudt, B. G., Torre, M. E., & Patel, L. (2018). Promise and provocation: Humble reflections on critical participatory action research on social policy. *Urban Education, 53*(4), 473–502.

Townsend, E. (2017). Social problems through an occupational lens. *Japanese Journal of Occupational Science, 11,* 12–27.

van Bruggen, H. E. (2017). Mind the gap: Addressing inequalities in health through occupation-based practices. In D. Sakellariou & N. Pollard (Eds.), *Occupational therapy without borders: Integrating justice and practice* (2nd ed., pp. 411–423). Edinburgh, UK: Elsevier.

World Federation of Occupational Therapists. (2006). *Position statement, human rights.* Retrieved from https://www.wfot.org/resources/human-rights

15

Occupational Therapy on the Move: On Contextualizing Citizenships and Epistemicide

Nick Pollard, Inés Viana-Moldes,
Hetty Fransen-Jaïbi, and Sarah Kantartzis

INTRODUCTION

Citizenship and the forms of societal organizations that make citizenship possible have emerged at different and quite independent points in history. As this book celebrates a southern epistemological perspective of occupational therapy, situated in Brazil, which has emerged from post-colonial history and movements against tyranny, this chapter will explore citizenship and occupation in a wider context than the traditional exposition that it must first begin with. While citizenship received a considerable exploration and focus in the original edition of this book, this was in the context of the evolution of social occupational therapy as a response to conditions such as structural poverty, economic and political barriers, and authoritarianism in Brazilian communities (see Section 1, Chapter 1). Across Latin America, as professional organizations celebrated significant anniversaries of their foundation during the middle of the decade, occupational therapy associations traced their distinctive historical origins, often against decades of social injustice and inequality that accompanied vertiginous economic development and that look toward the development of occupation as a human right and this right as an ethic of practice (Guajardo Córdoba & Galhiego, 2015). Further to this work from Latin America, the connection between citizenship and occupational therapy has been little explored in Anglophone professional literature and in occupational science. In English-language texts, the term "citizen" is generally used as an alternative to people or individuals, as in "senior citizens," and rarely in the sense of a citizen enacting rights or in the joint construction of a social and public world by citizens.

The authors of this chapter, the ENOTHE citizenship group, have critically explored some of the dominant influences on occupational therapists' partnerships with citizens, groups, and communities from perspectives on citizenship as a framing paradigm in order to recognize and problematize broader population needs. We have attempted to challenge assumptions within the dominant paradigms and frameworks leading our profession and develop an understanding of how occupation and health relate to citizenship, social justice, and human development. The four of us, all university educators in occupational therapy, bring together multiple citizenships, citizenship experiences, and belongings, geographically originated in Brazil and Spain, Ireland, Greece and Scotland, Tunisia and the Netherlands, and England, as well as living with and knowledge of several languages (namely Spanish, Portuguese, Dutch, French, Arabic, Greek, and English), all being fluent in at least two or three languages. These multiple citizenship configurations of our coexisting citizenship stories are built upon experiences of migration, transnationality, postcolonialism, cultural diversity, and socioeconomic and political realities, nourishing our reflections and debates about citizenship, occupation, and occupational therapy. As a group, working together since 2013, we have regularly reflected on our own positions as citizens in an increasingly globalized world and are engaged in the ongoing debate about how professional practice should address present and future contexts. Our contribution of this chapter will be framed by a critical reflection exposing multiple aspects of the concept of citizenship as an important paradigm for understanding broader issues, as well as for the strategic positioning and actions of citizens, societies, and occupational therapists. Citizenship is an evolving concept, dependent on cultural, socioeconomic, political, and historical contexts. It may be a helpful concept and lens, describing and questioning the social realities we live in, we are part of, and we are produced by.

While the concept of citizenship may be considered as the expression of an "ideal" (and so static) situation, such binary thinking both limits and simplifies our understanding. Citizenship is a contested and complex concept, fluid and used in multiple ways in time and place. We need to apply complex thinking to help us better understand and work with the processes and the contexts of the challenges of the world today and to prepare us for changes and for the understanding of their nature. Complexity thinking in this chapter is enacted in the presentation of and working with multiple perspectives and the process of weaving them together, linking viewpoints, different disciplines of thought, and levels of analysis.

Our (critical) discussion is based in two main elements. One is a historical-economic British perspective focusing on the development of capitalism, market-related principles, and colonialism through which Britain's economic privilege has influenced global history (Kabeer, 2002; De Sousa Santos, 2018a). The other is an epistemological perspective based in the work of De Sousa Santos (2015), a Portuguese sociologist, on epistemicide to address issues of citizenship related to power and powerlessness, decolonization and marginalization, and the (de)construction of knowledge. It aligns the assertion of citizenship rights with the philosophical roots of the profession in social reform and the perspectives of citizenship against the dynamic of social inequities and the thrust of the rest of this book. It concludes with some thoughts on the ethical responsibilities of professionals on the enablement of citizenship.

REFLECTIONS ON COEXISTENT CITIZENSHIPS

Civic Societies

Everywhere in the world where people live in groups, some form of social organization has to be contracted to enable survival, manage resources, prevent excessive conflict, and facilitate trading. While typically we consider civic society and the relationships of citizens in terms of nations, such organization also might be developed between groups of people who need no larger allegiances or else who may form confederations with similar groups, without government (Mann, 2005). The form a society takes stems from geographical, social, and economic forces combined with the effects of weather and topography on crops and farming, the accessibility of natural resources to mining techniques and wind or waterpower for processing materials, and the accessibility of routes for trade or for making war. Factors such as these determine how political systems develop and people organize processes such as trade, work, marriage,

storing foods and materials, and festivals—the features that shape a civil society through which a concept like citizenship is realized. Social existence has taken different forms throughout history according to local contexts and environments. Awareness of the coexistence of diverse societies and ways of living together simultaneously (or not) is needed to (re)think the complexities of citizenship.

The hunter-gatherer societies were (and still are in some limited situations today) characterized by their high mobility based on the abundance of resources available to survive (Ruiz, 2005). Issues and values relevant to their daily common life include action sympathetic to the environment so as not to deplete natural resources; not having fixed homes and only having a few, mostly exchangeable, possessions to facilitate personal mobility—which in turn emphasizes that generosity and reciprocity are valued over selfish acquisition and that barter strengthens social relations; population control to maintain balance with existing resources, through abortion and infanticide; and physical resistance to scarcity (Harris, 1994; Ruiz, 2005; Diamond, 2013). In these societies, there is gender division; the women take care of the children and gathering, while the men explore the environment and hunt animals.

New social orders emerge where hunter-gatherer societies, composed primarily of family or kinship groups, have transitioned to larger farming societies (Harris, 1994). Larger groups of people have to establish processes for living together that go beyond family affiliations, with more sedentary societies; more labor required to work crops, domesticate animals, and develop tools and pottery; and the emergence of surplus production and its storage. These features, evident in the Neolithic Revolution (Harris, 1994), required the organization of rights around the ownership of land, the buying and selling of products and labor, and many other aspects of emerging urban life.

In feudal societies, as well as those with limited industrialization, while many people may not be involved in day-to-day government and legal processes, the large majority of self-employed—artisans, farmers, tradespeople—are involved in everyday processes of creation with control over their work while also engaged in networks of collaboration across the society.

With the rise of industrial, capitalist societies, new forms of production and daily life emerged. Machines replaced artisan work and generated an increase in bureaucratic tasks as a new logic of production stimulated the meta-fragmentation of the workforce and its knowledge. Populations increasingly moved from the countryside to the cities, seeking better life opportunities.

The different forms of production of goods and services in different contexts have shaped human needs, thus characterizing the forms of reproduction and social and institutional relationships that have made the continuity of human societies, knowledge, and goods possible. Changes in the patterns of everyday life and different power relationships and social values (e.g., individualism, consumerism, and competitiveness) shape new orders of citizenship: in particular, citizens' alienation as social beings, with class stratification and domination (De Sousa Santos, 2015). These changes also produce diverse strengths in societies, such as more freedom for some groups, creating conditions for the development of knowledge, and technologies that connect people and make the exchange of information available. At the same time, these forces increase social inequities between people, groups, and societies (De Sousa Santos, 2010, 2015) and enable domination between and within peoples in which a subject or group of the population made use (and sometimes abuse) of official and symbolic power. This power determines the social scripts expected of some and allowed others, including the creation of social invisibilities, for example, for women, the working class, people with disabilities, or cultural minorities.

An awareness of the superdiversity (Vertovec, 2007) of societies, how different groups coexist and manage different ways of living together simultaneously (or not), is needed to critically explore the complexities of citizenship. De Sousa Santos (2010, 2015) has coined the term "epistemicide" to refer to the destruction of the knowledge and cultural experiences of peoples caused by European colonialism. In a way, this irreparable loss in any of the aforementioned spheres also conditions the co-construction of a planetary citizenship, insofar as the voices and knowledge of so many minorities (or majorities) have been silenced, invisible, absent, and even eliminated (De Sousa Santos, 2002). A dialogue entails a conversation with another person; without the other perspective, or if the other person is an oppressor who denies opportunities for free dialogue, the result is a monoculture, in which statements around citizenship and rights are merely a pretence (De Sousa Santos, 2015). These questions invite meta-reflection and moral debate related to the diversity of human existence. De Sousa Santos calls for a re-evaluation of the power dynamics in knowledge that offers equal social esteem to different modes of thinking—for example, questioning the assumption of the dominance of Western (particularly Anglophone) philosophy and science, which he terms "cognitive justice" (De Sousa Santos, 2007).

ANGLOPHONE PERSPECTIVES ON CONTEMPORARY CITIZENSHIP (EUROPE AND UNITED STATES)

An Anglophone and European perspective of modern citizenship is composed of three elements: civil rights to equal protection in law, political rights for participation in political decisions such as voting processes, and social rights to a level of basic well-being (Marshall, 1950). Western, and specifically English, examples have predominated illustrations of the development of citizenship through the historical position of the United Kingdom as being the first country to have an industrial revolution and of the contribution of British colonialism to the identity of the United States (Bendix, 1977).

Marshall (1950, pp. 10–11) points to the significance of this history in his outline of the elements of citizenship and presented what was the classic definition of citizenship made during the consolidation of the British postwar welfare state:

The civil element is composed of the rights necessary for individual freedom—liberty of the person, freedom of speech, thought and faith, the right to own property and to conclude valid contracts, and the right to justice. The last is of a different order from the others, because it is the right to defend and assert all one" rights on terms of equality with others and by due process of law. This shows us that the institutions most directly associated with civil rights are the courts of justice. By the political element, I mean the right to participate in the exercise of political power, as a member of a body invested with political authority or as an elector of the members of such a body. The corresponding institutions are parliament and councils of local government. By the social element, I mean the whole range from the right to a modicum of economic welfare and security to the right to share to the full in the social heritage and to live the life of a civilised being according to the standards prevailing in the society. The institutions most closely connected with it are the educational system and the social services.

However, since Marshall's elements (to which we shall return) and Bendix's midcentury account of nation building, these positions on citizenship have been assailed by various forces. The development of a neoliberal political order has been characterized by the privileging of free market values and global economic concerns as the determinants of international relations, with challenges to social rights, the last of these elements. Consequently, national welfare systems for citizens are challenged by austerity measures that respond to worldwide market forces. For example, while visiting the United Kingdom in 2019, neoliberal US President Donald Trump said that US–UK trade talks should include a condition that will open up the UK state health system, the National Health Service (NHS)—access to which is regarded as a fundamental citizenship right—to purchase by US businesses. A question about the political element of citizenship that has been confronting many people in Europe has been whether they are citizens of particular countries within Europe, a larger federal organization of states (the European Union), or some further reorganization of nationality within or outside this such as Catalonia, Scotland, or Wallonia.

Territoriality

Territoriality is therefore a significant aspect of citizenship, as it is of occupation; having a space in which to be, belong, and become is fundamental to human experience (Doroud, Fossey, & Fortune, 2018), and displacement can be a huge disruption of identity in terms of personhood as well as sociocultural and economic ties. Migration has been a constant feature of human societies throughout history, but with capitalism it has taken particular forms (colonization, slavery and trafficking, economic inducements and expropriation). Thus, it has been a major influence in enabling people to develop critical perspectives of their social position through the comparison of their experiences. While citizenship has traditionally suggested a relationship to a polity that is territorially bounded within a country, or a state within a federal republic, the development of globalized or transnational political, social, and economic relationships (Kreisi, 2013; Donaldson & Kymlicka, 2017) impacts many aspects of daily life through which citizenship may be expressed. Since World War II, former colonial empires have dissipated, while new superstates and federal bodies have emerged, such as the European Union. With these developments, legal opportunities for migration have increased for some, and thus cultural, family, and personal connections may cross many borders or be interdependent. It is possible to have multiple legal citizenships through living in different countries. Many other complex relations between the individual and the political and economic apparatuses of government have emerged with this degree of movement.

The emergence of larger political bodies such as the European Union has brought into question the issues of accountability for decision making affecting national and communal life and where and by whom this should be determined if it is to meet local concerns. An important element in other arguments around nationality and citizenship has been a popular nationalism around cultural identities that are supposedly under threat from the influences of migration. Examples include the English Democratic Party, Fidesz and Jobbik Magyarországért Mozgalom in Hungary, and the Alternative fur Deutschland. The popularity of these movements, mostly of the new right, but some of it from traditional socialist groupings, is partly reaction to the need for a flexible and mobile workforce (e.g., hotel workers, agricultural laborers, care workers, and

those with specialized skills in medicine and information technology) following the neoliberal global market. However, they also contain challenges to civil elements of Marshall's (1950) perspective, as well as the nation building of Bendix (1977).

Another aspect of territoriality, and a frequent element in the history of social groups, is the tendency to eliminate from sight or to exclude certain groups from everyday social life. This social practice enables societies to avoid everyday confrontation with issues that question or challenge structures that dominant powers uphold. Often, communities of neighbors exercise their collective power to veto the arrival of new groups in their midst through a discrediting discourse (e.g., conferring a dangerousness of the "other" on such groups, such as a negative impact on homeowners' property values), which justifies the establishment of social or territorial distances. In this way, certain groups are moved from the population nuclei toward the geographical and sometimes social periphery. Taylor (2016) explores how social exclusion and the absence of women's rights was at the forefront of British (and revolutionary French) agitation against developing capitalism during the late 18th and early 19th centuries, but working-class women underwent significant loss of social equality as they became marginalized through social and economic pressures. Other examples of this social phenomenon were people with leprosy who were established in isolated colonies; other populations have been excluded on the basis of "poverty," "madness," or religious or political "dissidence" with confinement in institutions, such as asylums, drug treatment centers, jails, slums, settlements, and their use as a colonized labor force.

These and other social mechanisms of exclusion that operate through lack of recognition (Fraser & Honneth, 2003) disable the participatory elements of citizenship and generate "discitizenship" (Devlin & Pothier, 2006; Fransen, Pollard, Kantartzis, & Viana-Moldes, 2015). As De Sousa Santos (2007) points out, not taking account of the knowledge of others is a reciprocal loss of knowledge, and the assumption that others are ignorant overlooks the impact this has on self-ignorance.

Citizenship, Capitalism, and Colonialism

De Sousa Santos (2018a, p. 15) refers to the forms of modern domination, "capitalism, colonialism and patriarchy," which constitute hetero-patriarchy and which are an essential part of the logic and mentality of today's world that underpins the discourse of equal citizens and equal rights. It is difficult to resist, because hegemonic power is not shared and operates on a pervasive, all-encompassing scale. There are innumerable examples of colonialisms in various spheres (cultural, economic, geographical, historical, scientific, idiomatic, and aesthetic colonialism, among others). Although their forms change over time, they continue to obey the overarching hegemonic power, in what De Sousa Santos (2018b, p. 1) calls "insidious colonialism" manifested through the everyday products people buy and a low-level sustained commentary in the media, in which colonialism becomes part of daily life.

Many of the concepts of modern citizenship arise from the long-running and historical social conflicts between peasants, working-class people, landowners, and employers. In the economies of Europe and North America, industrialization occurred alongside political, social, and economic changes and religious reformation, as the polity shifted from feudal systems to business-like administrations. A concern with doing, becoming, and belonging and the expression of being through forms of productivity has emerged through this development, but a dominant economic class from very early in its development ordered the form that it took. This class took a brutal and punitive view of any attempts from the lower orders to express their interest as citizens, that is, in having a role in and responsibility for the organization of their communities or societies, and hung, flogged, burned, or branded those who challenged them.

The early rise of capitalism was characterized by enclosures of common land, which deprived many people of their livelihood, a process that began in England from the late 1400s and spread through Britain into the 1800s (Petergorsky, 1994 [1940]; Linebaugh & Rediker, 2012). At the same time, entrepreneurs in colonial settlements in Ireland and in the new Atlantic trade with the American coast and islands bought the victims of these expropriations, indentured[1] and enslaved with the connivance of governments. Historically, modern cosmopolitan global society began with this development. However, colonialism also provided opportunities for cultural exchange between oppressed people. People from Europe discovered alternative ways of living among the indigenous people and slaves they worked with, and with them developed resistance and mounted challenges to the dominant rule (Linebaugh & Rediker, 2012). The development of the modern capitalist economy has contended with a persistently rebellious and diverse citizenry over the last 500 years. Consequently, it is ahistorical to consider citizenship only within a Western paradigm of industrial and capitalist development, as the strategies and ideas informing the rebellions frequently came from the non-Western experience of organized societies.

During the 1600s, several rebellions in the new Atlantic colonies were organized by mixed groups of English, Irish, African, and Indian slaves and indentured servants, some of whom formed groups of maroons[2] with the intent to establish their own free society (Linebaugh & Rediker, 2012). Eventually, the colonies and the English Parliament developed legal definitions of citizenship, afraid that the lucrative slave and sugar trade, and their own rule and possessions, could be lost. British citizenship stemmed from the principle of the "free born Englishman" who would have certain rights in any of the colonies, while slaves would have none. These measures, in the British-administered American and Caribbean colonies, were intended to separate English servants from the other slaves, although indentured servitude continued. British civil rights were accorded, therefore, by the powerful to divide a dangerous commonality and were not so much about freedom as a preventative to struggles for freedom (Linebaugh & Rediker, 2012), a rather different perspective to that of Marshall's elements.

CITIZENSHIP AND THE MANY-HEADED HYDRA

Citizenship may be a fluid concept that is as much about human connection as obligation within a political system. It is as much enacted from below as above, shaped by people as they work to live together, in response to changing conditions.

One example is of European colonization in New England, which was much more of an exchange of ideas than is often suggested in popular history. Europeans had to learn from their indigenous neighbors how to survive and in this encounter with social and cultural difference came to question their own culture and social relationships (Philbrick, 2006). Many of them went to live among the Native Americans, valuing their more egalitarian and freer lifestyle in preference to the restrictions of colonial religious communities, which themselves were philosophically often at odds with developments, including experiments with republican democracies, in the European states from which they came. Native Americans sometimes formed their own democratic political institutions to resolve issues between groups. Not having the degree of social differences found among Europeans, they often expressed criticism of

---

[1]Contracted to work off the debt of a migratory passage, or a judicial sentence, for a number of years, before being released by an employer.

[2]Maroons were usually former slaves who organized themselves into independent communities, often in remote areas.

the social acceptance of inequality among Europeans (Mann, 2005; Linebaugh & Rediker, 2012). Native American forms of liberty—*as they were perceived by the colonists*—may have contributed to modern ideas about democracy as the movement for American independence developed during the 18th century (Linebaugh and Rediker, 2012).

Another example of emerging citizenship can be seen in the arts and crafts variants of socialism from which occupational therapy emerged in the 19th century. William Morris envisaged a society that certainly emphasized doing, being, becoming, and belonging, but without any polity (1888) and therefore no convention of citizenship that might be associated with national identity. His *News from Nowhere* (1968) presented a citizenship that conformed with the picture presented by Donaldson and Kymlicka (2017, p. 843), as generally seen as a contractual relationship, which requires the capacity to "articulate, understand, evaluate, negotiate, and commit to linguistic propositions regarding the terms of social cooperation with your fellow citizens." This Morris (1888) derived from his understanding of changing social relations in the late Medieval (after 1380) period in the United Kingdom, a turning point in which a free commonality in the use of land and organization of agriculture and work was wrested from the nobility by more prosperous laborers. Some of the more successful workers became a rapacious new business class, who expropriated the land and threw its inhabitants into indentured labor in the new colonies that were being opened up. It was in the colonies that such people often found common cause with the free indigenous people they found there (Linebaugh & Rediker, 2012).

Linebaugh and Rediker (2012) reveal a global society that has developed over the last 500 years. It is even one in which people were able to consider themselves citizens of the world in the context of the antislavery movements that emerged from the link between capitalism, expropriation, slavery, and the multiethnic mass of sailors forcibly recruited to supply the labor in its fleets over 200 years ago. This mobile and rebellious "hydra" offered resistance to harsh conditions imposed by government and entrepreneurs, and which Linebaugh and Rediker (2012) suggest had a continuity stringing together many of the protest actions over a few centuries. Hydra was the epithet frequently applied to it by authorities across, and in the midst of, the Atlantic, at sea, or, for example, through piracy by former sailors and slaves, and on land through other alliances of servants, slaves, prostitutes, and laborers, all combinations of excluded groups without rights. For well over 100 years, it was repeatedly associated with the radical working-class movements of the English Civil War and the Masaniello rebellion against Hapsburg Naples (both in the

1640s), often combined with ideas and tactical expertise from African and Native American people and their experiences of slave rebellions. Aside from rebellions, "hydra" manifested itself in more permanent self-governing maroon societies (mostly composed of former slaves) and piracy. O'Leary (1999) felt that a legacy of this diversity, at least in the United States, had continuously and to the present time produced multiple identities and contested perspectives of citizenships and the patriotisms that are often bound to it.

As a consequence of such issues—which are contested not only in the United States but also in many other countries—the concept of global citizenship, which is more commonly familiar, has been applied to citizenship values in relation to the cultural diversity and migratory forces that characterize many societies. Global citizenship may range from the top-down promotion of a stable world order by a world government to a globally focused anarchism such as the anti-capitalist and anti-globalization movements (Oxley & Morris 2013), a present-day manifestation of the forces described by Linebaugh and Rediker (2012).

CRITICAL CONSIDERATIONS

Dahlgren (2006) suggests that fields for learning citizenship exist in a range of formal and informal public spheres or spaces where people communicate. This argument is supported by historians "from below" such as Linebaugh and Rediker (2012) and Taylor (2016), whose work underpins some of the arguments here. The forms of organization developed by ordinary people (e.g., trade unions, resistance around poaching, land rights or tree culling, or even organized sports activities) may address aspects of power with which they are in conflict over their control (the media, the judiciary, local government, public bodies). Other forms of local organization may emerge in the absence of powerful central government and institutions. For example, the contemporary development of solidarity organizations of citizens in Greece, organizing soup kitchens, pharmacies and clinics, groceries, time banks, and continuing education centers, occurred in response to the inability of central government to address citizens' and refugees' fundamental needs (Cabot, 2018). Many other forms of local organization are at the level of social activities through clubs and sports associations, and even casual conversation, through which the local social fabric is shaped and maintained (Kantartzis, 2013).

Consequently, the division between the public and the private sphere is blurry. The division of labor in the home, gender relationships, are aspects of personal and intimate life that may be played out through the way people publicly identify themselves and participate in community, society, or civic structures; the personal cannot easily be divided from the political, just as the struggle for women's rights has long determined (Taylor, 2016). The relationship between personal and political enables creative and emancipatory objectives to be developed around the everyday things that are directly meaningful to people (Doroud et al., 2018). However, there are risks of assuming that they are not open to manipulation and control by more powerful bodies. Ordinary and everyday issues like unpaid housework have been the long focus of the women's struggle (Taylor, 2016) and become the penetrating and intrusive focus of state terror in dystopias such as *We* (Zamyatin, 1993 [1921]) or *Nineteen Eighty-Four* (Orwell, 2013 [1949]) and in the totalitarian practices of Stalinism, Nazism (Turnbull, 2018), or Apartheid (Luthuli, 1963). *We* was also a critique of the early social application of Taylorism (Figes, 1996), the organization of occupation for efficiency scientifically adopted in the early years of the Russian Revolution—and which was also related to some of the underpinning of the science of activity analysis in the occupational therapy profession (Litterst, 1992). The position of the professional in assessing activity and function in everyday life is not only enabling but also potentially a source of maligned power, for example, in operating assessments for access to state benefits in order to restrict payments (Cousins, Pennings, Roberts, & Stafford, 2016).

As Marshall (1950) illustrated, there is a sociocultural and historical element in the enactment of citizenship; it concerns a way of being and acquires experiential narratives that may be localized and different to the larger theory and ideas of political forces but not unconnected with them. Dahlgren (2006) argues that while political opinions may often be prefabricated by professional commentators and retailed second hand in everyday conversation, the determination of "what is a reasonable expectation" and the formation of political strategies to meeting those ends may take other forms and actions, including unrest.

OCCUPATIONAL THERAPY, OCCUPATION, AND CITIZENSHIP

Grassroots Means for Citizenship

Despite its origins in the Christian socialism of the arts and crafts movement, occupational therapy did not become primarily a profession for social reformers but a clinical profession (Frank & Zemke, 2009); its paradigms focused on treatment within a medical understanding of conditions rather than a program of action to deal with their social and economic causes.

William Morris's arts and crafts writings (1973) suggest that community structures such as grassroots forms of organization are the arenas for working out these practical issues, such as setting up social facilities and community resources (Kallman & Clark, 2016). These are one form of the expression of citizenship and the development of mutually useful and reciprocal arrangements among communities. They can also take the form, in occupational therapy, of being part of the service learning, emergent role, or social occupational therapy interventions initiated with communities as described elsewhere in this book, but these interventions are often based on the spontaneous responses of communities to the needs of their fellows. An example of how such spontaneous, grassroots actions might operate is that of chain or bridgehead migration first identified by MacDonald and MacDonald (1964), in which first arrivals in a country enable other people from their home community to find a base and establish themselves in the host context through personal networks. These networks have become part of the diverse citizenship fabric of many societies and suggest that citizenship is a global phenomenon, at least for those in such networks, while for those in the host communities, they may be perceived as a threat to national identity notions of citizenship.

Sometimes the establishment of community history or local writing groups to celebrate specific cultures (Morley & Worpole, 2009) emerged from consciousness raising, which built on these and other developments. They were a part of a community arts movement that offered an alternative, inclusive, and extensive critical commentary from the bottom up through much of the last half century (Matarasso, 2011). For one author (NP), they were a means for occupational engagement in cultural politics through the critical expression of narratives (Pollard & Sakellariou, 2012; Ikiugu & Pollard, 2015; Pollard 2016a, 2016b). The sense of continuous anger and disenfranchisement arising from experiences of discitizenship (Devlin & Pothier, 2006) described by Matarasso through his analysis of community arts and its relationship to expressions such as UK riots in the 1980s and 2011 is something that has strong parallels to cultural, social, and economic and epistemic oppression in other parts of the world as described by De Sousa Santos (2010, 2015, 2018a).

On the whole, the use of capability theory, the interest in human rights to occupation delivered through not-for-profit and nongovernmental work suggested throughout this book, would suggest that occupational therapy discussions, for example, around service learning, role-emerging placements, social transformation, and community development work, have tended to focus on interventions delivered by professionals working with communities. The practical implementation of these interventions requires a broad understanding of some of the other aspects, such as cultural, economic, and environmental dimensions of citizenship, issues that so far have not been significant in Anglophone occupational therapy discourse, and an unpacking of the philosophical and conceptual nuances they contain. In the context of cultural diversity often encountered in Western countries, these complex issues often need to be unraveled; practitioners need to reflect on how and why they are coworking with populations and how their input may be experienced.

Occupational Therapy and Citizenship

Occupational therapists may recognize doing, being, becoming, and belonging (Wilcock, 1999; Hitch, Pépin, & Stagnitti, 2014a, 2014b) as the underpinnings of a relational and participatory citizenship (Doroud et al., 2018), from which many of the people they work with, for example, people with cognitive difficulties or physical disabilities, are disenfranchised through considerations of risk and physical, legal, or systemic barriers. This puts people with disabilities in a position of dependence and of imposition, in which their relationship to the mainstream is defined by its administrators, for example, occupational therapists (Cousins et al., 2016). The resulting relationship has been widely compared to that between the colonizing state and people in its occupied territories (Meekosha, 2011), characterized in terms of parent–child, with colonized people denied their full capacity (Rollo, 2016). The way in which citizenship is portrayed can unwittingly continue this relationship; citizenship becomes something to be extended to the disenfranchised, from the colonizer to the colonized, or to the rest of the world from the powerful and well-meaning West (Swanson & Pashby, 2016). Participation then becomes not so much a right of all citizens but patronage to those who are characterized as dependents. For example, there was also an epistemicide implicit in occupational therapist paradigms and interventions that maintained populations in a powerless position of lacking knowledge, whose voices and expertise were invisible (McCorquodale & Kinsella, 2015; Whalley Hammell, 2015; Palacios, 2017). In this sense, the main challenge to the profession is to advocate and collaborate to cocreate a common scenario, guided by the population needs and focused in occupational rights and social contexts, in dialogical partnerships with other social actors (Fransen et al., 2015).

In occupational therapy's Anglophone professional discourse around citizenship, the term "citizen" is often used interchangeably with "client" and "patient" and refers to the recipient of a service. We have briefly reviewed how this is expressed in current education standards. The American Occupational Therapy Association's (2009) model curriculum relates the "occupational needs of society" (p. 75) with the understanding that community is "the source of learning, health, and citizenship" (p. 138), since occupation is interdependent with the community. Occupational therapy students are to be expected to see themselves as part of that diverse community and to enact this through their education, for example, through service learning. The European 2008 Tuning document (TUNING, 2008) discusses the term "citizen" as part of a broader health discourse around the connection between social factors and health that had grown by the end of the 20th century, associated with a supportive role for occupational therapists working outside a traditional hospital setting. On the whole, however, Tuning's concept of citizenship is addressed through generic competences associated with the values that might be imparted through higher education of which professional training is part; the relationship between different aspects of disability and their effect on citizenship; opportunities for employment, social participation, and lifelong learning as a right; and ethnicity, migration, and participation. A section on "Participation, Citizenship and Governance in Europe" (TUNING, 2008, p. 168) relates these objectives within the context of the European Union, and a further section frames discussion of cultural competency within the ambit of the World Federation of Occupational Therapists' (2016, p. 57) concept of the "global citizen."

Any discussion of citizenship and its conceits has to take a critical account of historical and social contexts that underpin the views being upheld, and this must include the record of everyday experience. A useful concept relating to the participatory aspect of citizenship that seems to be frequently discussed in occupational therapy might be what De Tocqueville (2003, p. 284) called the "general activity" of the American society he observed; an enthusiastic involvement in political activity in a society without hierarchy extended into every aspect of social life. Thus, a person might not be very far up in the political structures but might be rewardingly active in a local community through the networks he or she may be a part of.[3] Dahlgren (2006) argues that citizen engagement suggests an agency through which the citizen develops his or her skills, capacity, and contribution to society, across all levels, not merely the political. Such a discussion might seem to favor the communitarian end of the triangle between liberalism, republicanism, and communitarian values, which often

---

[3]Kallman and Clark (2016) give a very useful historical run through the Western thinking over the last 200 years through which democratic governance, the set of relationships through which engaged citizenry may be facilitated, has evolved. We refer readers to this chapter.

define how citizenship as civic engagement is viewed (Hoskins, Abs, Han, Kerr, & Veugelers, 2012).

However, as Palacios (2017) argues, "intervening in" communities requires reading the context for intervention as it develops, but where communities are defined in capitalist, consumerist, and neoliberal terms, the basis for integrating or readapting people must be critically questioned. In line with the concept of epistemicide, Marmot et al. (2010) and Wilkinson and Picket (2010) suggested that communitarian values may be fragmented by neoliberal policies and their effects on diminishing social capital. Occupational therapists' work may be concerned with individual and community needs, but it is also carrying out a role of reprogramming those needs in ways that serve dominant structures. Recent health policies often concern risks arising from long-term systemic costs generated by unhealthy lifestyles and preventable disease. Typically, those who are at most risk of becoming unhealthy are those who are poorest and most marginalized, people who will lack access to other resources or amenities and who will have missed opportunities for education—those who are least likely to be able to inform themselves of risks and their avoidance.

CITIZENSHIP AND POLITICAL LIBERATION

Dagnino (2003) identified citizenship concepts as crucial to the struggle for political liberation and overcoming economic deprivation, poverty, and exclusion in Latin America during the 1970s and 1980s, the point at which social occupational therapy originated (Guajardo Córdoba & Galhiego, 2015). This issue was especially pertinent because of the social authoritarianism prevalent in many Latin American societies—tending to a view of the poor as having no rights, reinforced by the acceptance of the dominance of the market as the arbiter of principle, that what is right for the market is what is right, and anything else is an obstacle to its progress. Dagnino (2003) argues that the perception that embracing the market is a requirement for economic development had tended to undermine social reforms in Latin American countries. The effect that market determinism has is that social rights are displaced under the form of emergency action for needy groups of people, who remain needy and are never invested in sufficiently to obtain any handholds for climbing out of their position. When they intervene because the state has retreated from work with these people, nongovernmental organizations (NGOs) reinforce this situation because the state is often the means of access to needy populations, so NGOs need to cooperate with state agencies to do their work. The licence to do this depends on being perceived as acceptable partners. Any action is therefore limited and

unlikely to challenge the main causes of problems affecting marginalized citizens, since this would mean challenging the market-led principles of the state. While this situation is frequently encountered in countries in the global south, similar issues have developed in Northern Hemisphere countries through the implementation of market fundamentalist social policies that enforce austerity measures on the most needy in their societies (De Sousa Santos, 2018a). Food insecurity and homelessness are significant health issues in otherwise wealthy societies such as the United States and the United Kingdom (Marmot et al., 2010; Wilkinson & Pickett, 2010), countries that often celebrate their national philosophical and political contributions to ideas around democracy and the principles of citizenship.

As the World Health Organization's (WHO) work on the social determinants of health indicated (2008), there is often an intergenerational history of complex issues around the experiences of socioeconomic factors such as poverty, immigration, and disability, aspects of everyday life affecting millions of individual citizens who have to renegotiate their occupational roles as a result of their changing conditions. People often experience these problems as multiple disenfranchisements. The basis of their interaction with the social and political environment is changed by the changes in their material circumstances—the need to be dependent on welfare for the security of their right to a home, income, or access to services and even food is altered and contested: "they're ready to throw you off," blues performer Freddy King was singing in 1962 in the beginning of the black civil rights upheaval. As has been long and well understood in the popular culture of some populations of the United States, navigating these aspects of occupational performance in navigating benefits systems and welfare processes is essential to retaining the status one has as a citizen in a system that is tuned toward marginalization (Cousins et al., 2016). In an earlier paper, we explored some challenges for just one Somali cultural minority group in a UK city in balancing care needs with extended family responsibilities and the demands of the Western welfare system for conformity (Pollard, Kantartzis, Ismail, Fransen-Jaïbi, & Viana-Moldes, 2018). The welfare safety net in the United Kingdom, instead of assisting people in need, creates additional demands and dependencies that obstruct the meeting of needs of extended families—the Somali concept of family and the understanding of its requirements are not recognized.

Were concepts of citizenship to take account of different historical and cultural perspectives, then some of its expressions, such as occupational therapy (as a form of valuing participative doing), may also require some reexamination, even where it does address citizenship. While the origins of the profession in social reform have recently been celebrated in the United States, authors have acknowledged that a position alongside biomedicine drew its emphasis away from social factors and toward constructing health as an individual experience. Occupational therapy's future requires skills beyond measuring outcomes and gathering evidence, or even collecting information on client goals and performance (Baum, 2006). It must include confronting daunting complexity in the administration of social security systems and dealing with the consequences of structural inequality, as this is experienced by the people therapists are working with (Aldrich, Boston, & Daaleman, 2017).

CONCLUDING REMARKS: CITIZENSHIP AND ETHICAL AND MORAL RESPONSIBILITY

Every profession has an ethical and moral responsibility to critically and reflexively question their underpinning principles. To fail to do so may expose its members to engaging in processes that are harmful to the health of marginalized citizens and the wider social fabric. In their professional capacity occupational therapists often have to negotiate the system of social welfare on behalf of their clients or advocate on their behalf. Of course, there may be unrealistic expectations and limitations to what can be achieved, but if professionals feel unable to critique and challenge on justifiable grounds, there are serious concerns, not only about the function of their profession, but also about the worth of its core values. It potentially reveals partiality in favor of power, the heteropatriarchy, and the incompleteness of understanding of experience and a betrayal of the client relationship.

For example, international migration is leading to an increasing plurality of cultures making up many urban populations around the globe. Arguably, the experiences of occupational therapy colleagues around the world may prove directly relevant to local needs and also tell occupational stories that come from diverse cultural and global perspectives (e.g., Garcia-Ruiz, 2016). Professional, English-language literature tends to define citizenship through a culturally Western and Northern Hemisphere lens, which is shaped through socioeconomic privileges in relation to other parts of the world (Kabeer, 2002). If the Northern Hemisphere has developed spaces of superdiversity, everyone's story encompasses some degree of that diversity (Vertovec, 2007; De Sousa Santos, 2007). Consequently, occupational interventions that address these kinds of issues must be more than clinical; they require a social, dialogical, reciprocal approach to manage the interdependence of experience with contextual realities (Morrison, 2016).

A common feature in all these histories has been inequity. The relationship between combined historical, cultural, and economic factors on life quality is inscribed in the physical and mental health of people, and this combination is the focus of occupation-based intervention. As has been understood throughout much of the early modern period of history to the present, the health and welfare of people are related to their enjoyment of liberties in the form of the expression of citizenship—and discitizenship where this has been denied (Fransen et al., 2015). Whichever aspect colors the daily lives of communities, families, and individuals, the route to obtaining recognition, rights, and access to health and ensuring the broad range of conditions that promote health is through social occupational engagement.

In this chapter, we aimed to highlight perspectives of citizenship from different realities and explored with examples and illustrations traditional and less traditional perspectives of citizenship situated in a British history arising from exploitative capitalist and colonial development and perspectives based in the work of De Santos Sousa related to issues of the decolonization of knowledge and epistemicide. We are aware that more perspectives exist—for example, French writers would probably have another historical account on citizenship based in the importance of the French Revolution as a turning point in their history. This underlines how citizenship is contextualized, not only politically and geographically, but also through many distinctive characteristics that claims of universality would exclude. Faced with these contradictions, several stories of our history exist, told by different people in different contexts, making us aware of the partiality of all stories and the profound conviction that we all have limited knowledge (De Sousa Santos, 2010, 2012).

Citizenship is a valuable concept for considering the occupations of people coming together, but there can be considerable variation in how it is experienced and enacted. The movement of thinking in reflective dialogue (Morin, 2015) enables every party to understand the paradigm and the vocabulary of the other to some extent (Morin, 2015). To make this possible, it is important that there is the intention and the posture of cooperation, an equal stance in the power relationship. From this point of "coming together," moving forward toward a different or new solution that is acceptable for all may become possible, with its basis in decision-making processes and plural criteria (Morin, 2015). All truly human development must include the joint development of individual autonomy, community participation, and awareness of belonging to the human species (Morin, 1999). Occupational therapists and occupational scientists may seek to answer this complex issue by considering individual and collective narratives that connect occupation with autonomy and citizenship through doing as a daily routine. The base for occupational therapists' and occupational scientists' professional discourse on citizenship is in the plurality and diversity of everyday context, the needs of sharing ecologies (De Sousa Santos, 2012) about the coexistences, interdependencies, and interrelationships contained in the pursuit of doing, being, becoming, and belonging but aware of the colonizers' powers (Wilcock, 1999; Hitch et al., 2014a, 2014b). Inevitably, the concept of citizenship is political, civic, social, and personal. An occupational approach to citizenship therefore has to be fluid, receptive, reflexive, and critical about the power relationships.

REFERENCES

Aldrich, R. M., Boston, T. L., & Daaleman, C. E. (2017). Centennial topics—Justice and U.S. occupational therapy practice: A relationship 100 years in the making. *American Journal of Occupational Therapy, 71*, 1. doi:10.5014/ajot.2017.023085

American Occupational Therapy Association. (2009). *Occupational therapy model curriculum*. Retrieved from https://www.aota.org/~/media/Corporate/Files/EducationCareers/Educators/OT-Model-Curriculum.pdf

Baum, M. C. (2006). Centennial challenges, millennium opportunities. *American Journal of Occupational Therapy, 60*(6), 609–616.

Bendix, R. (1977). *Nation-building and citizenship: Studies of our changing social order*. Berkley, CA: University of California.

Cabot, H. (2018). The European refugee crisis and humanitarian citizenship in Greece. *Ethnos, 84*, 747–771. doi:10.1080/00141844.2018.1529693

Cousins, M., Pennings, F., Roberts, S., & Stafford, B. (2016). *Comparative systems of assessment of illness or disability for the purposes of adult social welfare payments second report (Carers)*. Mel Cousins & Associates. Nottingham: Nottingham University. Retrieved from http://eprints.nottingham.ac.uk/46567/1/Comparative%20systems%20of%20assessment%20of%20illness%20or%20disability%20for%20the%20purposes%20of%20adult%20social%20welfare%20payments%20-%20Carers.pdf

Dagnino, E. (2003). Citizenship in Latin America: An introduction. *Latin American Perspectives, 30*(2), 211–225. doi:10.1177/0094582X02250624

Dahlgren, P. (2006). Doing citizenship: The cultural origins of civic agency in the public sphere. *European Journal of Cultural Studies, 9*(3) 267–286. doi:10.1177/1367549406066073

De Sousa Santos, B. (2002). Para uma sociologia das ausências e uma sociologia das emergências [Towards a sociology of absences and a sociology of emergencies]. *Revista crítica de ciências sociais, Outubro* (63), 237–280.

De Sousa Santos, B. (2007). A discourse on the sciences. In B. De Sousa Santos (Ed.), *Cognitive justice in a global world: Prudent knowledges for a decent life* (pp. 13–45). Lanham, MD: Lexington Books.

De Sousa Santos, B. (2010). *Descolonizar el poder, reinventar el poder* [Decolonize power, reinvent power]. Montevideo, Uruguay: Trilce.

De Sousa Santos, B. (2012). *De las dualidades a las ecologías* [Of the dualities of the ecologies]. La Paz, Bolivia: Red Boliviana de Mujeres Transformando la Economía REMTE.

De Sousa Santos, B. (2015). *Epistemologies of the South: Justice against epistemicide*. London: Routledge.

De Sousa Santos, B. (2018a). ¿Unidad de las izquierdas? Cuándo, por qué, cómo y para qué [Unite the left? When, why, how and what?]. *Revista Conjeturas Sociológicas, Enero-Abril* (15), 10–59.

De Sousa Santos, B. (2018b). El colonismo insidioso [Insidious colonialism]. *Publico*. Retrieved from https://blogs.publico.es/espejos-extranos/2018/04/04/el-colonialismo-insidioso/

De Tocqueville, A. (2003). *Democracy in America: And two essays on America*. London: Penguin.

Devlin, D., & Pothier, R. (2006). Towards a critical theory of citizenship. In D. Pothier & R Devlin (Eds.), *Critical disability theory: Essays in philosophy, politics, policy and law* (pp. 1–22). Vancouver: UBC Press.

Diamond, J. (2013). *The world until yesterday: What can we learn from traditional societies?* London: Penguin.

Donaldson, S., & Kymlicka, W. (2017). Inclusive citizenship beyond the capacity contract. In A. Shachar, R. Bauböck, I. Bloemraad, & M. Vink (Eds.), *The Oxford handbook of citizenship* (pp. 838–860). Oxford: Oxford University Press.

Doroud, N., Fossey, E., & Fortune, T. (2018). Place for being, doing, becoming and belonging: A meta-synthesis exploring the role of place in mental health recovery. *Health & Place, 52*, 110–120.

Figes, O. (1996). *A people's tragedy: Russian Revolution 1891–1924*. London: Jonathan Cape.

Fransen, H., Pollard, N., Kantartzis, S., & Viana-Moldes, I. (2015). Participatory citizenship: Critical perspectives on client-centred occupational therapy. *Scandinavian Journal of Occupational Therapy, 22*(4), 260–266.

Fraser, N., & Honneth, A. (2003). *Redistribution or recognition*. New York, NY: Verso.

Frank, G., & Zemke, R. (2009). Occupational therapy foundations for political engagement and social transformation. In N. Pollard, D. Sakellariou, & F. Kronenberg (Eds.), *Political Practice of Occupational Therapy* (pp. 111–136). Churchill Livingstone: Elsevier.

Garcia-Ruiz, S. (2016). Occupational therapy in a glocalized world. In D. Sakellariou & N. Pollard (Eds.), *Occupational therapy without borders* (2nd ed., pp. 185–193). Edinburgh: Elsevier.

Guajardo Córdoba, A., & Galheigo, S. (2015). Reflexiones críticas acerca de los derechos humanos: Contribuciones desde la terapia ocupacional Latinoamericana. *World Federation of Occupational Therapists Bulletin, 71*(2), 73–80.

Harris, M. (1994). *Introducción a la antropología general* [General introduction to anthropology]. Madrid: Alianza Editorial.

Hitch, D., Pépin, G., & Stagnitti, K. (2014a). In the footsteps of Wilcock, part one: The evolution of doing, being, becoming, and belonging. *Occupational Therapy in Health Care, 28*(3), 231–246. doi:10.3109/07380577.2014.898114

Hitch, D., Pépin, G., & Stagnitti, K. (2014b). In the footsteps of Wilcock, part two: The interdependent nature of doing, being, becoming, and belonging. *Occupational Therapy in Health Care, 28*(3), 247–263. doi:10.3109/07380577.2014.898115

Hoskins, B., Abs, H., Han, C., Kerr, D., & Veugelers, W. (2012). *Contextual Analysis Report. Participatory citizenship in the European Union.* Institution of Education. Retrieved November 15, 2015, from http://ec.europa.eu/citizenship/pdf/report_1_conextual_report.pdf

Ikiugu, M., & Pollard, N. (2015). *Meaningful living through occupation.* London: Whiting and Birch.

Kabeer, N. (2002). *Citizenship and the boundaries of the acknowledge community: Identify, affiliation and exclusion.* IDS working paper 171. Brighton: Institute of Development Studies. Retrieved from http://www.ids.ac.uk/files/dmfile/Wp171.pdf

Kallman, M. E., & Clark, T. N. (2016). Democratic governance and institutional logics within the third sector (or, How Habermas discovered the coffee house). In M. E. Kallman & T. N. Clark (Eds.), *The third sector: Community organizations, NGOs, and nonprofits.* Champaign, IL: University of Illinois Press.

Kantartzis, S. (2013). *Conceptualising occupation: An ethnographic study of daily life in a Greek town* (PhD dissertation). Leeds: Leeds Metropolitan University.

King, F. (1962). *(The welfare) turns its back on you.* Federal Records 45-12499, lyrics by Lucious Weaver and Sonny Thompson. Cincinnati, OH: Federal.

Kreisi, H. (2013). Introduction – The new challenges to democracy. In H. Kreisi, S. Lavenex, F. Esser, J. Matthes, M. Bühlmann, & D. Bochsler (Eds.), *Democracy in the age of globalization and mediatization* (pp. 1–18). Basingstoke: Macmillan.

Linebaugh, P., & Rediker, M. (2012). *The many headed hydra. The hidden history of the revolutionary Atlantic.* London: Verso.

Litterst, T. A. E. (1992). Occupational therapy: The role of ideology in the development of a profession for women. *American Journal of Occupational Therapy, 46*(1), 20–25.

Luthuli, A. (1963). *Let my people go.* London: Fontana.

MacDonald, J. S., & MacDonald, L. D. (1964). Chain migration ethnic neighborhood formation and social networks. *Milbank Memorial Fund Quarterly, 42*(1), 82–97.

Mann, C. C. (2005). *1491: New revelations of the Americas before Columbus.* New York, NY: Alfred a Knopf.

Marmot, M., Allen J., Goldblatt, P., Boyce, T., McNeish, D., Grady, M., et al. (2010). *Fair society, health lives.* London: Marmot Review.

Marshall, T. H. (1950). *Citizenship and social class and other essays.* London: Cambridge University Press.

Matarasso, F. (2011). *All in this together: The depoliticisation of community art in Britain, 1970–2011.* Retrieved from https://mailout.co/articles/all-in-this-together-the-depoliticisation-of-community-art-in-britain-1970-2011-by-francois-matarasso/

McCorquodale, L., & Kinsella, E. A. (2015). Critical reflexivity in client-centred therapeutic relationships. *Scandinavian Journal of Occupational Therapy, 22*(4), 311–317.

Meekosha, H. (2011). Decolonising disability: Thinking and acting globally. *Disability & Society, 26*(6), 667–682.

Morin, E. (1999). *Seven complex lessons of education for the future.* Paris: UNESCO. Retrieved from https://unesdoc.unesco.org/ark:/48223/pf0000117740

Morin, E. (2015). *Penser global. L'humain et son univers* [Think global. The human and his universe]. Paris: Robert Lafonte.

Morley, D., & Worpole, K. (2009). *The republic of letters: working class writing and local publishing.* 2nd ed. Philadelphia: New City Press; Syracuse: Syracuse University Press.

Morris, W. (1888). *Signs of change.* London: Longman. Retrieved from https://www.marxists.org/archive/morris/works/1888/signs/index.htm

Morris, W. (1968). *Three works: News from nowhere, dream of John Ball and pilgrims of hope* (A. L. Morton, Ed.). London: Laurence & Wishart.

Morris, W. (1973). *Three works: A dream of John Ball; The pilgrims of hope; News from nowhere.* London, Lawrence and Wishart.

Morrison, R. (2016). Pragmatist epistemology and Jane Addams: fundamental concepts for the social paradigm of occupational therapy. *Occupational Therapy International, 23*(4), 295–304.

O'Leary, C. E. (1999). *To die for: The paradox of American patriotism.* Princeton, NJ: Princeton University Press.

Orwell, G. (2013 [1949]). *Nineteen eighty-four.* London: Penguin.

Oxley, L., & Morris, P. (2013). Global citizenship: A typology for distinguishing its multiple conceptions. *British Journal of Educational Studies, 61*, 301–325. doi:10.1080/00071005.2013.798393

Palacios, M. (2017). Reflexiones sobre las prácticas comunitarias: aproximación a una Terapia Ocupacional del Sur [Reflections on community practices: An approach to an occupational therapy of the South]. *Revista Ocupación Humana, 17*(1), 73–88.

Petergorsky, D. (1994 [1940]). *Left-wing democracy in the English Civil War: A study of the social philosophy of Gerrard Winstanley.* Stroud, UK: Alan Sutton.

Pollard, N. (2016a). A narrative of cultural occupational performance. *Cadernos Terapia Ocupacional, UFSCar, 24*(1), 191–203. doi:10.4322/0104-4931.ctoARF0649

Pollard, N. (2016b). Post-colonial occupational therapy: Perspectives from an old empire. *Revista Ocupación Humana, 16*(1), 70–83.

Pollard, N., Kantartzis, S., Ismail, M. M., Fransen-Jaïbi, H., & Viana-Moldes, I. (2018). The occupation of accessing healthcare and processes of (dis)citizenship in UK Somali migrants: Sheffield case study. *WFOT Bulletin, 75*, 27–33. doi:10.1080/14473828.2018.1434989

Pollard, N., & Sakellariou, D. (Eds.). (2012). *Politics of occupation-centred practice.* Oxford: Wiley.

Philbrick, N. (2006). *Mayflower: A story of courage, community, and war.* London: Penguin.

Rollo, T. (2016). Feral children: Settler colonialism, progress, and the figure of the child. *Settler Colonial Studies, 8*(1), 60–79. doi:10.1080/ 2201473X.2016.1199826

Ruiz, O. A. (2005). Cazadores y recolectores. Una aproximación teórica [Hunters and gatherers. A theoretical approach]. *Gazeta de Antropología, 21*(22), 1–9. Retrieved from http://www.gazeta-antropologia.es/?p=2771

Swanson, D. M., & Pashby, K. (2016). Towards a critical global citizenship? A comparative analysis of GC education discourses in Scotland and Alberta. *Journal of Research in Curriculum Instruction, 20*(3), 184–195.

Taylor, B. (2016). *Eve and the New Jerusalem: Socialism and feminism in the nineteenth century*. London: Virago

Turnbull, D. (2018). Regarding Hannah Arendt's valuable contribution to occupational science: Some tensions with her approach to philosophy, politics and science. *Journal of Occupational Science, 25*(2), 240–251.

TUNING. (2008). *Reference points for the design and delivery of degree programmes in Occupational Therapy*. The Tuning Project. Bilbao, Spain: Universidad de Deusto. Retrieved from https://www.unideusto.org/tuningeu/subject-areas/occup-therapy.html

Vertovec, S. (2007). Super-diversity and its implications. *Ethnic and Racial Studies, 30*(6), 1024–1054. doi:10.1080/01419870701599465

Whalley Hammell, K. R. (2015). Client-centred occupational therapy: The importance of critical perspectives. *Scandinavian Journal of Occupational Therapy, 22*(4), 237–243.

Wilcock, A. A. (1999). Reflections on doing, being and becoming. *Australian Occupational Therapy Journal, 46*(1), 1–11. doi:10.1046/j.1440-1630.1999.00174.x

Wilkinson, R., & Pickett, K. (2010). *The spirit level*. London: Penguin.

World Federation of Occupational Therapists WFOT. (2016). *Minimum standards for the education of occupational therapists* (rev. ed.). Retrieved from https://www.wfot.org/assets/resources/COPYRIGHTED-World-Federation-of-Occupational-Therapists-Minimum-Standards-for-the-Education-of-Occupational-Therapists-2016a.pdf

World Health Organization (WHO). (2008). *Closing the gap in a generation: Health equity through action on the social determinants of health: Final report of the Commission on Social Determinants of Health*. Geneva: Author.

Zamyatin, Y. (1993 [1921]). *We*. London: Penguin.

Theoretical, Practical, and Contemporary Scenarios in the Metuia/UFSCar Experiences of Developing Social Occupational Therapy

Roseli Esquerdo Lopes and Ana Paula Serrata Malfitano

The second section of this book, Sketches and Scenarios, presents contemporary themes that have challenged social occupational therapy, drawing on experiences with teaching, research and extension projects. An "extension project" is the name applied in Brazilian public universities to projects developed by the university in partnership with the community, government, and/or nongovernmental organizations. Here we highlight projects carried out by the Metuia Network at its nucleus, the Federal University of Sao Carlos (METUIA/UFSCar).

The Metuia Network[1] is an interinstitutional group of studies, education initiatives, and actions aimed at supporting the citizenship of everyone: children, adolescents, youth, and adults (young and old), whose social support networks are ruptured or in processes of rupture. It was created in 1998 by three academics in the occupational therapy departments of three Brazilian universities: Denise Dias Barros, University of Sao Paulo (USP); Roseli Esquerdo Lopes, Federal University of Sao Carlos (UFSCar); and Sandra Maria Galheigo, who was then at the Pontifical Catholic University of Campinas (PUCC) (Barros, Lopes, & Galheigo, 2002). The Metuia Network proposed the development of projects in the areas of university teaching, research, and extension projects in social occupational

therapy. These projects approach occupational therapy programs' interconnectedness with social services, culture, and education, as well as with health services (Barros, Lopes, Galheigo, & Galvani, 2005).

For over 20 years, numerous projects have been implemented by teachers, professionals, and students of occupational therapy in the different nuclei of the Metuia Network. Currently, the following nuclei are active: UFSCar, USP-Sao Paulo, the Federal University of Sao Paulo (UNIFESP), the Federal University of Espírito Santo (UFES), the University of Brasília (UnB), and one nucleus that aggregates the Federal University of Paraíba (UFPB) and the Alagoas State University of Health Sciences (UNCISAL). These are all Brazilian public universities with the same mission (education, research, and extension projects). The Metuia Network has outlined strategies that aim to contribute to the professional education of occupational therapists within the agreed-upon parameters of the field, as established by the World Federation of Occupational Therapists (WFOT). It is especially concerned with those strategies that are related to developing the humanistic knowledge and critical capacity of occupational therapists (World Federation of Occupational Therapists, 2016), planning interventions based on professional, ethical, and political aspects (Lopes, Malfitano, Silva, Borba, & Hahn, 2012). These strategies also aim at the production of knowledge in occupational therapy, understanding the need to consolidate specific knowledge in dialogue on

---

[1]*Metuia* is a word from the native Brazilian language of the Bororo ethnic group that means "friend, companion."

social practices with other practices in occupational therapy to achieve the institutionalization of the profession. The experiences of Metuia/UFSCar[2] have focused on the community territory as a privileged *locus* for carrying out social occupational–therapeutic practices. Territory can be defined as the geographical delimitation of a given region, but it also includes the local historical, socioeconomic, and cultural relationships and social exchanges (Oliver & Barros, 1999).

Therefore, the experiences described in Section II—which have been in development since 2005 in the municipality of Sao Carlos, a medium-sized city located in the interior of the state of Sao Paulo—address everyone as noted previously, but they tend to focus on a specific portion of the Brazilian population: mostly young urban people. The youth were not a random choice, as they represent a complex demographic for which there was only a small accumulation of experiences published in occupational therapy literature. We directed the work, especially the work producing social technologies dedicated to creating spaces for democratic participation and expanding the social networks and possibilities for young people. We use the term "social technologies" to refer to the application of theoretical knowledge constructed in partnership with the community. The specific purpose in São Carlos is to involve youth in building a meaningful present with future perspectives, individually and collectively. Projects always draw on the social participation and autonomy of the individuals involved[3] (Lopes et al., 2012).

Along these lines, Metuia/UFSCar implemented a practical experience aimed at the production of knowledge that occurs in the territory, which means the fostering/implementation of coexistence between professionals and youth to transform the professional approach away from approaches rooted in a medical/clinical and individual perspective. Nevertheless, the singularities of individuals are respected, in line with the project's principles concerning the pursuit of the radical exercising of democracy and the rights and duties deriving from citizenship (Lopes et al., 2012). To this end, the development of social resources and technologies in social occupational therapy has been an important aspect in reaching these integrated collective and individual goals, and this is what we present in Section II.

The ongoing experiences of Metuia/UFSCar enable the practice of public university extension activities, informing Brazilian society about the knowledge it produces, educating occupational therapists, and collecting research data at the undergraduate and graduate levels. It is worth noting that we have conducted several studies dealing with the poor youth and presenting the challenges associated with occupational-therapeutic practices in such cases, which will be presented in the following sketches and scenarios.

In surveys of the experiences and academic production associated with this practice (Lopes et al., 2006; Lopes et al., 2012; Malfitano, Lopes, Magalhaes, & Townsend, 2014; Pan & Lopes, 2019), three categories of discussion have emerged: (1) practices that avoid moral judgment of youth and their families; (2) articulation of individual and collective demands, based on socioeconomic and cultural contexts; and (3) networking practices to link social facilities, including political management, especially public schools (Malfitano et al., 2014; Pan & Lopes, 2019). Efforts have been directed toward a theory-linked practice that contributes to

> *professionals dedicated to tackling the situations of major vulnerability experienced in the Brazilian context, which presents extreme social inequality and for which professional, ethical and political competence is necessary. This dimension is constructed insofar as it reflects and theorizes the practices implemented in everyday work activities. Such actions are imbued with moral, cultural and class values and with rules of conduct that should be discussed and problematized from the perspective of an intervention in the social context that effectively works towards the greater autonomy of people, whether individuals or collectives. Thus, we seek to ground actions in new concepts, eventually aiming at discussing rights and seeking full citizenship for all.*
>
> (Lopes, Malfitano, Silva, Borba, & Hahn, 2010, p. 143)

To this end, the chapters in this section present scenes, histories, themes, reflections, and propositions

---

[2]The Metuia Network can be described as a group of teaching, research, and extension project activities in social occupational therapy composed of different universities and created in 1998. The term Metuia/UFSCar refers both to the Metuia/UFSCar Project core and to its METUIA Extension Program in partnership with community – social occupational therapy. They both are related to Metuia Laboratory, Department of Occupational Therapy and Postgraduate Program in Occupational Therapy (master and PhD courses), UFSCar.

[3]Most of these actions were funded by the National University Extension Program-PROEXT of the Higher Education Department (SESu/MEC). It started in 2005 with the project *Recreating Paths and Building Perspectives: Tackling Urban Violence Among Popular Class Adolescents and Youth*, whose actions were expanded in 2006 with the program *Youth, Violence and Citizenship in Urban Popular Groups: Collective Intervention and Social Development*. It was consolidated with the program Social Networks, Public Space and Citizenship: Policies and Actions with Youth.

that demonstrate the complexity of reality and the need for knowledge articulation to offer professional answers through the work that is being developed. Hence, this section begins with a chapter that synthesizes what we have so far proposed as "resources and technologies in social occupational therapy: actions with poor urban youth," coauthored by Carla Regina Silva and Patrícia Leme de Oliveira Borba. Chapter 16 points out that the importance of social technologies and the work of social occupational therapists do not lie in their mere existence, but in the fact that the existence of social technologies is a means for professionals to help tackle the harmful consequences that stem from social inequities; that is, they help enable occupational therapists to cope with the social questions posed in the lives of these young people.

Lívia Celegati Pan highlights almost 15 years of activities conducted in a school belonging to the public education network of the state of São Paulo, located in the municipality of São Carlos, listing multiple possibilities for occupational therapy practice to contribute to poor urban youth in public schools. Social occupational therapy has fostered strategies to help young people remain in school and, above all, to create socioeducational proposals that are based on democratic principles and that confront the status quo.

Letícia Brandão de Souza and Aline Cristina de Morais report on the experience of disseminating the Child and Adolescent Statute (the Brazilian legislation on the rights of children and adolescents) among children in public schools. How can the discussion about rights be transformed into playfulness? In an attempt to answer such a complex question, they describe play and the complexity of teaching children about the law.

Carla Regina Silva discusses education and, specifically, school through a personal experience permeated by the "nonplace" inside her. Silva refers to poor adolescents and youth who have a social "nonplace." Marc Augé (1992) challenges contemporary changes in a period he calls "supermodernity," which he defines as the carrier of excesses and changes in the spheres of time (agility, in various dimensions), space (breaking borders and migration), and ego (loneliness and isolation). In this created supermodernity, he notes the "nonplace" formed by the concreteness of depersonalized spaces, as well as by the relationships that individuals maintain in these places. Thus, this story demonstrates how institutions that are so central to young people's experiences can occupy "nonplaces" in their lives.

Also presenting us with a life trajectory, Patrícia Leme de Oliveira Borba and Beatriz Prado Pereira emphasize offense as one of the elements that traverses and leaves marks on these young people. They mention the challenges that social occupational therapists face when dealing with the structure of justice and injustice, specifically through socioeducational measures, and with the possibilities/impossibilities of action. They emphasize that "young offenders are first of all young people."

On this same theme, Giovanna Bardi discusses the social supports sought by young people on drugs. She points out the need for professional and institutional assistance to valorize the nonformal resources of the support network, remembering the necessity for approach and the understanding of the lives of others so that alternatives can be created and supported.

Along similar lines, Paulo Estevão Pereira focuses on the issue of drugs to make the same statement: it is another element in the everyday experience of stigmas and exclusion that permeates these young people's lives. Taking Hannah Arendt (1962) as a reference, he addresses the need to discuss "stateless people" and the condition of youth in our society.

Mayra Cappellaro describes episodes and traits in the lives of young girls from the urban periphery and the paths they follow, which are marked by the fact that they are women. Through an atypical story of someone who has found a leading role, she highlights the important factor of being a girl. This story foregrounds an important question that is addressed in different chapters of this section: What can the life history of children and youth contribute to the understanding of a given reality? Based on Pais (1999), the story addresses "life traits" rather than histories or trajectories of life, "because they are youngsters" (whose life experience is short). However significant the bonds formed between these individuals and the Metuia/UFSCar Project team, the research only touches on fragments of what they have lived. The methodological use of individual biographies and histories or trajectories of life stands out in the human sciences, in the midst of studies that focus on deepening the multiple experiences in the urban environment. According to Velho (2003):

> People, in their uniqueness, also became themes of anthropology, as they were perceived as individuals of a social action constituted from a network of meanings . . . with emphasis on a dynamic view of society and seeking to build connections between the micro and macro levels. (p. 16)

Studies using biographical sources can focus on different strands depending on their uses and interpretations. They present the possibility of being constituted as potential material that enables the history of life to exist and circulate, giving voice and ears to "subjective construction . . . through their personal reports . . . developing a narrative logic that seeks to provide meaning to what is told"

(Pais, 2005, p. 87). However, when decontextualized and isolated, the biographical sources can be constituted as an "illusion," not rooted in the "surface of social life," which demonstrates that the individual plays a plurality of roles and represents the respective social dynamics involved in them (Bourdieu, 1986). In other words, if the biography or history of life is analyzed in isolation, it does not allow connection with its social insertion and results in fragmented analyses (Malfitano, 2011). Therefore, the richness of the traits depicted here, in the form of words, can only be read in the light of the social and macrosocial contexts that make up the lives of these young people.

Gustavo Artur Monzeli discusses gender and sexuality as presenting elements to think about professional action and questions to what extent professionals of an institution, thinking about ourselves as occupational therapists, reproduce different violence in bodies and desires. He advocates "the expansion of life and the valorization of different ways of living," which are essential when seeking to do ethical work based on nonmoral judgment of the other.

Rafael Barreiro and Marina Jorge da Silva discuss two different "spaces" that are equally important to how young people live their lives in cities. According to Rafael Barreiro, virtual environments and the technological advances that alter them affect how people's relationships with digital platforms occur, highlighting the relevance of dealing professionally with the changes in everyday life that result from the incorporation of these devices in young people's lives.

Marina Jorge da Silva, reflecting on the importance of "place" and "circulation" in people's lives, reports an occupational therapy experience in a neighborhood square where most of the young people assisted by the Metuia/UFSCar team lived. She makes use of public spaces such as squares "as privileged *loci* of intervention for the experimentation of coexistence and sociability, where links of social and personal support networks are formed and resumed, with occupational therapists as possible mediators of this process."

Finally, Carolina Donato da Silva and Letícia Brandão de Souza report another experience in this square, designing the territory and community work and illustrating the artisanal action of germinating relationships and developing ties.

This mosaic of studies and practices in Section II concludes our illustration of social occupational therapy. They involve the production of knowledge, the development of reflections, and the implementation of actions that lead to the social insertion of all, conceived as social participation, that is chosen from the possibilities presented by everyday life.

REFERENCES

Arendt, H. (1962). *The origins of totalitarianism*. Cleveland, OH: World Publishing Company.

Augé, M. (1992). *Non-places: An introduction to anthropology of supermodernity*. Paris, France: Le Seuil.

Barros, D. D., Lopes, R. E., & Galheigo, S. M. (2002). Projeto Metuia – terapia ocupacional no campo social [The Metuia Project – Occupation therapy in the social sphere]. *O Mundo da Saúde, 26*(3), 365–369.

Barros, D. D., Lopes, R. E., Galheigo, S. M., & Galvani, D. (2005). The Metuia project in Brazil: Ideas and actions that bind us together. In F. Kronenberg, S. S. Algado, & N. Pollard (Eds.), *Occupational therapy without borders: Learning from the spirit of survivors* (pp. 402–413). London, England: Elsivier Science – Churchill Livingstone.

Bourdieu, P. (1986). L'illusion biographique [The illusion of the biography]. *Actes de la Recherche en Sciences Sociales, 62*(1), 69–72.

Lopes, R. E., Malfitano, A. P. S., Silva, C. R., Borba, P. L. O., & Hahn, M. S. (2012). Occupational therapy professional education and research in the social field. *WFOT Bulletin, 66*, 52–57.

Lopes, R. E., Malfitano, A. P. S., Silva, C. R., Borba, P. L. O., & Hahn, M. S. (2010). Educação profissional, pesquisa e aprendizagem no território: notas sobre a experiência de formação de terapeutas ocupacionais [Professional education, research and learning in the territory: Notes on the experience of occupational therapists training]. *O Mundo da Saúde, 34*(2), 140–147.

Lopes, R. E., Malfitano, A. P. S., Silva, C. R., Borba, P. L. O., Takeiti, B. A., Garcia, D. B., et al. (2006). Terapia Ocupacional Social e a Infância e a Juventude Pobres: Experiências do Núcleo UFSCar do Projeto METUIA [Social occupational therapy and poor childhood and youth: Experiences from UFSCar core of Metuia Project]. *Cadernos de Terapia Ocupacional da UFSCar, 14*(1), 5–14.

Malfitano, A. P. S. (2011). Experiências de Pesquisa: entre escolhas metodológicas e percursos individuais [Research experiences: Between methodological choices and individual paths]. *Saúde e Sociedade, 20*(2), 314–324.

Malfitano, A. P. S., Lopes, R. E., Magalhaes, L., & Townsend, E. A. (2014). Social occupational therapy: Conversations about a Brazilian experience. *Canadian Journal of Occupational Therapy, 81*(5), 298–307. doi:10.1177/0008417414536712

Oliver, F. C., & Barros, D. D. (1999). Reflexionando sobre desinstitucionalización y terapia ocupacional [Reflexions about desinstitutionalization and occupational therapy]. *Materia Prima - Primera Revista Independiente de Terapia Ocupacional en Argentina, 4*(13), 17–20.

Pais, J. M. (1999). *Traços e riscos de vida: Uma abordagem qualitativa a modos de vida juvenis* [Traces and risks of life: A qualitative approach about youth way of life]. Lisboa, Portugal: Âmbar.

Pais, J. M. (2005). *Ganchos, tachos e biscates: jovens, trabalho e futuro* [Informal and odd jobs: Youth, work and future]. Porto, Portugal: Âmbar.

Pan, L. C., & Lopes, R. E. (2020). Terapia ocupacional social na escola pública: uma análise da produção bibliográfica do Metuia/UFSCar [Social occupational therapy in public school: an analysis of the bibliographic production of METUIA/UFSCar]. *Brazilian Journal of Occupational Therapy, 28*(1), 207–226. Epub February 17, 2020. https://dx.doi.org/10.4322/2526-8910.ctoao1760

Velho, G. (2003). O desafio da proximidade [The challenge of proximity]. In G. Velho & K. Kuschnir (Eds.), *Pesquisas urbanas: desafios do trabalho antropológico* [Urban research: Challenges of anthropological work] (pp. 11–19). Rio de Janeiro, RJ: Jorge Zahar Editor.

World Federation of Occupational Therapists. (2016). *Minimum standards for the education of occupational therapists.* Retrieved from https://wfot.org/resources/new-minimum-standards-for-the-education-of-occupational-therapists-2016-e-copy

Resources and Technologies in Social Occupational Therapy: Actions with Poor Urban Youth[1]

Roseli Esquerdo Lopes, Ana Paula Serrata Malfitano,
Carla Regina Silva, and Patrícia Leme de Oliveira Borba

INTRODUCTION

As discussed in previous chapters of this book (see Chapters 1 and 5), the concerns of social occupational therapy are directed toward people who face difficulties of access to rights and social goods and to those who are in higher or lower levels of vulnerability. Social occupational therapy articulates a certain notion of citizenship and rights, with a focus in particular on situations arising from struggles related to the social question within the context of structurally unequal societies.

Social occupational therapy interventions draw from the work of French sociologist Robert Castel. According to Castel, situations of deprivation can be understood as resulting from the conjunction of two social life axes: relations of labor (ranging from stable employment to the complete absence of work, including precarious and intermittent occupations) and relational insertion (from inclusion in solid social networks to total social isolation). These two axes compose different zones in the social space: the integration zone, which implies access to permanent work together with solid relational supports; the disaffiliation zone, which combines the absence of work and social isolation, resulting in a double rupture of the networks of sociability and participation; and the vulnerability zone, which entails precarious work and relational fragility (Castel, 2000, 2003).[2] The boundaries between these zones overlap, and disaffiliation feeds on the dynamics that arise from precarious work and relational fragility—that is, vulnerability—which increases in situations of economic crisis, poverty, famine, violence, and war (public or "silent," as occurs in Brazil). On the other hand, a good social familial relationship can compensate for and/or mitigate the effects of disaffiliation in one's labor relations, just as a good labor situation often enables people to seek, via the market, the creation and/or expansion of closer social relations—that is, the economic dimension—which, in the case of the working classes, is based on access to work that, although fundamental, is not the sole factor determining a person's situation. For members of these classes, who are "always more or less poor" insofar as they do not control the means of production, social insertion synergistic actions offer the chance to exist in less vulnerable spaces (Lopes, 2007). In this context, social support networks can

---

[1]A previous version of this manuscript was published in Portuguese: Lopes, R. E., Malfitano, A. P. S., Silva, C. R., & Borba, P. L. O. (2014). Recursos e tecnologias em terapia ocupacional social: ações com jovens pobres na cidade [Resources and technologies in social occupational therapy: Actions with the poor youth in town]. *Brazilian Journal of Occupational Therapy, 22*(3), 591–602. http://dx.doi.org/10.4322/cto.2014.081, and in Spanish: Lopes, R. E., Malfitano, A. P. S., Silva, C. R., & Borba, P. L. O. (2016). Jóvenes pobres em la ciudad: cotribuciones de la terapia ocupacional social [Poor youth in the city: Contributions from social occupational therapy]. In S. Simó Algado, A. Guajardo Córdoba, F. C. Oliver, S. M. Galheigo, & S. García-Ruiz (Eds.), *Terapias Ocupacionales Desde El Sur: Derechos Humanos, Ciudadanía y Participación* [Occupational therapy from the south: Human rights, citizenship and participation] (pp. 321–340). Santiago de Chile: Editorial Universidad de Santiago de Chile.

---

[2]Robert Castel also describes a fourth social space combining the absence of work due to incapacity and a high social inclusion level: the social assistance zone of insured and integrated dependence.

be characterized dynamically and procedurally, where their presence, their absence, and major or minor disruptions in them are results of social existence modalities that range from autonomy to dependence.

Creating, expanding, and strengthening social support networks imply that people, civil society, and governments all act in these processes. Thus, population groups whose socioeconomic vulnerabilities impact on the deficits in their social insertion become the focus of social occupational therapy action, which aims at developing strategies for the creation and/or strengthening of social support networks for these populations with a view to their greater autonomy and social insertion, as in the case of poor urban youth.

POOR URBAN YOUTH

Youth has been the focus of numerous studies, discussions, and debates within civil society in many countries. It is a theme that is addressed in different fields of knowledge and that is the subject of various concepts. Previous research on youth has explored a variety of experiences of young people from different social, cultural, economic, and other perspectives (Freitas, 2005). Notwithstanding these different perspectives, there is an ever-present fundamental aspect that can never be overlooked when considering youth: the role of social class. The socioeconomic structure of society creates differences in the possibilities of young people's experiences. Access to social rights (which, in Brazil, include education, culture, and health, among others), material goods, and the possibility of insertion in the world of work are relevant elements when thinking about who these youths are, what their perspectives are, and their range of experiences transitioning to adulthood.

Social occupational therapy prioritizes a reading in which young people are understood in terms of their interactions with social processes and their insertion in the set of relations produced throughout history. Thus, a choice has been made in this chapter to apply a sociohistorical framework to address a specific group of young people who are in the most vulnerable socioeconomic situations. This is justified by the social conditions experienced in Latin America, which shows a high level of economic inequality (Comissão Econômica para a América Latina e o Caribe [CEPAL], 2013). According to Abad (2002), youth policies in Latin America were determined by social exclusion and the challenges of how to facilitate the processes of transition to adulthood and integration. Bango (1995) adds that the great challenge for Latin America in the 2000s was—and still is—to transform policies aimed at this group, both in terms of content and implementation,

actualizing the youth as people with rights and people with agency to inform their own development.

The United Nations chose 1985 as the "Year of Youth." At that time, specialized studies were commissioned, existing processes to establish national policies were strengthened, and new ones were initiated (Bango, 2008). In the 1990s, the Ibero-American Youth Organization (OIJ) was founded[3] with a view to strengthening policies aimed at young people in member countries (OIJ, 2010).

A new conceptualization of citizenship, informed by the struggles of social movements for democratic freedoms and the guarantee of rights, emerged in Brazil in the late 1980s. The federal constitution of 1988 changed the constitutional bases of social, civil, and political rights, incorporating a universalist agenda of social rights and protection into the legislation. From the standpoint of social rights, the question proposed was how this legal guarantee could be realized, considering that Brazil was still marked by profound inequalities regarding the enjoyment of these rights (Delgado, Jaccoud & Nogueira, 2008). The guarantee of rights for children and adolescents, legitimized as an "absolute priority," was an important focus of the Brazilian Child and Adolescent Statute (CAS) (Brasil, 1990), a piece of national legislation that pertains specifically to the child and adolescent population. Nevertheless, the CAS does not cover all young people, as it focuses on children (0 to 12 years) and adolescents (12 up to 18 years), whereas the Brazilian definition of "youth" refers to young people up to the age of 29.

At the beginning of the 2000s, the public policies directed toward this population showed precarious and insufficient coverage, quality, and results. "Preparation for the future" was their guiding philosophy, hence their focus on educational policies. But in reality, they were aimed at adolescents and children in special situations of "abandonment," "deviance," or "marginality"; therefore, these youths were, and often continue to be, the objects of focal actions of social assistance, restraint, or punishment by the state (Abramo, 2004).

Another aspect regarding the youth and the need for public policies has been the growth of violence in Brazil

---

[3]Comprising representatives of the Andean region, the Caribbean, Central America, South America, and the Iberian Peninsula, the OIJ seeks to promote and encourage efforts of its member states to improve the quality of the life of the youth in these regions and foster the strengthening of governmental structures for this population, and to promote coordination among institutions and sectors directly involved in integrated youth policies, among others (OIJ, 2010). Brazil became a member of this organization only in 2010.

and, especially, the indices on juvenile mortality (Castro, Aquino, & Andrade, 2009). Young people are associated with violence, both as perpetrators and as victims; from this perspective, the poor youth are more strongly associated with delinquency and crime[4] (Wailselfisz, 2011).

Although some Latin American countries are generally in a more stable macroeconomic position, there is still a need for an urgent response to social demands. This apparent stability has not allowed a solid reversal of historically constructed social inequality; despite our many riches, we remain poor. According to Grynspan (2010), the countries that have protected the mechanisms that regulate, redistribute, and promote the democratic state are better equipped to cope with financial crises and their aftermath. Thus, in this context and with an eye to exploring who these young people are and what social conditions exist for them, we will report on some experiences of social occupational therapy engagements with poor urban youth.

TECHNOLOGIES, STRATEGIES, AND EXPERIENCES WITH POOR URBAN YOUTH: SOCIAL OCCUPATIONAL THERAPY ACTIONS

Since 1998, the Metuia Laboratory team of the Occupational Therapy Department, Federal University of Sao Carlos (UFSCar) has been constructing a set of procedures and resources that have contributed to social occupational therapy actions based on the concepts of territory and community,[5] with a view to a locally based technical contribution and to face the challenges posed to those who work in the social field (Lopes et al., 2006; Lopes et al., 2010). Metuia members have engaged in activities that integrate university teaching, research, and partnerships between the university and the community, including public bodies.

---

[4]In the 1980s and 1990s, the complexity of urban violence and crime was reflected in the increased number of homicides as well as in serious violations of human rights (lynchings, summary executions, police violence, etc.). During this period, the following risk factors were associated with urban violence: being young (aged 15 to 29), being male, being of African descent, being poor, and residing in large urban centers and/or favelas. From 1980 to 2007, the death rate by homicide increased 167% among the young population (aged 15 to 24), whereas a growth of 17.8% was observed in the total population (Wailselfisz, 2011).

[5]Territory is defined as the geographical area of a given region occupied by a community, with the local historical constitution and the socioeconomic and cultural relations developed there also necessarily included in this concept. In this space, different forms of life and social exchanges are observed.

In the experience we have developed in the municipality of Sao Carlos, located in the interior of the state of Sao Paulo, Brazil, since 2005, we have addressed issues associated with the poor youth of a specific territory, an urban periphery. In this region of the city, aiming to assert the social rights of people and collectives, we chose to carry out interventions in two spaces: a center for leisure, sports, and shared activities dedicated to the youth, called a "youth center" (YC), and a public elementary and middle school. The occupational-therapeutic action conducted in these two institutional spaces is a theoretical-methodological approach that is in line with the principle of responsibility in the territory (Barros, Ghirardi, & Lopes, 1999). In this action, the professionals meet the target population in its territory, considering that it is necessary to promote a "decentralization" of the action, moving it from institutional and clinical settings to the spaces of everyday living.

In this context, addressing the poor Brazilian youth necessarily requires dialoguing with public schools, because that is where many young Brazilians can be found (Lopes & Silva, 2007). The school is a reference space for the youth, despite the historical and current difficulties the education system faces, with questions about its efficiency and the resources it uses to work with children and adolescents. For those who have left school, the community—that is, the place that provides formal and informal living support—becomes the meeting place. Therefore, seeking to also make contact with those young people who are no longer in school, we opted for the development of a practice in the community, specifically in the YC.

The experience accumulated by the Metuia/UFSCar Laboratory has produced social technologies that have been able to foster new possibilities of practice, integration, and articulation of macro- and micro-social actions.

We use the term "social technologies" to refer to the application of theoretical knowledge constructed in partnership with the community, avoiding the use of terms widely used in the health sector. From this perspective, the following interventions can be highlighted: *workshops/activities, dynamics, and projects*; *individual territorial follow-ups*; *articulation of resources in the social field*; and *dynamization of the support network*. Each of these interventions will be explored individually below.

Workshops/Activities, Dynamics, and Projects

Social occupational therapy uses these activities as mediators of its practice to approach, follow up, and understand the demands of the people and collectives to whom it directs its actions. In our experience, we have focused on the use of activities in group and/or collective spaces. By means of this instrument of practice, which should be mastered by occupational therapists, it is possible to understand the immediate environment of the target population, significantly increasing the possibility of creating bonds, and thus generating opportunities for professional action that contributes to the joint construction of plans and projects (Lopes, Borba, & Cappellaro, 2011). The use of these activities enables learning and the recognition of the needs of people and the development of their capacity to seek their own creative solutions to their problems. They create potential spaces of experimentation and learning, conceiving each participant as an active being in the process of constructing subjectivity—a being of praxis, action, and reflection.

The workshops (their activities, dynamics, projects, and products) allow a powerful range of actions that can be classified, understood, and applied with different purposes, such as the management of the techniques inherent to the proposition of the activity; the use and production of materials and resources; transit through various sectors (culture, art, sport, leisure, work, etc.); compliance with proposals previously prepared on pre-established themes and objectives (e.g., discussions about everyday life, life perspectives, exchanges of information about the world of work, educational processes focusing on rights and duties, and the protection network for children and adolescents in the city, among others); the needs and possibilities of everyday life; and different meanings that the target population can designate or apply according to their personal experiences—in this case, even if the proposals come with previously determined directions, they must be flexible enough to change based on the individual needs and perceptions of the individuals engaged in the activity (Silva, 2011). These devices facilitate closer contact with the adolescents, from which a comprehensive reading of individual and collective needs becomes possible. It also fosters greater contact and shared living between the participants themselves; it provides a pleasant space of sociability and exchanges that can move beyond the physical space of the workshop, transcending into the broader context of that community (Lopes, Borba, & Cappellaro, 2011).

As one of the ways to respond to the demands of the young people that attend the YC, the METUIA Workshops, so called by both the youth and the local staff, provide an open space for those who want to participate. The workshops favor the use of activities as a facilitating means of approaching the youths' world and addressing their rights, including the right to choose and the right to recognize oneself as a person that does, thinks, experiences, and desires. The ideas for the activities come from the youth themselves and from the professional team members; they can be specific activities, such as the construction of kites and masks, cooking, physical activities, group activities, and conversations, or longer-term projects, such as the

production of exhibits, soccer tournaments, and collaboration in the planning and execution of local and regional conferences on the rights of children and adolescents, among others. These "doings" enable exchanges and dialogues that become vehicles for inventions and creations for everyday life, for their own everyday lives. Figure 16.1 presents a photograph taken at the Metuia Workshops conducted in the YC.

Among the intervention modalities developed in a public school, we highlight the design and facilitation of group activities, in partnership with high school teachers of the disciplines of sociology and philosophy, with a view to resignifying and facilitating the understanding of class contents and the resulting reflective processes. Given the curricular content, dynamics were prepared based on different resources (audiovisual, expression, drama, and interactive games). The processes constructed during the meetings became a social technology to approach the adolescents and restructure the curricular content, focusing on themes associated with citizenship, social and human rights, and socialization and sociability processes, and with the denaturalization of the reality, violence, and prejudice experienced by these youths. The combination of the experimentation and the experience of those activities/resources and their articulation with the collective reflexive process enabled greater awareness on the part of the students with respect to the themes addressed, in the context of contemporary problems. In addition, it motivated discussion and apprehension of individual and collective ways of tackling these problems.

With regard to the school staff (principal and teachers), these actions have offered strategies to discuss the construction of educational proposals within the public

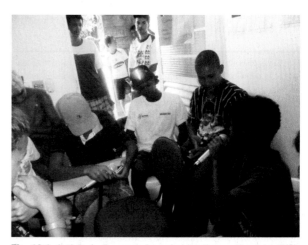

Fig. 16.1 Activity in the workshops held at the youth center (YC).

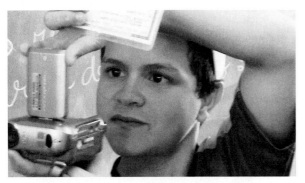

Fig. 16.2 Activity in the workshop held at the public school.

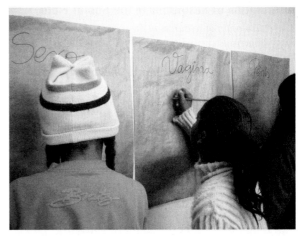

Fig. 16.4 Group dynamics and action in the public schools.

school, based on democratic principles that are closer to the needs and reality of the students and that challenge that status quo. Figure 16.2 shows a photograph taken at the Metuia Workshops conducted in a public school. Figures 16.3 and 16.4 show group dynamics and action at the YC and in a public school.

Individual Territorial Follow-ups

Individual territorial follow-ups are used in social occupational therapy as intervention strategies that enable real perception of and interaction with the everyday lives and life contexts of people, interconnecting their histories and pathways and their current situations and social networks. These follow-ups begin with a close listening to the demands of people, groups, or collectives, which are most often determined by the situation of vulnerability, social inequality, and lack of access to social services and essential goods, with the aim of developing joint processes (Lopes, Borba, Trajber, Silva, & Cuel 2011; Malfitano, Adorno, & Lopes, 2011). Figure 16.5 shows a photograph taken during these follow-ups.

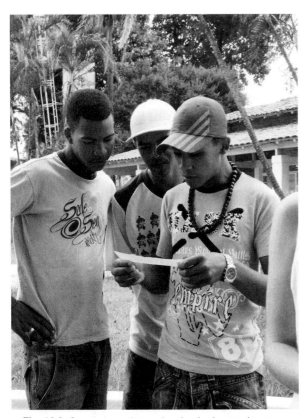

Fig. 16.3 Group dynamics and action in the youth center.

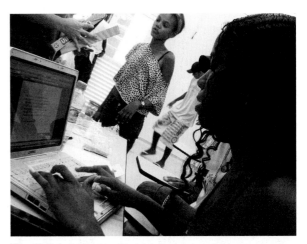

Fig. 16.5 Individual territorial follow-ups and the construction of possibilities.

Articulation of Resources in the Social Field

The *articulation of resources in the social field* consists of an array of actions carried out at the individual level, moving up to the group and collective levels, and eventually to the levels of politics and management. The strategy consists in managing the practices at different levels of assistance involving common goals and using the possible resources, understood as the financial, material, relational, and affective devices, either macro- or micro-social, to compose the interventions. Therefore, it is necessary to use intervention methodologies that are also included at these different levels to enable the identification, negotiation, and effective contribution of these resources. Figure 16.6 shows a snapshot of the search for this articulation.

The Dynamization of the Support Network

The *dynamization of the support network,* in the case of assistance to the youth, aims to map, disseminate, and consolidate all programs, projects, and actions aimed at this population group and/or its community to foster interaction and integration, articulate the different sectors and levels of intervention, and facilitate the effectiveness and direction of the strategies. Figure 16.7 presents a photograph taken at this intervention.

Since 2008, under the coordination of the Special Municipal Department of Children and Youth, professionals working in the municipality of Sao Carlos have been discussing the need for articulation between services and professionals working with children, adolescents, and the youth in the sectors of social assistance, education, culture, sports, justice, and health, among others. With this in mind, the "Network of Children and Adolescents of Sao Carlos" (ReCriAd) was created, and the Metuia/UFSCar

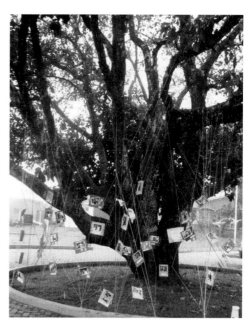

Fig. 16.7 Intervention at the Municipal Conference of Rights: Creation of the "Youth Tree."

Laboratory team was invited to advise on the planning and implementation of the project. Addressing intersectionality and interdisciplinarity (which are necessary for the construction of a network of social services that meet the needs of children and adolescents), four rounds of meetings were held in the five administrative regions of the municipality with the aim of creating a forum of intersectoral discussion on referrals and interventions. The intention was to establish and strengthen public spaces that could support the professionals involved in the delivery of the services, through the presentation and understanding of the objectives, methods, and actions effectively carried out. These actions addressed policy, focusing on the production of joint responsibilities for reflection and action, to provide responses to the young people's demands, be they individual or collective (Malfitano, Lopes, Borba, & Magalhães, 2014).

FINAL REMARKS

Given the enormous social inequalities faced by Brazil, as professionals and researchers we are aware of the limitations and time constraints of our interventions in a context that combines the education of occupational therapists with a view to knowledge production. However, the development of these projects offers us important elements and indicators, as well as strengthening the theoretical assumptions of the direction that the approaches and methodologies

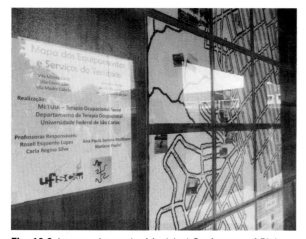

Fig. 16.6 Intervention at the Municipal Conference of Rights.

employed in the action with adolescents and the youth should contain: conditions for the promotion and appropriation of rights, the construction of relationships of respect, and the exercise of autonomy (Lopes et al., 2008).

The social technologies herein presented have been used by the Metuia Project for over two decades (Barros, Lopes, & Galheigo, 2007) and by the Metuia/UFSCar Laboratory, which is specifically dedicated to issues concerning poor urban youth, for the past 15 years. Our experience has fostered reflections on the work processes to be undertaken by occupational therapists in the social field, taking into account the professional, ethical, and political dimensions that compose their professional education and qualification. The following elements have become evident: time; the availability of professionals; agility and ethical and technical responsibility in the articulation between different actors and services; the constitution of a centered and knowledgeable reading of the social, subjective, individual, and collective realities; a wide repertoire for the daily proposition of activities, as well as the expansion of the concept of the activities; knowledge about and dialogue with the network of social resources pre-existing in the community and the city; and reflection on the limits of the professional relationship in the care and reception of social questions at the individual level. All these elements encourage us to reflect on the occupational-therapeutic actions in the social field and on the necessity for daily work directed at the urgency of effective changes of the—sometimes very hard—reality these young people experience.

In view of the complex difficulties encountered by services that assist the youth, coupled with the lack of actions that strengthen the articulation between referral services for this population in the territory in which we practice, the continuity of actions aims, in particular, to assist the public services and society in creating ways of responding to the demands of this population group through strategies that enhance partner services and foster articulation between them. In this way, we seek to ensure greater possibilities of offers and choices for this population, which experiences fragile opportunities to engage in significant life projects, closeness to informal and illegal work, and lack of schooling, all of which contribute to creating a situation of social and personal vulnerability.

The experiences of the Metuia Laboratory have demonstrated that the combination of a professional repertoire of knowledge about the rights of adolescents and youth, with an interdisciplinary approach and a dialogue in the field, can enable the creation of collective actions capable of provoking changes in their participants and in the often authoritarian relations that still rule the community and school spaces.

Collectively, we have learned—from the young people we have met and from our partners and local interlocutors—where these technologies can come into practical and conceptual existence and constitute tools of social occupational therapy practice. It is worth emphasizing that the importance of social technologies—that is, of occupational social therapy practice—does not lie in their existence but in the fact that their existence is a means that enables professionals to assist with coping with the harmful consequences arising from social inequality; that is, they help us deal with the social question's effects on the lives of these young people. The intention is to move toward widening the space of social occupational therapy practice in the public sphere and to produce greater participation with more freedom, autonomy, and solidarity.

REFERENCES

Abad, M. (2002). Las politicas de juventud desde la perspectiva de la relacion entre convivencia, ciudadania y nueva condicion juvenil [Youth policies from the perspective of relationship among sociability, citizenship and new youth condition]. *Última Década, Valparaíso, Chile, 10*(16), 119–155. doi:10.4067/S0718-22362002000100005

Abramo, H. W. (2004). Políticas de juventud en Brasil: nuevos tempos nuevas miradas [Youth policies in Brazil: New times, new perspectives]. In D. Krauskopf, H. W. Abramo, A. Paciello, O. Dávila, & E. Rodriguez. (Eds.), *Políticas de juventud en latinoamérica: Argentina en perspectiva* (pp. 33–43). Buenos Aires: Facultad Latinoamericana en Ciencias Sociales [Youth polices in Latin America: Argentina in perspective].

Bango, J. (1995). *Politicas de juventud em America Latina en la antesala del año 2000: logros, desafíos y oportunidades* [Youth policies in Latin America before 2000: Achievements, challenges and opportunities]. Montevideo: Organización Iberoamericana de Juventud.

Bango, J. (2008). Políticas de juventude na América Latina: identificação de desafios [Youth policies in Latin America: Identification of challenges]. In M. V. Freitas & F. C. Papa (Eds.), *Políticas públicas: juventude em pauta* [Public polices: youth in debate] (2nd ed., pp. 33–55). São Paulo: Cortez.

Barros, D. D., Ghirardi, M. I. G., & Lopes, R. E. (1999) Terapia ocupacional e sociedade [Occupational therapy and society]. *Revista de Terapia Ocupacional da Universidade de São Paulo, 10*(2/3), 71–76.

Barros, D. D., Lopes, R. E., & Galheigo, S. M. (2007). Novos espaços, novos sujeitos: a terapia ocupacional no trabalho territorial e comunitário [New spaces, new subjects: The occupational therapy in community and territorial work]. In A. Cavalcanti & C. Galvão (Eds.), *Terapia ocupacional - fundamentação & prática* [Occupational therapy: background and practice] (pp. 354–363). Rio de Janeiro: Guanabara Koogan.

Brasil. (1990). *Estatuto da Criança e do Adolescente* [Brazil's Statute of the Child and Adolescent]. São Paulo: Cortez.

Castel, R. (2000). As armadilhas da exclusão [The pitfalls of exclusion]. In: Belfiore-Wanderley, M., Bógus, L. & Yazbeck, M. C. (orgs). Desigualdade e a questão social [Inequalities and social question]. São Paulo: Educ, 2000, pp. 15–48.

Castel, R. (2003). *From manual workers to lage laborers: Transformation of the social question.* London & New York: Routledge Taylor & Francis.

Castro, J. A., Aquino, L. M. C., & Andrade, C. C. (2009). *Juventude e políticas sociais no Brasil* [Youth and socials policies in Brazil]. Brasília: Ipea.

Comissão Econômica para a América Latina e o Caribe (CEPAL). (2013). *Panorama social da América Latina* [Social view from Latin America]. Retrieved January 2014, from http://www.eclac.cl/cgi-bin/getProd.asp?xml=/publicaciones/xml/9/51769/P51769.xml&xsl=/tpl/p9f.xsl&base=/brasil/tpl/top-bottom.xsl

Delgado, G., Jaccoud, L. & Nogueira, R.P. (2008). Seguridade social: redefinindo o alcance da cidadania [Social security: redefining citizenship reach]. In: Instituto de Pesquisas Econômicas Avançadas (IPEA), *Políticas sociais: acompanhamento e análise*, Instituto de Pesquisas Econômicas Avançadas (IPEA), 17(1), 17-40. Retrieved June 2019, from: https://www.ipea.gov.br/portal/images/stories/PDFs/livros/bps_completo_1.pdf

Freitas, M. V. (2005). *Juventude e adolescência no Brasil*: *referências conceituais* [Youth and adolescence in Brazil: Conceptual guides]. São Paulo: Ação Educativa. Retrieved June 2019, from http://library.fes.de/pdf-files/bueros/brasilien/05623.pdf

Grynspan, R. (2010). Desenvolvimento, crescimento e superação da pobreza: desafios impostos pela crise internacional [Development, growing and overgrowing poverty: Challenges posed by the international crisis]. In M. F. P. Coelho, L. M. S. Tapajós, & M. Rodrigues (Eds.), *Políticas sociais para o desenvolvimento*: *superar a pobreza e promover a inclusão.* Ministério do Desenvolvimento Social e Combate à Fome. Brasília: UNESCO.

Lopes, R. E. (2006). Terapia ocupacional social e a infância e a juventude pobres: experiências do Núcleo UFSCar do Projeto METUIA [Social occupational therapy and poor youth: Experiences from Núcleo UFSCar Core of METUIA Project UFSCar of METUIA Project]. *Cadernos Terapia Ocupacional UFSCar, São Carlos,* 14(1), 5–14. Retrieved June 2019, from http://www.cadernosdeterapiaocupacional.ufscar.br/index.php/cadernos/article/view/162/118

Lopes, R. E. (2007). Redes sociais de suporte [Support social networks]. In M. B. Park, R. F. Sieiro, & A. Carnicel (Eds.), *Palavras-chave em educação não-formal* [Key-words of non-formal education] (pp. 249–250). Holambra: Ed. Setembro; Campinas: Centro de Memória da Unicamp.

Lopes, R. E., Malfitano, A. P. S., Silva, C. R., Borba, P. L. O., & Hann, M. S. (2010). Educação profissional, pesquisa e aprendizagem no território: notas sobre a experiência de formação de terapeutas ocupacionais [Professional education, research and learning in the territory: Notes from an experience of occupational therapy education]. *O Mundo da Saúde, São Paulo,* 34(2), 140–147. Retrieved June 2019, from http://www.saocamilo-sp.br/pdf/mundo_saude/75/140a147.pdf

Lopes, R. E., Adorno, R. C. F., Malfitano, A. P. S., Takeiti, B. A., Silva, C. R., & Borba, P. L. O. (2008). Juventude pobre, violência e cidadania [Poor youth, violence and citizenship]. *Saúde e Sociedade,* 17(3), 63–76. doi:10.1590/S0104-12902008000300008

Lopes, R. E., Borba, P. L. O., & Cappellaro, M. (2011). Acompanhamento individual e articulação de recursos em terapia ocupacional social: compartilhando uma experiência [Individual support and resources articulation in social occupational therapy: Sharing an experience]. *O Mundo da Saúde,* 35(2), 233–238. doi:10.15343/0104-7809.20112233238

Lopes, R. E., Borba, P. L. O., Trajber, N. K. A., Silva, C. R., & Cuel, B. T. (2011). Oficinas de atividades com jovens da escola pública: tecnologias sociais entre educação e terapia ocupacional [Activities workshops with public school youngsters: Social technologies between education and occupational therapy]. *Interface (Botucatu),* 15(36), 277–288. http://dx.doi.org/10.1590/S1414-32832011000100021

Lopes, R. E., & Silva, C. R. (2007). O campo da educação e demandas para a terapia ocupacional no Brasil [The field of education and demands for occupational therapy in Brazil]. *Revista de Terapia Ocupacional da Universidade de São Paulo,* 18(3), 158–164. doi:10.11606/issn.2238-6149.v18i3p158-164

Malfitano, A. P. S., Adorno, R. C. F., & Lopes, R. E. (2011). Um relato de vida, um caminho institucional: juventude, medicalização e sofrimento sociais [Life story, institutional path, medicalization and social suffering]. *Interface, Botucatu,* 15(38), 701–714. doi:10.1590/S1414-32832011005000042

Malfitano, A. P. S., Lopes, R. E., Borba, P. L. O., & Magalhães, L. V. (2014). Lessons from the experience of Brazilian occupational therapists engaged in social policy making and implementation: Building a dialogue with Canadian occupational therapists. *Occupational Therapy Now,* 16, 10–12.

Organização Ibero-Americana De Juventude (OIJ). (2010). *Sobre OIJ* [About Ibero-American Youth Organization]. Retrieved December 10, 2010, from http://www.oij.org

Silva, C. R. (2011). *Percursos juvenis e trajetórias escolares*: *vidas que se tecem nas periferias das cidades [tese]* [Youth routes and school trajectories: Lives that are woven in the outskirts of cities]. 330f. (Tese Doutorado em Educação). Programa de Pós-Graduação em Educação da Universidade Federal de São Carlos UFSCar, São Carlos. Retrieved June 2019, from https://repositorio.ufscar.br/bitstream/handle/ufscar/2268/4064

Wailselfisz, J. J. (2011). *Mapa da violência 2011 – os jovens do Brasil* [Violence's map of 2011: Young people from Brazil]. Brasília: Instituto Sangari.

17

Social Occupational Therapy in School: Experiences with a Student Association

Lívia Celegati Pan

From the perspective of social occupational therapy (Barros, Ghirardi, & Lopes, 2005), the Metuia/UFSCar Project team has been conducting discussions on youth and education. The Metuia/UFSCar Project team carries out projects based on the principles of public higher education in Brazil, which establish the nexus between university teaching, research, and extension activities. These projects are carried out in partnership with several public bodies and communities, with work teams composed of lecturers and professors, occupational therapists, researchers, and undergraduate and graduate students (Lopes, Malfitano, Silva, Borba, & Hahn, 2012). This chapter provides a report on an experience in a public school. As Lopes, Silva, and Borba explain in another chapter of this book, the aforementioned team has been undertaking actions in public schools in the municipality of Sao Carlos, state of Sao Paulo, since 2005.

As one of the actions of the Metuia/UFSCar Project, the author has been developing an experience in a public school since 2015; this chapter describes some theoretical-practical reflections that originated from that action. This experience has been developed jointly with undergraduate students of the Occupational Therapy Program at the Federal University of Sao Carlos (UFSCar), specifically through actions aimed at the members of the student association (SA) of the school in the periphery of the city. In the context of basic education in Brazil, student associations are organizations created by students that represent the student body of a school and aim to promote dialogue between students and professionals at the school, as well as with the community, seeking to foster the interests of the student body regarding both didactic and academic activities, such as leisure, sports, and culture. Thus, student associations can become an important space for learning responsibility, exercising citizenship, and advocating for rights (Instituto Sou Da Paz, 2002). We therefore considered the SA, the target of our interventions, as a "collective subject"; it is connected by a common purpose since it consists of individuals who share particular subjectivities. In the expanded scope of Metuia/UFSCar action in public school (primary/secondary school), student organizations are considered important for the construction of a democratic and democratizing school. Because we believe it is important for students to get involved with SAs and that they present a potential to become a space for participation in school and experimentation with political and democratic processes essential for the exercise of citizenship, the actions herein reported were undertaken with a view to strengthening these associations.

For youths who do not have reference to democratic spaces of personal representation in their everyday lives, awareness of the importance of participation is not innate, but rather a process that must be constructed gradually, often from scratch, beginning with the perception of its possibility. We believe that school is a fundamental environment for this learning and that occupational therapists are qualified to undertake this process because of their general professional education, which is aimed at understanding, assisting, and respecting diversity. Within the context of this experience, these attributes helped us play the role of articulator for the different individuals that compose the school, and of mediator of conflicts that arose due to the diversity of interests inherent in democracy.

The author of this chapter began her participation as an occupational therapist at the school associated with this experience in 2014 with a broader proposal, in line with what had previously been presented by Lopes, Silva, and Borba. At that time, some members of the SA were contacted to introduce participants for the specific action that would begin in 2015. Our first initiative as occupational therapists working there was to conduct a survey on how several school actors understood the role played by the SA. Regarding the members of the SA, many of them did not know exactly what the organization was and participated because of teachers' referrals or an invitation from the

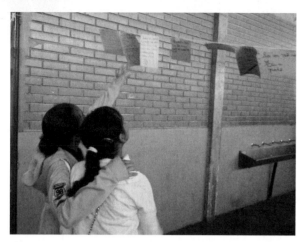

Fig. 17.1 Students in an intervention developed jointly with members of the Student Association during school break.

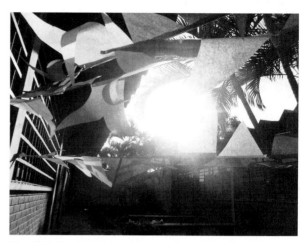

Fig. 17.2 Banner flags made together with members of the Student Association for the *Festa Junina* (Junefest).

teacher responsible for the group (the supervisor). They did not recognize themselves as a collective and were largely inactive with respect to the various school issues they experienced. Concerning the school staff and the supervisor, we perceived a relationship of guardianship and often fear and insecurity regarding what the students could propose and do if they were organized more autonomously. As for the other students in the school, there was a general feeling that the SA was "useless."

A process of sensitizing the whole school to the potentialities of this organization was then undertaken based on a mobilization strategy of the SA members. They were invited to participate in workshops on activities, dynamics, and projects (Lopes, Malfitano, Silva, & Borba, 2014) conducted during the periods opposite to those of their teaching schedule. The workshops addressed the importance of collective organization for the construction of a democratic society and the possibilities of doing this in the school, using spaces of representation. The workshops also addressed the desires the students projected for the school and the possible ways of achieving them.

This process is illustrated in Figure 17.1.

Despite the initial enthusiasm with which our proposal was received, the students became discouraged throughout the year, justifying their absence and turnover with other commitments such as courses and responsibility for the care of younger siblings or household chores. In our analysis, another factor that may have influenced this decrease in attendance was the behavior of the supervisor, a teacher whose recurrent interference with the students' schedules, imposition of how the SA should be conducted, and demand for the students' participation generated some conflicts that had to be mediated by our team.

Nevertheless, in what Martins and Dayrell (2013) call a disorganized organization, the students engaged in some actions, especially in the preparation of two commemorative celebrations in the school: *Festa Junina*[1] (see Figure 17.2) and Halloween. These initiatives were important because they demanded joint collaboration among the members of the SA and enabled the learning of negotiation skills, since it was necessary to build dialogues and agreements with the school board to organize the parties. In addition, these were important moments of integration and socialization between all the school community members—students, teachers, and staff—who positively received the work of the SA, whose members were then able to perceive what could be undertaken through their work, initiative, and organization.

In this context, it is worth mentioning a relevant process that occurred at the end of 2015 with the participation of public school students in Brazil. That year, the public power of the state of Sao Paulo (the most populous and richest in the country) had proposed a restructuring of public schools, particularly of high schools, aimed at optimizing spaces and resources, which in effect would lead to students being transferred to other schools. In disagreement with this decision, some schools started a movement, mostly organized by students, occupying school buildings. This process expanded throughout the state, reaching a total of over 200 school units that were occupied for up to

---

[1]The *Festa Junina* is a popular cultural event in Brazil associated with the celebration of days of Catholic saints. Brought by the Portuguese settlers, it is celebrated in June and includes a traditional dance known as *Quadrilha* (square dance), regional foods, games, and plays.

55 days, and only ended with the withdrawal of the proposal by the state government (Campos, Medeiros, & Ribeiro, 2016). The students occupied the school premises around the clock, holding debates and cultural activities. This movement needs to be emphasized because, on the one hand, it gives us insight on how important spaces of participation are for youths, and on the other hand, it indirectly influenced our work the following year. Even with the students' victory, there were aftereffects in the school daily routine. Because student associations are potent places for the organization of student movements, some attempts to restrict more propositional organizations were made by the governing body responsible for public high schools. One of the strategies was that the student societies would be assigned precompleted projects to complete with no emphasis on student interest or autonomy.

In this context, we began 2016 with a proposal to meet with the SA members regularly during the class period, and the school board released the students at certain times so that we could collectively work out ways to put their proposals into practice. An agreement was made with the school board that the students could participate in the activities of our project provided that these activities were conducted during the periods opposite to those of their classes, which hindered the participation of the youths, who had other responsibilities to tend to during those times.

In spite of the many ideas presented by the youths, they were discouraged by the imposition and/or direction that SAs at public schools must carry out the projects prioritized by the educational governing body; such projects did not dialogue with the students' realities and everyday life and, according to them, did not correspond to their interests. Moreover, it was noticed that the board of that SA was not composed based on the students' organization and that decisions on admission to the organization were ultimately made by the supervisor. Considering interest in participation to be a fundamental issue for a collective organization, in parallel with our work with the students, we initiated dialogue with this supervisor with the aim of starting an electoral process for the SA the following year. Even with these obstacles, the students were able to organize some of their proposals: the celebration of some commemorative dates such as World Environment Day, Mother's Day, Father's Day, and Independence Day, as well as a party for *Festa Junina* and a children's party in celebration of Children's Day.

In 2017, following the process of sensitizing the school staff—especially the supervisor—to the importance of holding SA elections to legitimize the association and encourage student involvement, an electoral process was achieved for the first time with the candidacy of two groups. Although the process of choosing the students that would compose each of the groups was still influenced by the supervisor, it was an enriching experience for the students as it created opportunities for them to think about proposals that benefited the school as a whole, and not just a particular group, and also fostered the importance of debating ideas. The work of the students elected that year once again encountered institutional obstacles: due, on the one hand, to the projects sent by the educational governing body to be carried out by the members of the SA and, on the other hand, to the demands received by the supervisor and conveyed to the students for such projects to be conducted. Even with the demotivation that plagued the students throughout the year (because it did not make sense for them to develop projects that were not consistent with their interests), they managed to organize commemorative events similar to those held in previous years.

In 2018, it was possible to strengthen the electoral process. The SA managers who had been elected in 2017 organized a campaign to mobilize other students so that they approached the SA, and this action was developed in all classrooms. The campaign emphasized the SA as a space of representation and the purpose and importance of student participation and concluded with an invitation for students to think about the possibility of running for a position in the next election; it resulted in the registration of two groups. During the election campaign process, our team offered support to the competing groups by conducting activities that triggered reflection and discussion on the collective demands of the students and the school as a whole. Our activities supported the preparation of action plans for each of the groups and the joint construction of strategies to publicize their proposals, such as the creation of posters to be posted in the school corridors, electoral stickers to be delivered to the students, and the preparation of speeches about their proposals to be delivered in the classrooms. Some events of this period are highlighted next.

One group consisted mostly of students considered to be undisciplined "screw-ups," whereas the other group was composed of the "best students" in the school. It gradually became evident that the supervisor supported the latter, which generated conflicts among those involved. Occupational-therapeutic intervention in this situation occurred as mediation on three levels: first with the students, explaining the democratic character of the elections, which would be decided by the students of the school; second with the supervisor, reflecting on the harm that her explicit preference would cause, with even greater consequences if the other group won, considering that she would have to work with them; and finally, mediation between the students and the supervisor.

After the elections ended with the victory of the "bad" students, many times we had to play the role of mediators once again: with the teachers, dialoguing about the importance of those students taking on this role, favoring them to occupy other "positions" in school, and breaking the stigma they carried; with the elected members of the SA, dialoguing about the different aspects of the positions they would be occupying and about the strategy they would have to adopt, including the adjustment of their behavior to gain the confidence of the school staff and to succeed in conducting their projects; and with the students of the losing group, dealing with the conflicts that arose from differences of opinion and the need for consensus.

Throughout the year, the members of the SA, focusing their efforts on the students' interests and with the support of our team, managed to organize soccer and table tennis tournaments between the classes—a longstanding general demand of the students that had not yet materialized—by negotiating with the school board. Other important achievements included the reactivation of the school radio station, with music during the breaks; the creation of a Facebook page, which, in addition to publicizing the actions of the SA, would be a channel of communication with other colleagues and the community; articulation with all students to decide how to use the funds granted to the school; and the organization of a schedule of activities to be conducted together with the teachers in the last weeks of the academic year, generating different spaces of communication between all school participants. We believe that these achievements were the result of the processes undertaken in previous years, as well as of the process developed that year, with the election of a group that organized autonomously and conducted projects based on the students' interests. The expected continuity of the SA's work shows that it is possible to sustain this experience by promoting actions aimed at the involvement of other students in the SA, constructing a student assembly so that all students can have their demands met and their proposals analyzed, and including the members of the SA in the school planning so that they can participate in broader institutional decisions.

The experience herein reported is understood as an ongoing process that is still under development, and some issues have led to reflections that deserve attention. For instance, we could see that one of the students' greatest desires was for parties and sports tournaments. This may be related to the lack of investment in public policies for the youth (Lopes et al., 2008), which ends up limiting the spaces of leisure and life sharing for young people, especially for those who do not have the financial resources to access private spaces, for whom school is one of the few potential spaces for such activities. Similarly, the students'

recurrent demand for parties, while indicating the difficulty in thinking about broader proposals that impact school organization to make it more democratic, also evidences the scarcity of spaces of sociability for these youths. Therefore, the importance of these initiatives is understood since they enable the school to be a space of significance and construction of more horizontal and dialogical relationships. The organization of these actions by the students themselves may favor self-esteem, sense of value, self- and mutual respect (Sennett, 2004), and the feeling of belonging to the school institution. They also enable the school and its different participants to recognize their demands and those of their public and their surroundings, such as leisure programs aimed at young people in all their diversity and spaces for life sharing, facilitating the creation and expansion of proposals.

It is also worth mentioning the possibility of learning about issues related to the exercise of citizenship and, in consonance with Martins and Dayrell (2013), to the scope of education, and also, with Lopes and Malfitano (2017), to the scope of social occupational therapy, through the learning of collective experience, ways of solving conflicts and making choices.

Finally, we emphasize the importance of the use of intervention methodologies based on the interests of the individuals to whom the actions are directed, placing them at their center in an active and participative way, thus allowing interventions to be, in fact, meaningful from their point of view, enabling them to recognize themselves in the process (Lopes, Borba, Trajber, Silva, & Cuel, 2011).

FINAL REMARKS

The experience herein reported grew out of a belief in the potential of student associations to create democratic and democratizing spaces in public schools. We aimed to highlight the difficulty in developing practices that focus on the participation of young people in countries such as Brazil, particularly (but not only) those from the lower social strata, who are often seen as problems and not as carriers of a future that should interest everyone. This difficulty also occurs due to the structures of school institutions, which are mostly hierarchical and authoritarian. With the identification of these potentialities, we intend that other practices in this sense be visualized and explored by professionals in school institutions.

We believe in the possibility of an education based on democracy and geared toward citizenship education, but this requires a transformative praxis. Therefore, we consider fundamental the presence of professionals in school institutions who commit themselves to and engage in actions based on this perspective. As described in this chapter, it is a long course that demands skills for dialogue and mediation and, from our point of view, can be performed by occupational therapists. The experience herein reported was also a means of raising awareness and training for this.

Occupational therapists seek to create strategies that increase the possibilities of individual participation. School occupies—or should occupy—a central place in the everyday life of children and youths. In the case of the poorest stratum of this population, school is often the only possible place in its social context for this to occur. Therefore, engaging in creative and diverse strategies for participation in school, including political participation, and mediating processes to expand it, is a possible assignment for social occupational therapists. In the practice of social occupational therapy, it is important that professionals be attentive to the diversity of demands arising from the multiple life situations of individuals and to the possibility of professional practice as articulators and mediators of micro-political processes, aiming widely at the exercise of citizenship.

REFERENCES

Barros, D. D., Ghirardi, M. I. G., & Lopes, R. E. (2005). Social occupational therapy: A socio-historical perspective. In F. Kronenberg, S. Simó Algado, & N. Pollard (Eds.), *Occupational therapy without borders: Learning from the spirit of survivors* (pp. 140–151). London: Elsevier Science - Churchill Livingstone.

Campos, A. M., Medeiros, J., & Ribeiro, M. M. (2016). *Escolas de Luta* [Fight schools]. São Paulo: Veneta.

Instituto Sou Da Paz. (2002). *Guia Grêmio em Forma: material para formação de grêmios estudantis* [Guide guild shaped: Material for formation of student groups]. Rio de Janeiro: Instituto Sou da Paz.

Lopes, R. E., Adorno, R. C. F., Malfitano, A. P. S., Takeiti, B. A., Silva, C. R., & Borba, P. L. O. (2008). Juventude pobre, violência e cidadania [Poor youth, violence and citizenship]. *Saúde e Sociedade, São Paulo, 17*(3), 63–76.

Lopes, R. E., Borba, P. L. O., Trajber, N. K. A., Silva, C. R., & Cuel, B. T. (2011). Oficinas de atividades com jovens da escola pública: tecnologias sociais entre educação e terapia ocupacional [Activities workshops with public school youngsters: Social technologies between education and occupational therapy]. *Interface: comunicação, saúde e educação, Botucatu, 15*(36), 277–288.

Lopes, R. E., & Malfitano, A. P. S. (2017). Social occupational therapy, citizenship, rights and policies: Connecting the voices of collectives and individuals. In D. Sakellariou & N. Pollard (Eds.), *Occupational therapies without borders: Integrating justice with practice* (pp. 245–256). Edinburgh: Elsevier.

Lopes, R. E., Malfitano, A. P. S., Silva, C. R., & Borba, P. L. O. (2014). Recursos e tecnologias em Terapia Ocupacional Social: ações com jovens pobres na cidade [Resources and technologies in social occupational therapy: Actions with the poor youth in town]. *Cadernos de Terapia Ocupacional da UFSCar, 22*(3), 591–602.

Lopes, R. E., Malfitano, A. P. S., Silva, C. R., Borba, P. L. O., & Hahn, M. S. (2012). Occupational therapy professional education and research in the social field. *WFOT Bulletin, 66*, 52–57.

Martins, F. A. S., & Dayrell, J. T. (2013). Juventude e Participação: o grêmio estudantil como espaço educativo [Youth and participation: The student council as educational space]. *Educação & Realidade, Porto Alegre, 38*(4), 1267–1282.

Sennet, R. (2004). *Respeito: a formação do caráter em um mundo desigual* [Respect: The formation of character in an unequal world]. Rio de Janeiro: Record.

18

The Caravan for the Promotion of Rights: Disseminating and Discussing the Child and Adolescent Statute (CAS) in Schools

Letícia Brandão de Souza and Aline Cristina de Morais

INTRODUCTION

This chapter presents the "Caravan for the Child and Adolescent Statute (CAS): Promoting Rights and Articulating Actions," a project funded by the Brazilian Ministry of Education in 2013, after being proposed in response to a public call for proposals. This project arose from the understanding of the CAS as an important legal framework for the construction of new paradigms for this population, which is now recognized as a rights holder (Malfitano, Lopes, Brandão, & Morais, 2013).

The project originated from a partnership between the Metuia/UFSCar Laboratory and the Special Municipal Secretary for Children and Youth of the municipality of Sao Carlos, state of Sao Paulo, Brazil, established in 2008. This partnership is rooted in an action strategy called the Network of Children and Adolescents (ReCriAD) aimed at fostering and constructing a collaborative network, integrating and coordinating services and professionals from different sectors (social welfare, education, culture, health, etc.) that work with children, adolescents, and youth in the municipality. Thus, among other actions, the ReCriAD offered training on the CAS, and the present project focused on its dissemination and discussion in some local public schools.

The CAS is an outcome of social movement actions advocating for children's and adolescents' rights, which took place in the context of the struggle for democratization in Brazil and for state accountability regarding social demands. The debates of the 1980s in opposition to the dictatorship informed the democratic constitution. Two years after the birth of the constitution, the specific law about children and adolescents was enacted based on democratic principles, such as replacing the punitive logic of the Penal Code for Minors (created in 1927, revised in 1979). It removed the approach of the old legislation to those who were not "family children," that is, for children who were abandoned, in need, or in conflict with the law, and added the idea of rights for all children and adolescents in the country (Lopes, Silva, & Malfitano, 2006).

The CAS establishes the universalization of rights for Brazilian children and adolescents, ensuring basic rights for all and providing for integral protection and the implementation of an array of services that allow access to and guarantee these rights (Vogel, 1995). It states, "It is the duty of the family, community, society in general, and the government to ensure, with absolute priority, the realization of rights relating to life, health, food, education, sport, leisure, professionalization, culture, dignity, respect, freedom, and family and community living" (Article no. 4), recognizing the "peculiar condition of children and adolescents as people under development" (Article no. 6, Brasil, 1990). Therefore, the Brazilian legislation recognizes childhood and adolescence as a priority for investment in social policies from a universalist perspective and establishes the need to create services to be rendered by the state and society (Brasil, 1990).

Although there have been initiatives, studies, and some outlining for the constitution of a public policy dealing with this area, "fragmented experiences, with weak power of impact and dissemination unfavorable to the creation of consistent elements of a new political culture in the formulation of actions" still predominate (Sposito & Carrano, 2003, p. 35). In this legislative context, which provides a new legal framework for this population—which, conversely, faces inequality in Brazilian society—various experiences have been developed aiming to either reproduce the status quo or, in contrast, create new public spaces following the principles of the new law (Sposito, 2007). Aligned with the latter direction, the proposal for the dissemination of the CAS was developed based on recognizing the need to disseminate and discuss the rights ensured by this statute, both with society in general and directly with the child and adolescent population. Another aim of this project was to offer information that could compose actions promoting meaningful education and enabling the formation of critical citizens able to discuss their social rights and duties.

THE CARAVAN FOR THE CHILD AND ADOLESCENT STATUTE

The choice of the school environment for the execution of this project was linked to the perception of the relevance of this institution for children and youth, taking into account the universalization of the right to education, which should be a fundamental concern for occupational therapists in their actions with this population (Lopes & Silva, 2007). Considering that social occupational therapy aims at strengthening social support networks, coping with existing social inequalities, and achieving the guarantees of social rights (Barros, Ghirardi, & Lopes, 2002), the school should be understood, like other socioeducational institutions, as a relevant social device that may or may not allow certain groups to access educational and cultural experiences and/or better life conditions (Lopes et al., 2011).

The aforementioned project was developed with children aged 6 to 10, totaling 152 classrooms and approximately 4,500 students from 13 public state elementary schools located in the municipality of Sao Carlos (Sao Paulo state, Brazil). We prepared activities appropriate to the children's ages, engaging in play activities followed by dialogues to highlight the concepts of "rights and duties," "system of guarantees," and "legislation," among others.

In the planning stage of the intervention, two play activities were prepared based on participatory methodologies that consider children to be active individuals in the teaching-learning process. These activities—"rights brigade" and "dance of guarantees"—aimed to foster interest in these themes among the child and juvenile public (see Figure 18.1).

Because it allows participants to experience the concepts in a concrete way, the first activity was used especially with the younger students, aged 6 to 8. In this activity, we first presented a story about a bridge, already drawn on the classroom floor. After that, some guidelines were provided: (1) *cross the bridge*—everyone has the right to do it; (2) *be creative*—you are not allowed to use your feet; (3) *be different*—you cannot imitate any of the last three children to have crossed it; (4) *free pass*—after crossing the bridge for the first time, you have the right to come and stay on the bridge, even using your feet; and (5) *lifeguard*—it is guaranteed that everyone will be safe during the crossing.

Thus, the children sat, crawled, crossed it on the laps of others, and supported themselves, among other methods they found to make the crossing.

The second activity, which required greater abstraction, was directed mainly at children aged 9 to 11. A large space was opened between the desks, and everyone was invited to stand in a circle in the center of the classroom. The children were asked to think of a song they liked and dance to it, first with their eyes closed, in silence, and using only their fingers; gradually, other parts of the body could enter the dance, following our guidelines, increasing the possibilities of experiencing different movements in the play activity (see Figure 18.2).

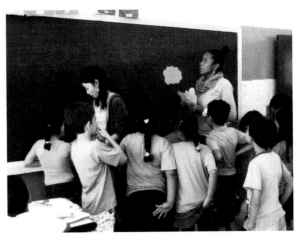

Fig. 18.1 Activities: "Rights bridge" and "dance of guarantees".

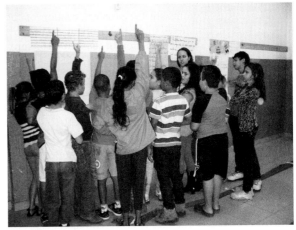

Fig. 18.2 Intervention during the Collective Pedagogical Work Class (CPWC)

Following the plan, we discussed the activities performed, the limitations and guarantees of the law (CAS), the duties and rights involved, and how this information related to the facts of the school environment, further extending this reflection to other spaces of life. It was possible to perceive the development of the discussion and the understanding of the concepts covered beyond the definition of each word related to the law (CAS) and their socially pre-established senses. It achieved the objective of constructing a collective notion about the principles of the law, while children were thinking about daily life and approaching the concept of rights and the system of guarantees. Thus, it was urged that the discussion should address the CAS, referring to its complexity and, simultaneously, to its approximation to the experience, the knowledge repertoire brought by the children, and their everyday life. The aim was to illuminate the concept of citizenship, emphasizing the link between individual, collective, social, and cultural dimensions.

In many instances, there were changes in the environment that could be interpreted as "disorganization" generated by the activity. However, we knew that proposals that stimulate the use of the body along with the activity tend to generate noise and a certain "disorder" in the local norm (in that case, the classroom). In these situations, we noticed that the teachers tended to interfere mandatorily, aiming to restore "order," which hindered the experience and the possibilities of problem solving intended by the ongoing proposal. When this "disorder" occurred without the intervention of adults, we observed that the children tended to solve intercurrences more autonomously (see Figure 18.3).

After witnessing this first phase conducted directly with the children, some teachers suggested another stage of the work directed exclusively at them. Thus, in view of the possibility of expanding the social actors to disseminate the CAS in association with the problematization of the network of services offered to the child and juvenile public, and with the positive participation of the school, we proceeded to an intervention during the "Collective Pedagogical Work Class (CPWC)"[1] with professionals from 10 of those public schools, which enabled direct contact with over 200 teachers, as well as with other education professionals from the public school network of Sao Carlos (see Figure 18.4).

We began by presenting the project and results achieved with the children, followed by reflections on cases and situations present in the school that were pervaded by the

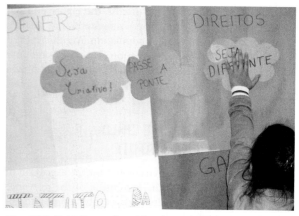

Fig. 18.3 Guidelines of activity through discussion of rights and duties

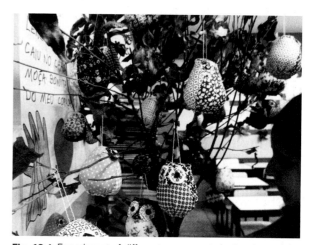

Fig. 18.4 Experiment of different movements in the play activity

issue of rights; these examples were suggested by teachers, pedagogical coordinators, principals, and other participants. Based on the elements brought up in each reflection, propositions of referrals were raised, with discussion of which paths and partnerships could facilitate teamwork to ensure the rights of students. We discussed the practical feasibility of the CAS, and the teachers repeatedly voiced the belief that this legislation brought more problems than solutions to the school, demanding permissive action with children to "speak only of rights," "exempting them from the social function of demanding the fulfillment of duties." At times, we reflected on these and other matters that pervade a superficial or decontextualized reading of the CAS, which is still quite present in our society, generating misconceptions that are used to explain complex social problems. Quite often, it was mentioned that we

---

[1]The CPWC is a time dedicated to the collective planning of activities at school, discussion of experienced situations, and teacher training.

should speak more of duties than of rights with the children, reasoning that they were not fully aware of their responsibilities. Based on the work developed, it was interesting to note that, at least at the theoretical level, there was a change in the view of some professionals regarding the CAS and the debate on rights and duties.

Reflections on the current situation, especially on the new familial and social conformations and the old institutional dynamics, assisted with overcoming the idea that these rights "destroyed the quality of public education." Another challenge was to stop blaming a single instance for all the problems of the school, which were sometimes the responsibility of the students or their families and other times the fault of the school staff or the state. We sought to perceive the complexity of the issues presented and identify the responsibility of each instance, as well as the best way of intervening so that the potential of all these actors could be used.

FINAL REMARKS

Despite the 25-year existence of the CAS, the challenge of its implementation and interpretation remains, insofar as many children and adolescents still have their rights violated in view of the context of social inequality in Brazil (Mendez, 2006). Therefore, it is extremely important for society to create propositions in social occupational therapy aimed at favoring the institution of public spaces and the composition of actions in education that foster access to information, contributing to bringing themes often silenced to the public arena.

In the brief report herein presented, the use of play was a way and a methodology for the articulation of transversal educational contents that are part of the school context, aiming at knowledge constructed during the activity process. More than offering answers and ready solutions, our aim was to stimulate reflection on new action alternatives that are aligned with each other to form a network more capable of addressing children's and youths' demands.

Considering that occupational therapists are professionals focused on discussing forms of social inclusion for different social groups, discussion on the CAS involving the child and juvenile public is a priority demand in Brazil. Specifically in social occupational therapy—which in the experience of the Metuia/UFSCar Project has chosen the public school as a priority space for working with children, adolescents, and youth belonging to urban popular groups—the development of social technologies to approach contemporary issues has been a theoretical and methodological challenge that entails understanding the social function of collective discussions in the dimensions that affect the life of individuals. In this experience, it is

important to centralize the discussion of the CAS legislation in the school environment, with the participation of students and teachers, acting for the dissemination of information on the subject. It is expected this discussion will result in better conditions for understanding children's and youths' situation and the possibility that access to public civil actions may be provided when their rights are not guaranteed. Thus, reflecting on public policies, knowing the specific legislation, and constructing proposals for action in the public sphere are demands for the practice of occupational therapists, who act as articulators in the social context (Malfitano, 2005). It is expected that occupational therapists can contribute to the development of knowledge and intervention methods that offer comprehension and action related to the social condition of Brazilian children and youth.

REFERENCES

Barros, D. D., Ghirardi, M. I., & Lopes, R. E. (2002). Terapia Ocupacional Social [Social occupational therapy]. *Revista de Terapia Ocupacional da Universidade de São Paulo, 13*(3), 95–103.

Brasil. (1990). *Estatuto da Criança e do Adolescente* [Child and Adolescent Statute]. São Paulo: Cortez.

Lopes, R.E., Borba, P.L.O., Trajber, N.K.A., Silva, C.R., & Cuel, B.T. (2011). Oficinas de atividades com jovens da escola pública: tecnologias sociais entre educação e terapia ocupacional [Activities workshops with public school youngsters: Social technologies between education and occupational therapy]. *Interface - Comunicação, Saúde, Educação, 15*(36), 277–288.

Lopes, R. E., & Silva, C. R. (2007). O campo da educação e demandas para a terapia ocupacional no Brasil [The field of education: Possible contributions of occupational therapy in Brazil]. *O campo da educação e demandas para a terapia ocupacional no Brasil, 18*(3), 158–164.

Lopes, R. E., Silva, C. R., & Malfitano, A. P. S. (2006). Adolescência e juventude de grupos populares urbanos no Brasil e as políticas públicas: apontamentos históricos [Youths of Brazilian's urban popular groups and the public policies: Historic appointments]. *Revista HISTEDBR On-line, 23*, 114–130.

Malfitano, A. P. S. (2005). Campos e núcleos de intervenção na terapia ocupacional social [Intervention fields and cores in social occupational therapy]. *Revista de Terapia Ocupacional da Universidade de São Paulo, 16*(1), 1–8.

Malfitano, A. P. S., Lopes, R. E., Brandão, L., & Morais, A. C. (2013). Caravana do ECA: Promovendo Direitos e Articulando Ações (p. 18) [Caravan for the Child and Adolescent Statute (CAS): Promoting rights and articulating actions] [Activity report]. Ministério da Educação, Secretaria de Ensino Superior: Programa de Extensão Universitária - PROEXT. Relatório de Atividade de Extensão.

Mendez, E. G. (2006). Evolución histórica del derecho de la infancia: ¿Por que uma historia de los derechos de la infancia? [Historical evolution of the right of the childhood: Why a history of the rights of the childhood?] In ILANUD, ABMP, SEDH, & UNFPA (Eds.), *Justiça, adolescente e ato infracional* [Justice, adolescente and offense] (pp. 7–23). São Paulo: ILANUD.

Sposito, M. P. I. (2007). Introdução – Espaços Públicos e tempos juvenis [Introduction – Public spaces and juvenile times]. In M. P. Sposito (Ed.), *Espaços públicos e tempos juvenis: um estudo de ações do poder público em cidades de regiões metropolitanas brasileiras* [Public spaces and juvenile times: A study of actions from public policy in cities of metropolitan Brazilian regions] (pp. 5–43). São Paulo: Global.

Sposito, M. P., & Carrano, P. C. R. (2003). Juventude e políticas públicas no Brasil [Youth and public policies in Brazil]. *Revista Brasileira de Educação, 24*, 16–39.

Vogel, A. (1995). Do Estado ao Estatuto – Propostas e vicissitudes da política de atendimento à infância e adolescência no Brasil contemporâneo [From state to statute – Proposals and vicissitudes of the politics of care for children and adolescents in contemporary Brazil]. In F. Pilotti & I. Rizzini (Eds.), *A arte de governar crianças: a história das políticas sociais, da legislação e da assistência à infância no Brasil* [The art of governing children: The history of social policies, legislation and children assistance in Brazil] (1st ed., pp. 299–346). Rio de Janeiro: Instituto Interamericano Del Nino, Universidade de Santa Úrsula, Amais Livraria e Editora.

19

Youth and Education: The Path Constituted by the Nonplace[1]

Carla Regina Silva

This chapter presents the scholarly path of a young man named Charles.[2] His experience has been understood through individual and territorial follow-up(s) (Lopes, Malfitano, Silva, & Borba, 2014). It can be defined as a procedure applied by occupational therapists trying to promote individual needs in the social context. The potentiality of these tools depends on the occupational therapists' reality reading ability and their ethical and technical responsibility. To achieve the individual and territorial follow-up, articulations of different resources are involved, including families, communitarian services, and public agencies. However, it is also important to recognize the limitations of occupational therapists' actions.

KNOWING CHARLES

Charles is a young white man, aged 23, who was born in Piripá, state of Bahia, but has lived in Jardim Gonzaga, a district of São Carlos, state of São Paulo, since he was very young. He is shy but enjoys making people laugh. He is introverted, has a lot of friends, and really likes football. He lives with his mother, Josefina (aged 49), and his younger siblings. He has 10 siblings and 10 nephews and nieces. His five older siblings are illiterate; Charles was the first of Josefina's children to start going to school. His father died when he was 12 years old, and he has a lot of respect for his mother, whom he considers a fun and present

person. Josefina does not seem to demand that her children study or work, an attitude that is relativized by the context.

According to Charles, Jardim Gonzaga is a good, simple neighborhood that has a lot of hardworking people and where he loves living. From his perspective, people should understand that a poor neighborhood does not need to be considered dangerous. He appreciates the fact that people organize themselves to make their situation better, although he has never participated in the residents' organizations. A huge concern for the people of the community is the police, whose abuses of power are countless, including violent entrances into people's houses in search of drugs, and conducting searches of anybody, from babies to the elderly. Charles once had the experience of being mistaken for a drug dealer. The police officers grabbed him and pushed him several times against a wall in daylight. They also slapped him and insulted his mother using bad, rude words, which revolted him.

Charles' profile is remarkable compared to other young men from the same area. A pastor from an evangelical church noticed Charles' characteristics and invited him to participate in services and be part of a course run at a farm belonging to the church that does spiritual work with young people who have had chemical dependencies. The pastor praised Charles, saying that he is a decent young man who does not use drugs, valorizing his moral qualities, and relating them to religious principles. Those same virtues that the pastor recognized have effectively helped Charles in his development, as Charles felt very proud and capable, certain that he was on the right path.

THE SCHOLAR'S PATH

Charles' struggle to adapt at school was remarkable. He remembers that when he was 6 years old, he started his studies and had some difficulties in the first year, but he managed to continue. However, he failed the second and

---

[1]This text is one of the outcomes of the research that resulted in *Youth Routes and Scholar Paths: Lives That Are Designed in the Suburbs* (Percursos juvenis e trajetórias escolares: vidas que se tecem nas periferias das cidades), a doctoral thesis defended by the author in the postgraduate education program at the Federal University of São Carlos (UFSCar) in 2011 under the supervision of Professor Roseli Esquerdo Lopes.

[2]This name is a pseudonym.

third grades and, as a consequence, he went to an acceleration classroom. As it offered a less rigorous evaluation, this path was touted as a way of finishing two grades in one year. He completed elementary school when he was 11 years old, a year later than the norm.

In his opinion, a good teacher is one who is concerned about whether the student is learning and who is patient and interested in explaining until the students genuinely understand:

> When I was studying, all my teachers respected me, but not all of them taught me. The History teacher was one of the most boring as he used to teach little and only once. The Math teacher was the worst because she arrived, delivered the books and sat down on the chair. When she decided to give a test, it was a surprise for us because she did not teach anybody to make the calculations. Everybody got zero but we did not complain. The Portuguese teacher was excellent because she was fun and used to teach very well, so she became our favorite teacher. As soon as we called her, she sat down next to us to teach.

Charles speaks clearly and deliberately: with the help and interest of his teachers, he achieved satisfying results. However, he stopped his studies when he was in sixth grade:

> I was discouraged because I didn't want to go to school anymore, I enjoyed staying on the street with my friends. Because of the absences, I lost my place, stopped studying and failed that grade. The following year, I decided to go back to school, but I resolved to stop again in the middle of the year and I have never returned.

His family did not require him to return to school. He had achieved a higher educational level than his siblings, parents, and friends, who had mostly stopped their studies earlier than him.

In 2007, the Metuia/UFSCar program "Youth, Violence and Citizenship in Urban Community Groups: Collective Intervention and Social Development" had as one of its central focuses[3] the continuity of its actions in public education. The program was based on the understanding of the importance of schools in helping young people face the challenges in their lives.

About 40 young people went to the local community center (currently it is a CRAS),[4] mainly men aged 12 to

29 who belong to low-income families or are in situations of extreme poverty, many of whom were directly involved with the illegal drug trade. The actions developed, as well as other actions, stimulated the reinsertion of these young people in school. As well as individual and territorial monitoring, many dynamics and activities were proposed and debates encouraged so that some young people could return to school. Charles, then aged 20, was one of those young men who registered to take his sixth-grade equivalency through Education for Youth and Adults (EJA), an evening class.

One of the strategies used in the project aimed at increasing the participation of educators and other professionals from the school to improve these young people's chances of obtaining educational success. This proposal was presented to the principal and the teachers of the school, who were made to understand that as a result of the persistent work of the project to encourage these students to return to school, some of them had registered, and the aim now was to help them in this process of rehabilitation. Having heard this, one of the school leaders responded, "So, is it your fault?" judging the situation negatively and prejudicially since they had to receive "those young people" in the school. It was in this context that Charles returned to his studies. He felt displaced in that school despite knowing several students from his neighborhood. He did not feel that he belonged in that place, and he did not believe he would be able to learn.

Charles represented the stereotype of "dawg," wearing loose clothes and speaking in slang, displaying his lifestyle and his appearance. He is the representation of a determined social group that, in general, does not have their educational needs addressed in our society (Lopes, Malfitano, Silva, & Borba, 2010; Silva, 2011; Borba, 2012). Charles was always a well-behaved student, polite and obedient of the rules, but he did not have the discipline to study. Despite finding difficulties with the content, he did not develop a routine for his studies. In the reality of shared classes (because of the lack of teachers and their absences), Charles stopped studying again. He remains convinced of the necessity of studying, but outside the classroom:

> The school I want is not different from what it is, but I would like the rules to be followed, I would like teachers to teach better. I see the lack of rebuilding: classrooms without doors, windows without glass, and there are also those people who jump the walls of the school to date or to fight. There is a lack of security in the

---

[3]With support from a public grant, and in partnership with the Municipal Office of Social Assistance and Citizenship (SMCAS) and the public school, the university extension activities were developed in a Center of Reference from the Social Assistance (CRAS) and in a public school.

[4]This is a service instituted by the National Policy of Social Assistance in Brazil.

schools. The school I want is not different from the schools now, but I just would like that students respect other people and teachers and that teachers respect students.

THOUGHTS ABOUT THE NONPLACE

Charles' path helps to understand how the exclusion of access to education is perpetuated as all the experiences at school produce rejection of the educational sphere, an introjection of his nonplace at school or in any associated environment. The necessity of earning money is the central factor causing young people to consider a minimal level of education to be sufficient. In such cases, the priority of material reproduction is seen to be incompatible with the education institution. However, in Charles' case, it is possible to observe that dropping out of school was not justified by the need to work, because in his path, working activities are irregular, informal, and short term. Charles is part of a group of young people who neither work nor study, which in 2014 represented 29.6% of young people aged 15 to 29 (Instituto Brasileiro de Geografia [IBGE], 2014). In 2013, 23.4% of those who neither work nor study were aged 18 to 24 and 21.3% were aged 25 to 29, and 70.3% of girls fell into these categories (IBGE, 2013).

Charles does not have what Bourdieu (Nogueira & Nogueira, 2006) calls familiar *ethos*,[5] being predisposed to valorize and motivate educational knowledge. This refers to a system of implicit values deeply internalized, indirectly more than directly, which is capable of contributing not only to Charles' cultural capital but also to his attitudes toward school. This is an important element to reach academic success and a differential determining his insertion into the school dynamics, including the discipline necessary to study. Charles expresses his origins in his appearance and the way he conducts himself in his corporal *hexis*.[6] The stereotype of "dawg" carries the social stigma of a young poor boy from the suburbs who causes fear and insecurity and is associated with violations even before any action. He and his group are not welcome in that school.

Before Charles abandoned the school, it had not taken responsibility for his education. The educational institution presents a system of values, some of which are veiled and incorporated into the hierarchical relation established among its participants. The use of values and morals is

inherent to education; historically, they have always been intertwined. However, in the process of educational democratization, with the establishment of universal educational policies, it is important to consider the judgments poor young people are subjected to, as Charles was, for example.

Although the investment of Charles' family was insufficient, how can only the family be responsible for determining his poor educational formation? It must be remembered that in Brazil, a historical delay in relation to access meant that entire generations did not have access to education. As education is considered a basic right for everybody, the question about Charles dropping out of school is a social problem, not only his family's. It brings about an immeasurable social loss due to the waste of human life that it produces.

To start with, it is necessary to scrutinize the judgment and reproduction processes instituted throughout the educational system. The democratic school—beyond its organization mechanisms, educational space management, and amplified decision-making process—needs to break and overcome its methods of distinction, coercion, and exclusion.

One of the paradoxes of what is called the "democratization of schooling" is that only when the working classes, who had previously ignored or at best vaguely concurred in the Third Republic ideology of "schooling as a liberating force" (l'ecole liberatrice), actually entered secondary education, did they discover l'ecole conservatrice, schooling as a conservative force, by being relegated to second-class courses or eliminated.

(Bourdieu, 1996, pp. 143–144)

If the investment in Charles' education was not prioritized either by the family or by the school, his socialization and formation, beyond formal education, were constructed in his groups of friends and peers, who live in the daily entangled dynamic of that territory. Other codes, rules, relations, experiences, information, and contents will be learned from them and again incorporated into his constituted existence. This aspect of Charles' path deserves emphasis: above all, his socialization with teenagers and young people involved in the illegal drug trade must be emphasized, considering it as a broad and complex network of economic activity in Brazil and abroad, which is related to other formal and legal business. He was not part of this network, and his path demonstrates an exception that confirms the rule. This young man takes part in a dual process, sometimes contradictory, as he suffers pressure and social stigmas as if he were involved with crime. He receives enforcement approaches from the police at the same time that he is banned from some activities in his

---

[5]This refers to the character, trained posture, and readiness to satisfy the demands, in this case, of school.
[6]For Bourdieu, *hexis corporelle* is a set of properties associated with the use of the body in which the class position of a person is exhibited (Nogueira & Nogueira, 2006).

group of friends, particularly those related to illicit acts. His involvement with the evangelical church can be seen as the result of this partial relation of belonging and the search for self-affirmation, which is not always fruitful. It must be observed, in this case, that morality does not come from his adherence to religion; on the contrary, Charles was identified to have, according to the pastor's evaluation, certain characteristics compatible with determined religious precepts.

The themes that emerge from Charles' life feed a debate about spaces of socialization and sociability beyond family and school. The question refers to the role and the potential of actions of these spaces in the fight for hegemony.[7] If education discriminates, evaluating students from a prestigious perspective, abandoning the democratic and transforming role, and not assuming its authentic and formative function to provide access to human culture, then it does not do anything more than maintain the status quo. The educational spaces outside school are also responsible for the task of interfering in reality, not only adapting to it. It is not possible to accept the exempted position of somebody who has an educator role, whoever this person is; the same happens to the student who not only is passive but also has a view of the world that should be rescued, understood, and redefined (Freire, 2000).

Key concerns for social occupational therapists should be inclusive formal and informal educational spaces; the defense of quality, public, free schools for everybody as a nonnegotiable social right; the guarantee of equality for nonprivileged groups (or any other that has their rights denied); and the construction of actions and strategies to address the rupture of the educational system and overcome its inherent reproduction, discrimination, and repression. Social occupational therapists can contribute their own theoretical and methodological framework for a better comprehension of these problems and action that transforms them, allowing subjects to improve their lives by staying on the school path.

School represents the most efficient public means to engage democratic processes capable of promoting social change, such as by promoting the social inclusion of poor young people instead of reproducing their exclusion and stigmatization. School can be a source of social support in youths' lives, especially when it is linked to other public social services. Together, the network, including civil society, would allow advances in meeting this population's needs, guaranteeing rights already enacted in society.

REFERENCES

Borba, P. L. O. (2012). *Juventude marcada: relações entre o ato infracional e a escola pública de São Carlos - SP* [Youth marked: Relations between the infraction act and the public school of São Carlos]. 250f. (PhD thesis in Education). São Carlos, SP, Brazil: Postgraduate Program in Education, Universidade Federal de São Carlos.

Bourdieu, P. (1996). *Distinction – A social critique of the judgement of taste* (N. Richard, Trans.). Cambridge, MA: Harvard University Press.

Freire, P. (2000). *Pedagogia da indignação: cartas pedagógicas e outros escritos.* [Pedagogy of indignation: Pedagogical letters and other writings]. São Paulo: Editora UNESP.

Gramsci, A. (2010). Textos selecionados. In A. Monasta (Ed.), *Antonio Gramsci* (Paolo Nosella, Trans.). Recife: Fundação Joaquim Nabuco, Editora Massangana.

Instituto Brasileiro de Geografia (IBGE). (2013). *Síntese de Indicadores Sociais 2013* [Synthesis of social indicators]. Brazilian National Household Sample Survey. Retrieved February 2015, from http://www.ibge.gov.br/home/estatistica/populacao/condicaodevida/indicadoresminimos/sinteseindicsociais2013/

Instituto Brasileiro de Geografia (IBGE). (2014). *Série Estudos e Pesquisas: Síntese de Indicadores Sociais 2014 – Uma Análise das Condições de Vida da População Brasileira (indicadores selecionados)* [Studies and Research Series: Synthesis of social indicators 2014 – An analysis of the living conditions of the Brazilian population (selected indicators)]. Retrieved February 2015, from http://www.ibge.gov.br/estadosat/temas.php?sigla=al&tema=sis_2014

Lopes, R. E., Malfitano, A. P. S., Silva, C. R., & Borba, P. L. O. (2010). *Escola, adolescência e juventude em grupos populares: cidadania, direitos e políticas públicas* [School, adolescence and youth in popular groups: Citizenship, rights and public policies] [Research report] (p. 203). Laboratório METUIA: UFSCar: CNPq: FAPESP. São Carlos (São Paulo – Brasil)

Lopes, R. E., Malfitano, A. P. S., Silva, C. R., & Borba, P. L. O. (2014). Recursos e tecnologias em terapia ocupacional social: ações com jovens pobres na cidade [Resources and technologies in social occupational therapy: Actions with the poor youth in town]. *Brazilian Journal of Occupational Therapy, 22*(3), 591–602. doi:10.4322/cto.2014.081

Nogueira, M. A., & Nogueira, C. M. M. (2006). *Bourdieu & a educação* [Bourdieu & education] (2nd ed.). Belo Horizonte: Autêntica.

Silva, C. R. (2011). *Percursos juvenis e trajetórias escolares: vidas que se tecem nas periferias das cidades* [Youth paths and school trajectories: Lives that are woven in the outskirts of cities] (PhD thesis in Education) (p. 330). São Carlos, SP, Brazil: Postgraduate Program in Education. Retrieved January 2019, from https://repositorio.ufscar.br/handle/ufscar/2268

---

[7]For Gramsci (2010), hegemony is a set of dominance and direction functions exercised by a dominant social class over another or over a group of classes due to historical process. Thus, the hegemonic fight refers to the process of disarticulating the dominant interests—articulated among them, but not inherent to the dominant ideology—and rearticulating them around popular interests, with consistency, cohesion, and coherence from a world conception elaborated from a philosophy.

20

Paths of Life and the Marks of the Juvenile Justice System

Patrícia Leme de Oliveira Borba and Beatriz Prado Pereira

The case described in this chapter unfolded from processes associated with the workshops of activities, projects, and dynamics and the individual territorial follow-up, one of the key elements of the structuring axis of social occupational therapy (Lopes, Malfitano, Silva, & Borba, 2014). This experience was conducted by the team of the Metuia Laboratory, Department of Occupational Therapy, Federal University of Sao Carlos (UFSCar), in two social institutions: a youth center and a public school located on the outskirts of the municipality of Sao Carlos, state of Sao Paulo, Brazil. The Metuia team has been conducting interventions with youths in the region that have developed into social and research activities at different levels (Lopes, Malfitano, Silva, Borba, & Hahn, 2012). Action in these spaces has also allowed us a clearer understanding of reality, with its potentialities and limitations, but above all, it has led to the formation of strong bonds with multiple young people.

In this chapter, the narrative of an adolescent reveals the complex and conflicting relationships experienced with his neighborhood, his family, and the legal assistance system that occurred at a particular time of his life. Writing this story required quite a few years of follow-up, many meetings mediated or not by activities and dialogue, collective efforts to integrate activities of university partnership with the community and research, and—above all—the opening up of this young person to share his life, dreams, desires, and thoughts with us.

JAGUAR

The young man's brother nicknamed him Jaguar. He likes it, because his real name is a combination of a Portuguese name and an English name that is hard to pronounce and even harder to spell. At 19, no longer so young, and with a muscular body, he is very concerned about his physical build and appearance; this can be observed in the way he carefully chooses his clothes, fragrances, and accessories. He has lots of friends, is always accompanied, and often has many friends over. He speaks very little about his personal life, his offense, or the illegal drug trade in his neighborhood, which also takes place in his house.

In terms of personality, Jaguar shows a certain shyness mixed with a mysterious, secretive tone. He was initially quiet during the Metuia workshops (Lopes et al., 2014) that we coordinated at the youth center; however, after joining our team, he became important to the group. At times, he helped with the planning of the workshops and was quite engaged in the organization of the soccer championship—one of our actions. He contributed suggestions and opinions and presented ways that the activities could be carried out. He seemed to be particularly interested in the proposal of kite building, for instance, which is an activity with some relation to his everyday life, and when audiovisual resources such as cameras and video recorders were used.

Jaguar lives with his mother, father, and four siblings, all male; he is the second oldest. They live in an alleyway off the main street of a neighborhood where drug dealing occurs explicitly. In this place, there is a high concentration of *bocas*—drug trafficking spots where drugs are sold and spread through the neighborhood according to the logic common to any trade. The presence of men and children playing cards in the surroundings of his house was very common. The unsuspecting might look at that situation and view the game only as a form of entertainment and occupation, which in part it is, but it is also part of the drug trafficking business, since the game tables are located at strategic points of the *favela* (shantytown), or at the entrances of the *bocas*. Therefore, the game is a way to disguise what is implicit and control what is explicit. As Jaguar's house is an important *boca*, the frequent presence of many people playing cards in the entrance area is justified.

As a result of Jaguar's offense, the juvenile justice system imposed a social-educational measure called Assisted Freedom (AF), which he had to comply with for six months when he was 15 years old. As mentioned in Chapter 12, "Social Occupational Therapy, Offenses, and School: Complex Plots in Fragile Relations," in Brazil, when adolescents (aged 12 to 18) commit a crime, they may have to comply with social-educational measures prescribed by legislation. In the case of AF, a social assistance service is designated to follow up with the adolescent to promote an educational intervention focused on personal assistance through guidance, maintenance of family and community ties, schooling, and insertion into the labor market and/or enrollment in vocational, formative courses (Morais & Malfitano, 2016).

This offense resulted from a police roundup of his home when he, concerned with his mother, took responsibility for the drugs seized, which belonged to her, and he was physically assaulted by the police officers. His family is involved with drug trafficking, specifically his mother, who, in an attempt to mitigate the situation in which she had involved her son, explained to the judge that Jaguar had problems with his health (episodes of epileptic seizures) and was taking medication.

Jaguar speaks very little about his offense because he does not like to "remember matters of the past." He did not spend time in prison in the juvenile justice system but instead was released and picked up by his mother on the day of the incident. He served 5 of the 6 months of his AF because he injured his foot, which prevented him from carrying out the rest since he commuted on foot or used a bicycle, even though he received bus tickets for this purpose. He said he had been summoned by letters sent by the service team demanding that he return, but even so, he did not serve the measure completely. He told us his attitude did not come to anything; that is, neither he nor his family suffered any consequences, confirming the opinion reiterated by many young people that AF "really does not come to anything."

Jaguar reports that he did not like the individual appointments scheduled as part of the AF because he did not want to talk about his life; he said the professionals asked him too many questions. However, it was through the AF that he became interested in the fitness center—one of the activities offered by the program—but because it is one of the activities most sought by adolescents, he was unable to join it, so instead he sought out his own resources to start physical activity near his home.

Jaguar's inclusion in school was an issue often raised by our team. Concurrent with the workshops held at the youth center, we offered another workshop at the school Jaguar attended, but he generally only attended at the beginning of the school year; he would drop out of the course each year. His school failure started when he was 11 years old, and he failed to complete the elementary degree two more times. He never actually flunked it but would quit his studies before that happened. Because of his age/school grade gap, he was entitled to enroll in Youth and Adult Education (EJA), but he also abandoned this educational program, which aims to offer basic education to adolescents and adults who were not able to complete their studies and/or did not have access to elementary/middle school at the appropriate age. At the age of 18, he resumed his studies with difficulties, failing the EJA once again but no longer evading it.

His is a school trajectory marked by difficulties and failures, but as Jaguar insisted on enrolling and resuming his trajectory, he demonstrated perseverance and that he believes that school is important. Jaguar told us that he used to fool around a lot: he did not like school or being in the classroom, he did not do his homework, and he joked with his classmates. He also told us that he and his friends used to jump over the school wall and that they came and went from the school building whenever they wanted and did not obey the established rules.

Most young people who commit offenses, like Jaguar, are expelled from school. Once they have entered the legal justice system, they have great difficulty in rejoining school, even though they are obliged to do so by the judge of the childhood and youth court and by the program of socio-educational measures (Borba, Lopes, & Malfitano, 2015). The compulsory insertion in school ordered by AF measures does not necessarily translate into effective action on the part of the justice system, as the responsible educational institutions are forced to commit to ensuring permanent access for these youths in school. In this sense, in the development of this process and at the edges of it, it becomes evident that the prescribed AF is weakened by the powers and logic inherent to the school system, which has well-established methods for delaying and/or preventing the admission of these youths, and when the school cannot prevent their admission, it instead expels them as soon as they enter (Borba et al., 2015; Lopes, Sfair, & Bittar, 2012).

When referring to his recent "past," Jaguar once told us he did not associate the role of school with the future, but this is different from how he understands it today; he now considers that it entails a better life situation, which is similar to the way most young people in Brazil think (Pereira & Lopes, 2016). Thus, he intends to complete his studies and find a job. This change in his discourse coincides with the advancement of age; today Jaguar is 19 years old, and his participation in school has occurred over the last 2 years, during his late adolescence and early adulthood, from the age of 18. One of the hypotheses raised to explain this change of attitude could be the effect of our team's individual territorial follow-up, which introduced into his daily life the presence of people who value studying and believe in the possibility of life transformation through it. On the other hand, our immersion in the contexts of the neighborhood and our understanding of Jaguar's life allowed us to construct another explanatory nexus: there is an age limit at which adolescents realize they cannot be incorporated by the illegal drug trade, which is a highly exclusionary system. This exclusion occurs when a person does not show the necessary expertise to carry out this activity. Jaguar demonstrates a lack of this expertise, either because of his excessive shyness or because he lacks knowledge about basic mathematical operations, which are vital to this type of trade. When faced with the reality that he could not follow this path, he began to appropriate the discourse that personal transformation could occur through school, and that has been creating generations that believe that personal transformation can occur through school.

Lagging behind, facing difficulties, and reproducing the social discourse of human/individual success through education, Jaguar continued in school, taking the EJA, which corresponds to the final years of the basic education. Jaguar may remain in this space not because of a conscious choice or a real desire but because he has not been offered another short-term option. This is an inference, though; the brevity of this story makes it difficult to affirm what his desires and projects are, but they surely exist, and are not few. However, we have confirmation of his action: he goes to school every day. Thus, action becomes more important than words, so we hope that the school and whatever territories he is in will welcome this action, at least this time.

SOCIAL OCCUPATIONAL THERAPY AND OFFENSES

We live in a young world, in a society that is structured and oriented toward profit and consumption, in a country with high levels of social inequality whose government shows countless weaknesses and difficulties in providing its citizens with what is constitutionally guaranteed. As a result, important violations of rights occur on a daily basis, and many Brazilian adolescents fail to be recognized as victims of inequality but are instead held responsible for various forms of social ills, especially those related to situations of urban violence (Lopes et al., 2008). Unfortunately, this situation is not a concern only in Brazil; as is well known, given the increased inequality worldwide, this situation exists even in countries whose social protection systems advanced in the 20th century (Castel, 1995; Sennett, 2004).

From the perspective of human rights, the United Nations International Convention on the Rights of the Child (UNICEF, 1959), the Brazilian constitution (Brasil, 1988), and Brazilian Child and Adolescent Statute (CAS) (Brasil, 1990) contain a comprehensive view of the rights of children and adolescents, considering them as citizens. Despite the clarity of the national and international norms of assigning rights to children and adolescents, Brazil has witnessed a pattern of disregard for the most elementary human rights in relation to this population group, especially when it comes to those from the poorest social strata (Lopes et al., 2008).

It should be noted that the frequently assumed association between poor youths and crime cannot be seen as a causal nexus; common sense rejects this oversimplification given the complex and diverse actions engaged in by both the poor and offenders, which demonstrates that this direct association denotes prejudice and stigmatization (Borba, Malfitano, & Lopes, 2015). In this context, we join Feltran (2008) in the defense of juvenile offenders who, instead of being considered deviant, should be understood, according to the CAS and the national legal system, as individuals who, although partly responsible for their actions, share that responsibility with the institutions that should guarantee their complete education and the protection of their fundamental rights.

Social occupational therapy is based on conceptions that address the strengthening and creation of social support networks in both the individual and collective spheres. To constitute individual territorial follow-ups, according to the methodology derived from social occupational therapy (Lopes et al., 2014, Lopes, Malfitano, Silva, & Borba, 2016), the main structuring axis in question should operationalize the follow-up of these youths based on the logic of territorialization, which means to be in the territory where people are. That is, professionals need to be geographically closer to those they intend to know and care for, and they should use community resources in which cultural values and social practices can be used as parameters in their practice, even in instances when coping with them is imposed. In this exercise of listening, investigating, and understanding, the occupational therapist contributes to the young people emerging in unique ways, through their interests and skills, joys and difficulties, networks of relationships, and strategies of survival, as well as through their offenses. From these spaces of reflection, one can understand the reality into which the youths are inserted and, through this more effective approach, attain conditions to recognize the paths that compose their trajectories and be able to assist them with coping with their realities and to create alternatives.

Above all, juvenile offenders are young people, and crime is one of the events in their lives. By looking solely at the offenses, it becomes impossible to understand their conduct, because their individual histories are unknown and disregarded. On the other hand, it is possible to understand the offenses, and even the reasons for their involvement, if we situate them within their life history, whose events are located within a network of relationships and exchanges cohering with the meanings established by society. This is a challenge for occupational therapists and for a society that intends to move in the direction of more justice and respect. As conceptualized by Sennett (2004), respect costs us nothing, but it is currently lacked deeply in society.

REFERENCES

Borba, P. L. O., Lopes, R. E., & Malfitano, A. P. S. (2015). Trajetórias Escolares de Adolescentes em Conflito com a Lei: subsídios para repensar políticas educacionais [School trajectories of adolescents with offenses: Subsidies to rethink educational policies]. *Revista Ensaio: Avaliação e Políticas Públicas em Educação, 23*(89), 937–963. doi:10.1590/S0104-40362015000400006

Brasil. (1988). Constituição da República Federativa do Brasil de 1988 [Federal Constitution from Brazil of 1988]. Diário Oficial da União, 5 de outubro de 1988. Brasília: Brazilian Federal Government.

Brasil. (1990). *Estatuto da Criança e do Adolescente* [Brazil Statute of the Child and Adolescent]. Lei no. 8069. São Paulo: Imprensa Oficial do Estado.

Castel, R. (1995). *Les metamorfoses de la question sociale: une chronique du salariat* [From manual workers to wage laborers: Transformation of social question]. França: Folio.

Feltran, G. S. (2008). *Fronteiras de tensão: um estudo sobre política e violência nas periferias de São Paulo* [Frontiers of tension: A study of politics and violence in the peripheries of São Paulo]. 336f. Tese (Doutorado em Ciências Sociais) - Universidade Estadual de Campinas, Campinas. Retrieved February 2019, from http://bdtd.ibict.br/vufind/Record/CAMP_d25ccc41896a464ccd04c4098dc0d5e7

Lopes, R. E., Adorno, R. C. F., Malfitano, A. P. S., Takeiti, B. A., Silva, C. R., & Borba, P. L. O. (2008). Juventude pobre, violência e cidadania [Poor youth, violence and citizenship]. *Saúde e Sociedade, 17*(3), 63–76. doi:10.1590/S0104-12902008000300008

Lopes, R. E., Malfitano, A. P. S., Silva, C. R., & Borba, P. L. O. (2014). Recursos e tecnologias em Terapia Ocupacional Social: ações com jovens pobres na cidade [Resources and technologies in social occupational therapy: Actions with the poor youth in town]. *Cadernos Brasileiros de Terapia Ocupacional, São Carlos, 22*(3), 591–602. doi:10.4322/cto.2014.081

Lopes, R. E., Malfitano, A. P. S., Silva, C. R., & Borba, P. L. O. (2016). Jovens pobres nas cidades: contribuições da terapia ocupacional social [Poor youths in the cities: Contributions of social occupational therapy]. In S. S. Algado, A. G. Córdoba, F. C. Oliver, S. M. Galheigo, & S. García-Ruiz (Eds.), *Terapias Ocupacionales Desde El Sur: Derechos Humanos, Ciudadanía y Participación* [Occupational therapies from the South: Human rights, citizenship and participation] (pp. 321–340). Santiago de Chile: Editorial Universidad de Santiago de Chile.

Lopes, R. E., Malfitano, A. P. S., Silva, C. R., Borba, P. L. O., & Hahn, M. S. (2012). Occupational therapy professional education on research in the social field. *WFOT Bulletin, 66*, 52–57. doi:10.1179/otb.2012.66.1.021

Lopes, R. E., Sfair, S. C., & Bittar, M. (2012). Adolescentes em medidas socioeducativas em meio aberto e a escola [Teenagers and socio-educational measures at open environments and at school]. *Cadernos Terapia Ocupacional da UFSCar, 20*(2), 217–228. doi:10.4322/cto.2012.023

Morais, A. C., & Malfitano, A. P. S. (2016). O terapeuta ocupacional como executor de medidas socioeducativas em meio aberto: discursos na construção de uma prática [Occupational therapist as socioeducational measures executor in open environment: Speechs to practice construction]. *Cadernos Brasileiros de Terapia Ocupacional/Brazilian Journal of Occupational Therapy, 24*(3), 531–542. doi:10.4322/0104-4931.ctoAO0727

Pereira, B. P., & Lopes, R. E. (2016). Por que ir à Escola? Os sentidos atribuídos pelos jovens do ensino médio [Why go to school? The meanings assigned by secondary education students]. *Educação & Realidade, Porto Alegre, 41*(1), 193–216. doi:10.1590/2175-623655950

Sennett, R. (2004). *Respect: The formation of character in an age of inequality.* Reino Unido: Penguin Books.

UNICEF. (1959). Fundo das Nações Unidas para a Infância. Convenção Internacional sobre os Direitos da Criança.

21

Social Occupational Therapy and the Support Contextures: An Experience Beyond Formal Devices

Giovanna Bardi

I first met Pedrinho[1] in 2009 when I was a graduate student participating in an extension project (in a partnership between the university and the community, with the participation of students and academic staff) at the Metuia Federal University of Sao Carlos (UFSCar) Laboratory. This project is designed to provide occupational therapy interventions to youth who attend a public school in a neighborhood on the outskirts of São Carlos. When I met Pedrinho, he was 15 years old. He stood out among the other teenagers because of his high level of participation, capacity for critical analysis, and diverse skills, which included drawing and painting. His appearance was striking, with makeup, bracelets, necklaces, hair styled in cornrows, and painted nails. Staff at the Metuia UFSCar Laboratory referred to suspected use of drugs and prostitution.

Two years later, after confirming the fact of his drug use, we met again for a specific purpose: I proposed that he take part in my master's research,[2] developed for the Graduate Studies Program in Occupational Therapy at UFSCar. This experience, which focused on Pedrinho's formal and informal social support networks—that is, individuals he thought he could count on in times of difficulty arising from drug use—has led to numerous reflections pertinent to the field of social occupational therapy practice with individuals undergoing some process of vulnerability, especially those who choose to use any type of nonprescribed drug. The proposal I made to Pedrinho was very direct

(there was a history between us that allowed this kind of relationship): I would accompany him for approximately a year to understand how he had been coping with drug use in his daily life and whom he could count on when there were troubles. As he was very fond of taking on new challenges, he promptly agreed.

My first intention for the follow-up was to gather ethnographic content (Nakamura, 2011). For this purpose, I circulated in the spaces where Pedrinho took me, going to his house and those of some of his friends, squares in the neighborhood (Figure 21.1), cybercafés, the community library, bars, and the Assemblies of God Pentecostal Church. Above all, I walked up and down hillsides alongside one, two, or more teenagers who joined us. I systematically recorded these activities in field diaries, describing them densely with the greatest wealth of detail possible (Gomes, 2008).

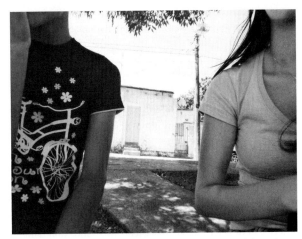

Fig. 21.1 Pedrinho and the researcher on a park bench

[1]To ensure the collaborators' privacy and follow ethical research principles, the names used in this study are pseudonyms. In the case of Pedrinho, the name was chosen by the collaborator himself.
[2]For further information, see the full master's thesis: "Life Stories on the Periphery: Youths and Their Interrelationships," supervised by Ana Paula Serrata Malfitano (Bardi, 2013).

In the first months of field research, I gathered a good deal of information about Pedrinho's relationship with drugs (Figure 21.2). He and his mother, Lucia, with whom I established close contact, explained when his cocaine use had started, for what reason, and under what circumstances (place, company, etc.). This information is of importance, but that was not the focus of my thesis, nor will it be the focus of this chapter. Other facts of equal importance were shared, such as Pedrinho's disastrous experience in a therapeutic community after being referred by the municipality's Psychosocial Care Centers for alcohol and drug users (CAPSad[3]). I will also not dwell on the details of this experience or on the outcome of this story but rather on the fact that, after he left the therapeutic community, he had not been integrated, as a user, into any formal assistance network or maintained "the vows" of abstinence that he had made while hospitalized in the therapeutic

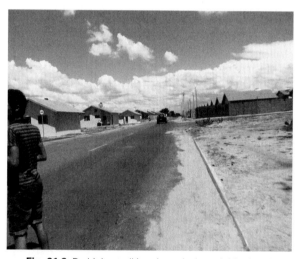

Fig. 21.2 Pedrinho walking through the neighborhood

community. Pedrinho never clearly explained his reasons for not adhering to the CAPSad, but he quite often commented that he did not like professionals because they did not understand him. Let us bear this in mind during the following reflections.

Regarding formal social networks, specifically about drugs, his only identified experience was involvement in the therapeutic community and hospitalization through CAPSad. It was clear that these two experiences did not mean much to him in terms of support or assistance in times of difficulty, because he did not turn to these networks when he needed help. Nevertheless, Pedrinho had demonstrated that he knew how to draw on the benefits of his connection with this formal network if advantageous to him.[4]

Pedrinho's social networks were more evident in the informal/affective field. Through the narrated stories and observation, it was found that he had important support from his mother and sister.

He also had religious assistance provided by two different beliefs: *candomblé*[5] and Pentecostalism (Protestant Christianity), which, in his own words, were both sources of great support (Bardi & Malfitano, 2014). This was the first important insight provided by the research: the need to dwell on the relationships that are constructed in the territory, to understand how and why they occur, what is sought, and what is found. Pedrinho allowed me a unique opportunity to learn about his experiences; his moving between two religious temples that were, in some ways, very different; and his access to different types of support afforded by each. He moved fluidly between the two religions and seemed to be aware of the "benefits" that each could bring, seeking them at specific times depending on his needs. There was nothing strange or incoherent about it, as some people expressed.[6] Fábio, the *candomblé* priest of the *terreiro* attended by Pedrinho, helped him many

---

[3]The Psychosocial Care Centers (CAPS), among all the devices for mental health care, have strategic value for Brazilian psychiatric reform and are beginning to demonstrate the possibility of organizing a network substitutive to the psychiatric hospitals in Brazil. The CAPS have the functions of providing clinical assistance to individuals with severe and persistent mental disorders in daily care, thus avoiding hospitalization in psychiatric hospitals; fostering the social inclusion of individuals with mental disorders through intersectoral actions; managing admission to the mental health care network in its area of activity; and providing support to mental health care in the basic health network. Specifically, CAPSad, the Psychosocial Care Centers for alcohol and drugs, are strategic devices for the care of patients with "addiction" and/or abuse of alcohol and other drugs (Brasil, 2005).

[4]I once had the chance to witness Pedrinho requesting bus tickets from the social worker of the community center in his neighborhood, claiming to use them for trips to the CAPSad. After receiving the tickets, he told me that, in fact, they would be used to go downtown to settle some pending issues.

[5]Candomblé is an Afro-Brazilian religious tradition practiced in Brazil and in other Latin American countries. It means "dance in honor of the gods." Candomblé originated in Salvador, Bahia, Brazil, at the beginning of the 19th century, when the first temple was founded. It was developed during the African slavery in Brazil during the 16th and 17th centuries.

[6]Several people with whom I had contact, such as one of Pedrinho's neighbors and the minister of the Pentecostal church he attended, mentioned the fact that he was a follower of two different religions as if it were an incoherent or confused attitude.

times when he was depressed due to problems he experienced in relation to drug use; he talked to him openly about it and other matters, maintaining a relationship of understanding and closeness. Fábio reported several situations when he welcomed Pedrinho after long days of drug use; in the terreiro, Pedrinho could wait until the effects of the drugs wore off, take a shower, eat, and only return home after he had recovered. A similar closeness was commented on by the minister of the Pentecostal church and his wife. Pedrinho visited their house when he needed some advice, and he felt comfortable doing it even (and especially) when he was under the influence of drugs. In my observation, the support that really seemed to help Pedrinho did not focus directly on problems associated with drugs, did not attend to classification of types of use, and did not focus on abstinence strategies; rather, these supportive interactions gave him a chance to be truly listened to. Thus, a challenge is posed for occupational therapists: they may be more effective when their actions take into consideration the life contexts of the people; when they apply an authentic, compassionate approach; and when they address the demands of both individuals and their society (Lopes, Borba, & Cappellaro, 2011). The notion of "territory" is equally important. Territory means the place where people have meaningful connections for their lives (Barros, Ghirardi, & Lopes, 2005). Attending to territory involves the need to overcome specialized spaces of professional action, with skills to recognize the habits, forms of communication, customs, rules, and ways of life, among other aspects, of population groups with which they interact in relations of otherness (Bardi, Monzeli, Macedo, Neves, & Lopes, 2016). In the case of Pedrinho, this territorial action was of great importance because he has limited engagement with formal institutions of care. As previously mentioned, according to his own words, the formal institutions he attended did not have the necessary approaches to help him; furthermore, he expressed that there were not enough human resources or time to respond to his demands. Approaching Pedrinho, and so many other adolescents who are otherwise viewed as "unapproachable" by society, is only possible if practitioners focus on the contexts in which they live, conduct an in-depth reading of individual and collective needs, and consider culture and subculture, from which people cannot be separated (Lopes, Malfitano, Silva, & Borba, 2014). Thus, the possibilities of understanding adolescent experiences that extend the explanation for drug use beyond a presumption of guilt and individualization could be established. This would then guide one's focus to understanding that the choices and conditions of citizens are continually influenced and shaped by socioeconomic processes. From this perspective, social occupational therapists can and should,

as a top priority, be responsible for assisting with the inclusion of marginalized/vulnerable young people in spaces and places (physical and social) that they wish to access.

When recognizing the occupational therapist's role and responsibility in strengthening the social support networks of citizens who are in positions of social vulnerability, it becomes increasingly imperative to examine and understand social networks from the perspective of others. Knowledge about social networks must be specific to the individual. In my study, it was the understanding of social networks based on a macro reading that revealed Pedrinho's demands. The intention is to understand the relationships between his condition and his life—not to view those relationships as instruments for measuring factors or risks—that are in line with the dominant social context of thinking about "drugs," creating a view of drug use based on individualization and guilt.

In this sense, instead of first prioritizing the identification of potential service gaps and possible institutions that could provide care and treatment, I recommend that occupational therapists step back and first learn whom, or what services, the young person is currently drawing on and what help is being accessed. This shift in clinical reasoning may foster a richer understanding about individual life contexts and the ways in which people live and develop personal strategies during times of difficulty. In this way, subjectivities of daily life are acknowledged and valued. Accordingly, by gaining an understanding of formal and informal relationships that an individual considers to be positive, occupational therapists are enabled to support people in their efforts to either strengthen existing support or co-construct other new and supportive relationships in the territory. Individuals with whom occupational therapists work are not only situated in formal social contexts or in institutions; consequently occupational therapists may need to supplement the institution by working in real places of life.

The need to develop knowledge and different ways of care is advocated. This knowledge should effectively contribute to occupational therapists' intervention when working with people who use drugs. All citizens should be able to have access to health services and be supported to enhance possibilities of treatment that respect their choices and positions related to the treatment, as proposed by the Brazilian Harm Reduction guidelines (Brasil, 2001). At the same time, it is necessary to reflect on what strategies might be employed to help people, which implies using critical analysis to recognize that the role of health services in complex problems, like drug use, is necessarily intersectoral. In this context, social occupational therapy is recognized as presenting a solid possibility of contributing to this field through its territorial action (in other words, by being where people are), dialoguing directly with social networks. It is expected that close consideration of personal histories can contribute to new proposals for professional action. At a macro-social level, considering personal histories and social networks could contribute to the formulation of social policies that are more consistent with the reality of people who use drugs, and the suggestions of the individuals themselves to resolve their social issues can be heard.

REFERENCES

Bardi, G. (2013). *Histórias de vida na periferia: juventudes e seus entrecruzamentos* [Life stories on the periphery: Youths and their intercrossings]. São Carlos, SP, Brasil: Dissertação de Mestrado, Universidade Federal de São Carlos, São Carlos, SP, Brasil.

Bardi, G., & Malfitano, A. P. S. (2014). Pedrinho, religiosity and prostitution: The managements of an ambivalent young man. *Saúde e Sociedade, 23*(1), 42–53.

Bardi, G., Monzeli, G. A., Macedo, M. D. C., Neves, A. T. L., & Lopes, J. S. R. (2016). Oficinas socioculturais com crianças e jovens sob a perspectiva da Terapia Ocupacional Social [Socio-cultural workshops with children and youth from the social occupational therapy perspective]. *Cadernos de Terapia Ocupacional da UFSCar, 24*, 811–819.

Barros, D. D., Ghirardi, M. I. G., & Lopes, R. E. (2005). Social occupational therapy: A socio-historical perspective. In F. A. Kronenberg (Ed.), *Occupational therapy without borders: Learning from the spirit of survivors* (pp. 140–151). London: Elsevier Science/Churchill Livingstone.

Brasil. (2001). Ministério da Saúde [Health Minister]. *Manual de Redução de Danos* [Harm reduction manual]. Brasília: Coordenação Nacional de DST e AIDS.

Brasil. (2005). Ministério da Saúde [Health Minister]. *Reforma psiquiátrica e política de saúde mental no Brasil* [Psychiatric reform and mental health policy in Brazil]. Brasília: Secretaria de Atenção à Saúde. Coordenação Geral de Saúde Mental. Documento apresentado à Conferência Regional de Reforma dos Serviços de Saúde Mental: 15 anos depois de Caracas.

Gomes, M. P. (2008). *Antropologia: a ciência do homem: filosofia da cultura* [Anthropology: Man's science: philosophy of culture]. São Paulo: Contexto.

Lopes, R. E., Borba, P. L. O., & Cappellaro, M. (2011). Acompanhamento individual e articulação de recursos em Terapia Ocupacional Social: compartilhando uma experiência [Individual support and resources articulation in social occupational therapy: Sharing an experience]. *O Mundo da Saúde, São Paulo, 35*(2), 233–238.

Lopes, R. E., Malfitano, A. P. S., Silva, C. R., & Borba, P. L. O. (2014). Recursos e tecnologias em Terapia Ocupacional Social: ações com jovens pobres na cidade [Resources and technologies in social occupational therapy: Actions with the poor youth in town]. *Cadernos de Terapia Ocupacional da UFSCar, São Carlos, 22*(3), 591–602.

Nakamura, E. (2011). O método etnográfico em pesquisas na área da saúde: uma reflexão antropológica [The ethnographic method in health researches: An anthropological thinking]. *Saúde e Sociedade, 20*(1), 95–103.

22

Poor Youth and the City: Violated Rights, Denied Spaces

Paulo Estevão Pereira

This chapter draws on the field research that composed my master's dissertation in occupational therapy, entitled *"Hey! Are you kidding me?" – As Said by Poor São Carlos Youth About Themselves and the Theme of Drugs*, completed at the Federal University of São Carlos, São Paulo, Brazil, under the supervision of Dr. Ana Paula Serrata Malfitano (Pereira, 2012).

Social occupational therapy seeks to understand people's everyday interactions, getting to know the various forms and intensities of their bonds with others, as well as their vulnerability with regard to social support networks and the world of work, which can be precarious (Barros, Ghirardi, Lopes, & Galheigo, 2011). The aim of social occupational therapy is to position individuals to take charge of the realities they experience in their lives and to foster possibilities for the chance to transform these lived realities. In this way, occupational therapists are coresponsible, along with the person with whom they are working, for taking measures to target social changes that are identified as necessary. From this perspective, social occupational therapy action is characterized by a confluence between describing/understanding situated realities and carrying out directed actions that are aimed at improving lived realities.

Guided by the perspective of social occupational therapy while undertaking my master's study, I sought to unveil and understand the realities experienced by impoverished young people living toward the periphery of a medium-sized city in the state of São Paulo, Brazil. My focus was on developing an understanding of the place of drugs and drug use in the context of the young people's lives, asking questions such as: What role did drugs play in the daily lives of young people? However, while immersed in the research field, I became privy to more complex and rich understandings of situations, beyond drug use, that placed young people in vulnerable situations. The theme of

"drugs," which I had presumed would be central to the analysis, actually emerged as a secondary theme. Instead, factors such as formal and informal restrictions on the use of the city and its spaces, human rights violations, lack of access to material and cultural assets, and precarious access to the work environment (which itself was equally precarious when obtained) were revealed to be instrumental to understanding lived realities and vulnerability. For instance, while this study showed that drug use and trafficking did indeed place people in positions of vulnerability, it became evident that constant violations of their rights affected them even more severely. External factors of vulnerability appeared to be less obvious but to affect them even more severely.

The young people who were a part of this study seemed to feel like outsiders within their own city. General relations among citizens are implicitly influenced by social class divisions that are evident through division of territory and use of space. It is argued that there are implicit territorial conflicts arising from the dynamics of the city, which impacts relations with impoverished young people. Based on perceived associations of danger associated with this group of youths (Lopes et al., 2008), they may be restricted from full entry to and participation in some areas. These restrictions lead them to circumscribe their spaces of social exchanges to their own neighborhood and to other neighborhoods that are also on the periphery of the city. Gustavo and Silas (pseudonyms) provide examples of these territorial conflicts and demonstrate the hidden logic in this relationship between impoverished youth and the city.

Gustavo is 15 years old. He lives close to the youth center where I conducted my research. During our interview, I asked him if he had ever been banned from entering places such as shopping centers or stores. This question arose from a conversation we had about prejudices he perceived experiencing as a young man living on the periphery of the city. He told me:

> Only once at the mall, because I was not carrying my ID. But I went in anyway, I snuck in. The security guard did not even see me getting in. After seven, there was a big line at the entrance, because a lot of people were going (there) on Saturday, so they would not let me in. Then I sneaked in.

In this situation, prejudice is evident. Entry to places intended for mass consumption is prevented or impeded, and the requirement to produce identification is not typically required of other young people. There is a violation of the rights of these young people, and there does not seem to be any public opposition or questions arising regarding this type of conduct by people in positions of authority. Impoverished young people are judged based on their clothes, their appearance, and the means of transportation they take to the mall. The lines to enter the mall and the control of IDs by the police are specifically for the poor youth. What does the requirement of having an ID mean when it comes to determining whether a young person "can" or "cannot" enter a mall? How does carrying an ID distinguish young people from each other? For some people, it means everything.

When writing about the condition of stateless persons after World War I—people totally destitute of their civil rights, not recognized by any state, and not subject to any law that protected them as a result of the peace treaties signed between the winners and losers on that occasion—Hannah Arendt (1985) considers the relativity of the Universal Rights of Man according to the revolutionary ideology of the 18th century, which presents these rights as inalienable and inherent to every human being. She states that this group of stateless persons were deprived of their civil rights and became "Earth's leftovers" (p. 300). The very condition of being understood as human beings was lost. Nobody wanted them or cared about them; they were perceived as a problem and as a nuisance to be eliminated. As Arendt writes, "It seems that a man who is nothing more than a man loses all the qualities that make it possible for others to treat them as a man" (p. 334). In that social and historical environment, human rights were conceived a priori as inalienable and inherent to the condition of being human. For this reason, human rights had not been constituted in formalized law. However, this experience shed light on the fact that human rights are contingent on the existence and enforcement of political injunctions, the signing of treaties, and the establishment of agreements. The author concludes:

> Equality, in contrast to everything that relates to mere existence, is not given to us, instead it results from human organization, and thus it is guided by the principle of justice. We are not born the same; we become equal members of a group by virtue of our decision to guarantee each other equal rights.
>
> (Arendt, 1985, p. 335)

I draw on Arendt's reflections on the "stateless" to reflect on the previous excerpt. The General Register of Brazilians (the identity card) is the document that attests to the identity of its bearer, with a photo and fingerprints. It is the document that, along with the birth certificate (in the case of native Brazilians), guarantees that its bearer is recognized by the state as a Brazilian citizen. In the previous example, by requiring the presentation of an ID as a way to screen young people and allow or not allow them to enter the shopping center, local security guards echo the treatment of the stateless persons described by Arendt, albeit on a much smaller scale. If they are not carrying their ID, they are not recognized by the security guards as citizens, and therefore they may be prevented from entering a public place, even without them having done anything to justify this impediment.

"Because a lot of people were going on Saturday" was the defense for regulating the circulation of "these young people" (specifically poor youth) in spaces intended for the general public. An assemblage of poor youth is certainly understood as being synonymous with danger, as was demonstrated by the Brazilian media's wide coverage of the case of "Rolezinhos" in 2013. In that instance, youth from the outskirts of big cities used the Internet to arrange large gatherings in shopping malls with the intention of having fun. This mass of young people sparked interventions by police and armed security from shopping malls, mobilizing political action and public opinion. These events feed the argument that measures must be re-established for controlling bodies to contain the potential for violence that is considered to be inherent to young citizens, specifically the young and poor. Given that scenes of this kind are not questioned as part of the dominant public discourse, even if they are witnessed by the population who enter the shopping centers freely, the poor young people find themselves isolated, without having people in authority or public influence who will speak on their behalf to protect their rights. In an attempt to circumvent the imposed rules, they find circumscribed solutions: "Then I sneaked in."

Such forms of control and rights violations of poor young people are not limited to the more central public places. Unfortunately, these practices are reproduced within liberal social contexts that are intentionally designed to work with this group of young people and espouse rights of citizenship and social participation.

The following extract taken from my field diaries exemplifies this:

Field diary, Oct, 05, 2010.

> *I arrive at the Youth Centre at 2:00 p.m. I will begin the interviews today and wait for the arrival of Daniel, with whom I will conduct the first interview, scheduled for 2:30 pm. While waiting, I talk to METUIA staff and to some Youth Centre employees. Soon, two boys arrive. One of them is recognized by the METUIA occupational therapist, and he is happily welcomed by all. However, he does not stay for the activities, he is asked to go back to his house and provide a 3×4 photo to make his card without which he cannot attend the Youth Centre. Even though he was welcomed, he had to come back the next day.*

The young man from the previous example (here referred to as Silas) was returning to the center after a period of imprisonment for involvement in drug trafficking. He had been released from jail a few days earlier. "He was a boy worth investing in," said an employee of the youth center. At any rate, due to recent "behavior problems" of some young people inside the youth center and subsequent confrontations with team members, an identification card system was instituted; without an ID, the youth could not enter or access services. As a result, all youths were required to bring a recent 3×4 photo and register at the secretary's office. It is noteworthy that this measure was taken by the youth center coordinators despite dissuasion from the local Metuia team, who encouraged reflection on the primary role of the service—namely, to function as an arena for youth empowerment and a freely accessible space for youth participation in a broad sense (Malfitano, Lopes, Magalhães, & Towsend, 2014). Returning to the episode with Silas, he certainly had no card since it was a recent request. Therefore, this well-liked young man, who was "worth investing in," and in a moment of personal fragility (a fresh start), had to go back to his house and find a 3×4 photo to gain the right to access the space that used to openly welcome him.

Public institutions that aim to systematize their activities in this way end up molding themselves in the institutional image (Barros, Lopes, & Galheigo, 2007), creating a "user profile" more in accordance with institutional logic than with the needs of that population. In breaching the rights of young people or not allowing the exercise of these rights to maintain order, a reproduction of disrespect, discrimination, and vulnerability is achieved. A space that was originally designed to ensure the inclusion and participation of young people (Metuia, 2008) adopts measures of differentiation between those who can and those who cannot attend it. Thus, a public facility aimed at vulnerable young people paradoxically contributes to increasing this vulnerability by alienating certain youths who do not meet the standards, and who will most likely find membership/belonging in other circumstances instead. This paradox was a primary concern of Metuia's UFSCar work with the youth center team to unveil contradictions and to build effective participation mechanisms for those young people.

FINAL CONSIDERATIONS

The scenarios of Gustavo and Silas bring to the surface conflicts that pervade our society regarding society's relationship with young people from lower classes. This population is systematically excluded from access to culture, leisure, and activities of consumption due to societal perceptions of personifications of violence and danger, which result in subjection to control of bodies and use of space. Young people from lower classes are excluded from fully accessing the city in which they reside, with the clear and objective demarcation of the spaces in which they are allowed to be: their neighborhoods of residence, on the outskirts, or in other neighborhoods that are more or less distant from the downtown but certainly on the periphery of the city.

What Gustavo and Silas denounce in stressing the restrictions on their mobility in the city is precisely the perverse logic behind the relationship between poor youth and the city, which involves public actions that effectively control private actions. These controls are justified and corroborated through notions of common sense. For instance, poor youth tend to be viewed unilaterally by the general population as being involved in drug use and trafficking, often with tragic consequences. This acts as a rationale for government measures that are directed at "taking these young people off the streets" and offering them worthier alternatives for life-building projects. Certainly, such measures are commendable and necessary, since a lack of prospects for many young people brings them closer to drug use and trafficking. However, the perverse logic lies in the fact that the city itself and society itself exacerbate the vulnerability experienced by youth by excluding them from participation in and enjoyment of material and symbolic goods and by restricting their mobility to certain areas of the city. This results in less access to culture, leisure, and education opportunities, which, paradoxically, create a need for inclusion policies. The greatest tragedy is that this logic continues to act invisibly; it is just as invisible as these vulnerable young people become when they are excluded from engaging in full citizenship in our cities.

REFERENCES

Arendt, H. (1985). O declínio do Estado-Nação e o fim dos direitos do homem [The decline of nation-state and the end of the rights of man]. In H. Arendt (Ed.), *Origens do Totalitarismo* [Origins of totalitarism]. Rio de Janeiro: Documentário.

Barros, D. D., Lopes, R. E., & Galheigo, S. M. (2007). Terapia ocupacional social: Concepções e perspectivas [Social occupational therapy: Conceptions and perspectives]. In A. Cavalcanti & C. Galvão (Eds.), *Terapia Ocupacional: fundamentação e prática* [Occupational therapy: Background and practice] (pp. 354–363). Rio de Janeiro: Guanabara Koogan,

Barros D. D., Ghirardi M. I. G., Lopes R. E., Galheigo S. M. (2011). Brazilian experiences in social occupational therapy. In F. Kronenberg, N. Pollard, & D. Sakellariou (Org.), *Occupational therapy without borders – Volume 2: Towards an ecology of occupation-based practices* (1st ed., pp. 209–215). Edinburgh: Elsevier.

Lopes, R. E., Adorno, R. C. F., Malfitano, A. P. S., Takeiti, B. A., Silva, C. R., & Borba, P. L. O. (2008). Juventudes pobres, violência e cidadania [Poor youth, violence and citizenship]. *Saúde & Sociedade, São Paulo, 17*(3), 63–76. doi:10.1590/S0104-12902008000300008

Malfitano, A. P. S., Lopes, R. E., Magalhães, L., & Towsend, E. (2104). Social occupational therapy: Conversations about a Brazilian experience. *Canadian Journal of Occupational Therapy, 81*(5), 298–307. doi:10.1177/0008417414536712

METUIA. (2008). *Projeto político pedagógico para o Cenro da Juventude da região sul de São Carlos* [Political pedagogical project for the youth center of the south region of São Carlos]. São Carlos: Federal University of São Carlos.

Pereira, P. E. (2012). *"Aí! Tá me tirando?!" – O que dizem jovenspobres de São Carlos sobre si mesmos e a temática das drogas* [Hey! Are You Kidding Me – As said by poor São Carlos youth about themselves and the theme of drugs.] (Master's dissertation), Postgraduate Program in Occupational Therapy, São Carlos, SP. Brazil. Retrieved May 2019, from https://repositorio.ufscar.br/bitstream/handle/ufscar/6851/4142.pdf?sequence=1

23

Overcoming Invisibility: Carla's Story[1]

Mayra Cappellaro

In an approach to the everyday scenes of a neighborhood on the outskirts of the municipality of Sao Carlos, state of Sao Paulo, Brazil, I developed a study that was included in my master's thesis entitled *Where Are the Girls? Everyday Life and Traits of Low-Income Female Young People from the Perspective of Social Occupational Therapy*. My participation in that location began during my undergraduate studies through participation in university teaching and extension activities conducted by the Metuia/UFSCar Project team.[2]

The study aimed to investigate who these female youths are, how their everyday life occurs in the local community, what their family and neighborhood relations are, how they access public spaces, their circulation in the city, their leisure activities, their family care responsibilities, their work and income opportunities, their school trajectory, and their experience regarding violence—in short, how their everyday lives are constituted. The concept of *life traits* of female youths living in urban peripheries was used. Reference to this concept can be found in Pais (1999), which addresses life traits rather than histories or trajectories of life, because they are young people (whose life experience is short) and, however significant the bonds formed between these individuals and the Metuia/UFSCar Project team, the research only touches on fragments of what they have lived.

The study was based on the concept of individual territorial follow-ups[3] developed by social occupational therapy (Barros, Ghirardi, & Lopes, 2005), as well as on techniques belonging to ethnographic research, aiming to apprehend and reconstitute the life traits of female youths living in a peripheral neighborhood. Weller (2005) addressed the issue of female youth and coined the concept of *female invisibility* to make explicit the absence of female youths in political-cultural contexts, alerting us to the fact that in studies on both youth and feminism, there is a large gap with regard to female juvenile manifestations. Weller adds that the few references to young female adolescents found in scientific research are associated with affectivity and sexuality or with socially precocious maternity.

The initial motivation to conduct research with this group was directly associated with my deepening interest in the theoretical and practical issues around low-income youths, which was cultivated during my undergraduate studies in occupational therapy at the Federal University of Sao Carlos (UFSCar) and through my participation in the Metuia/UFSCar Project. Since 2008, I have been part of the Metuia/UFSCar Project team, conducting activities in a peripheral neighborhood of the city, as well as with the

---

[1]This text grew out of the research that composed the master's thesis of the author, supervised by Professor Roseli Esquerdo Lopes, Graduate Studies Program in Occupational Therapy, Federal University of Sao Carlos (UFSCar).

[2]The Metuia Project was established in 1998 as an interinstitutional group to engage in actions in the field of university teaching, research, and extension in defense of the citizenship of populations undergoing processes of disruption from social support networks. Activities of this project include intervention programs in occupational therapy, in their interconnections with the sectors of social assistance and welfare, culture, education, and health care (Barros, Lopes, & Galheigo, 2007). Currently, named Metuia Network, there are six active nuclei in seven different universities in Brazil.

[3]The definition and further elucidation on the concept of individual territorial follow-ups can be found in "Individual Follow-up and Articulation of Resources in Social Occupational Therapy: Sharing an Experience" (Lopes, Borba, & Cappellaro, 2011).

Pro-adolescent Program.[4] Most of the interventions of this team occurred at the Elaine Viviani Youth Center, where a workshop on activities, projects, and dynamics[5] (Lopes, Malfitano, Silva, & Borba, 2014) entitled "Girls' Space"[6] was offered under my charge.

During these years of activity on the periphery of Sao Carlos, I have been able to observe that the presence of girls and female young people and youths has always been very scarce and, occasionally, almost nonexistent. In this sense, with the assistance provided by the Elaine Viviani Youth Center team, we were able to propose a specific workshop for this population. Initially, we conducted interviews with girls aged 15 to 24 years living in neighborhoods near the youth center to find information that would support the workshop proposal. The main objectives were to approach these girls, create a space of belonging and life sharing, and help them construct projects in their lives by expanding their personal repertoires and social support networks. Based on the information gathered in the interviews, we continued to configure the work design. Weekly afternoon 3-hour meetings divided into themes were then established. The following themes were addressed: media

imposition of beauty patterns, sexuality, relationships, sexually transmitted diseases (STDs), violence, drug trafficking and abuse, cultural diversity, gender (differences and violence), and life projects. Affective bonds were established through the proposition of mediating activities for the relationships between our team and the girls, which provided greater openness of access to information about the components of their lives, dreams, thoughts, beliefs, everyday living, and broader issues that arose from the specificity of working with this population.

"Girls' Space," the name adopted by the group, was consolidated through this modality of a workshop and held for 18 months, but the low attendance and the prevalence of younger girls (aged 11 to 13 years) generated many reflections and a good deal of anguish and restlessness. As the intervention developed with this population, the question "Where are the girls?" became increasingly present because, despite having conducted the interviews with a specific age group (15 to 24 years) and having proposed a space of life sharing based on the input of the interviewees, these girls were still not present in the youth center.

During the study, we relied on individual territorial follow-ups inspired by ethnographic studies—see Caria (2003) and Feltran (2008, 2010)—and proposed by social occupational therapy. Individual territorial follow-ups were carried out with six young girls over 2 years. Each follow-up occurred at different times and spaces (some of those girls continued to be followed by the Metuia/UFSCar Project team), respecting the needs and individualities of each girl. Communication occurred in several ways: text messages, online social networks, phone calls, casual encounters, and scheduled meetings depending on availability, but with at least one weekly meeting. We were guided by the methodology proposed by social occupational therapy, which considers that only through the creation of a bond of trust and respect is it possible to compose strategies for constructing the actions required in the course of individual territorial follow-ups (Lopes, Borba, & Cappellaro, 2011).

According to our close contact and bond with the community, we concluded that girls living in urban peripheries are mostly housed, responsible for the care of their children and/or siblings and household chores, and that they are subjugated to all sorts of violence, from parents and then from partners, and sometimes even from their mothers or stepmothers. School is still the only door that opens the possibility of leveraging this situation, because there they exist beyond their bodies. They have fragile support networks, but these networks at least allow them some circulation; however, the central role of these girls' lives is directly associated with reproduction and domestic responsibility. From a very early age, their dreams are shaped

---

[4]This program, which was funded by the Brazilian Ministry of Social Development and Fight Against Hunger, linked to the federal government, offered activities for young people aged 15 to 17 years who were recipients of the *Bolsa Família* Program or referred by the Special Social Protection. It focused on strengthening family and community life sharing, reintegration of adolescents in school, and their permanence in the education system. It included the development of activities that stimulate social life sharing, citizen participation, and general training for the world of work. The youths were organized into groups, called collectives, and the collectives were monitored by a social adviser, who was supervised by a reference technician housed in the Reference Centers for Social Assistance and Welfare, a social assistance service. The Pro-adolescent Program opened in Sao Carlos in 2008 with 12 collectives located in the outlying districts of the city.

[5]According to Silva: "these workshops are spaces comprising a social grouping in which proposals associated with doing and human action are established aiming to promote shared learning. The active character of individuals is emphasized in this process, as well as the dynamic character of these relational experiences: between participants, space, materials, memory, sensations, that is, between everything that is being done at the moment of this experience" (Silva, 2007, p. 213).

[6]The terms "boy" and "girl" were used on purpose and shared with the Metuia/UFSCar Project team, not only to avoid the gender-neutral term "young people" and its derivatives, but also with the intention of bringing the readers closer to these individuals, attracting their gaze and persuading them to show more sympathetic feelings toward those who come from less favored contexts, perhaps as it seems natural to us in the treatment of our siblings, children, nieces and nephews, and grandchildren (Lopes & Garcia, 2004; Trajber, 2010).

and the desire/reality of motherhood prevails, because they are imprisoned in the world of nature and a culture that subjugates them (Beauvoir, 2015); the exception is not becoming pregnant, not having a husband/partner, and that is all (Cappellaro, 2013).

In this context, we met Carla,[7] a girlish woman, warrior, questioner, and revolutionary, but who seldom accessed the public space reserved for young people of her neighborhood; at the time, she went to school and worked. She was born in Sao Carlos and has always lived on the outskirts of the city. Her parents had divorced when she still was a child, and she had little contact with her father. Her mother told us that she played the role of father and mother: she worked outside the home, but she also cooked, washed and ironed clothes, and educated. Carla has two siblings from her parents' marriage: an older brother and a younger sister. Her father has married three more times and has had one child with each of his partners, but Carla has no contact with her half-siblings. She underwent basic education in a school near her home. As she was already 16 years old and the family's financial situation was unstable, Carla gave up her studies and started working. She worked in a library at a university making photocopies of books for students and teachers. She liked the world of books and, even while working, decided to resume her studies. She used to work days and study nights. She completed her freshman year of high school (the last stage of basic education in Brazil) but gave up twice during her sophomore year. She told us that she could not concentrate, felt very tired, and had no motivation to continue attending school. She somehow managed to continue her studies and, when we met her, she was in her senior year of high school. She even thought about taking the exams to go to college but gave up because her career as a rapper was taking up space in her life.

Carla's interest in rap began in her early adolescence. Her older brother used to listen to rap a lot and had a group that performed at parties in the community. She accompanied her brother to all the concerts and rehearsals and fell in love with the expressive power of music, and that particular kind of music. At the age of 14, she began attending gatherings of girls who enjoyed rap and decided to put together a female rap group. They wrote lyrics and composed songs and decided to perform at an event in the community. She tried to stay and encourage the band, but of the five participants, three became pregnant and one was arrested. Carla was alone but determined not to give in:

At first there was some discrimination on the part of some people because I was just a little girl and I was among many boys, but thank God, my brother never treated me indifferently, but always demanded more from me, saying that I had do my best.

(Field notebook notes)

According to Carla, despite being a predominantly male and sexist environment, she continued to attend concerts. At the end of one of these shows, Carla was taken by the police to the Integrated Service Center of Sao Carlos (NAI)[8] with the justification that "it was neither time nor place for a girl to be." Her mother was notified by the authorities and took her daughter home, disgusted with the treatment Carla had received.

Carla used to accompany her older brother and, one day, received an invitation to help compose his musical group's songs. It was her opportunity to express what she thought and felt. She remained in this group for a year, and they managed to record an album:

It was with the Verso Consciente *[Conscious Verse: the name of the musical group] that we anchored our forces and were able to record a demo and soon the second album will be released. And despite being the only girl in the group, I write my parts in the songs.*

(Field notebook notes)

Concurrently with her participation in this group, Carla began to get increasingly involved with the city's hip-hop movement, especially with the collectives Hip Hop Sanca and Frente Nacional de Mulheres no Hip Hop (National Women's Front in Hip-Hop). She has been very active in the movement, participating in congresses, conferences, concerts, and demonstrations in several cities. With the support of the municipal government of Sao Carlos, the Hip Hop Sanca collective has promoted, for some years, Sanca Hip-Hop (a festival of hip-hop in one district of Sao Carlos, also known as Sanca). This event gathers many youths from the city who make or attend presentations and can reflect on issues such as race, gender, prejudice, and human rights. Carla has become a figure in the community and has overcome the invisibility of being a woman, a female youth, and a resident of the periphery. Today, she has a solo album with songs of her own and has often been sought out by the audiovisual media to discuss matters associated with feminism, rap, and hip-hop. Through rap, hip-hop, and the support of other girls empowered in the fight against toxic masculinity, she has been able to tread a path different from those of the other girls with whom she lives or has lived. Being critical of the system, she never knew why or what led her to engender these paths, but she

---

[7]Only the name is fictitious.

[8]This service was part of the social-juridical system and was directed at adolescents of the city that commit an offense.

attributed this to being able to experience not being discriminated against (in her family nucleus), enjoying and not being afraid of dreaming, and being able to pursue, to have thirst for knowledge, and to allow herself to live. At the end of the individual territorial follow-up, Carla composed a rap to tell, in her words, her life traits, struggles, and achievements:

Since I was little, involved, learning to take care of myself.

I suffered prejudice because I was a woman, but I've never let it overwhelm me.

Rap has taught me what to do, so that many would change their way of looking at things,

And that women also have an active voice and we make things happen.

We just need to go and fight that, everything starts to move.

Respect is the key to breaking down barriers, got it?

Today I am respected and have my place with my folks . . .

It's been almost seven years in this damn rush,

Concerts, writing, rap, parties, and political advocacy.

More than music and rhyme, it's a way out for me,

It has to have feeling and it must have truth.

Many more ideas, and has to act with wit.

Born and raised in the interior of Sao Paulo, "Sanca city,"

Cidade Aracy is my village . . .

The periphery continues to show that it's got talent, and that is not just drugs and crime, there is another segment!

Culture, art, leisure, we fight for this not to die . . .

More than woman and MC, my struggle is daily, because we have hope in this peace that seems like utopia.

More freedom of speech!

This has no price . . . That's why I keep singing the life and overruling the bad MCs.

(Carla, 2012)

Based on the social-anthropological framework, the Metuia/UFSCar Project has been conducting theoretical and practical efforts to encompass through social occupational therapy the theme of the marginal population, which Castel (1994) calls the leftovers. With this framework, we seek to understand the various forms of interaction occurring with individuals or collectives, their relationship of trust and respect, the vulnerability of social networks, and

the precariousness of the work in which they are immersed. When we analyze the specific context of girls living in the peripheries in Brazil (or indeed of girls from any walk of life impacted by toxic masculinity), we observe how much we lack the strategies to actually achieve our aims. Despite the deepening of the global debate on feminism and gender issues, we observe that much of the still-marginalized female population remains largely or virtually uninformed about these issues, reproducing a patriarchal structure that pushes women away from the autonomy necessary for social participation, and the actions to overcome the invisibility imposed on them (Beauvoir, 2015). Therefore, social occupational therapy in Brazil has become quite significant in assisting girls living in urban peripheries and in the creation of working methodologies with this population that encourage the overhaul of this negative panorama to which they have been doomed. Likewise, social occupational therapy has contributed to the field of knowledge to assist with the promotion of public policies that minimize the historical effects of oppression and violence against women.

REFERENCES

Barros, D. D., Ghirardi, M. I. G., & Lopes, R. E. (2005). Social occupational therapy: A socio-historical perspective. In F. Kronenberg, S. S. Algado, & N. Pollard (Eds.), *Occupational therapy without borders: Learning from the spirit of survivors* (pp. 140–151). London: Elsevier Science – Churchill Livingstone.

Barros, D. D., Lopes, R. E., & Galheigo, S. M. (2007). Terapia ocupacional social: concepções e perspectivas [Social occupational therapy: Concepts and perspectives]. In A. Cavalcanti & C. Galvão (Eds.), *Terapia Ocupacional - fundamentação & prática* [Occupational therapy: Fundamentals and practices] (pp. 347–353). Rio de Janeiro: Guanabara Koogan S. A.

Beauvoir, S. (2015). *The second sex*. London: Vintage Publishing.

Cappellaro, M. (2013). *Cadê as meninas? Cotidiano e traços de vida de jovens meninas pobres pela perspectiva da terapia ocupacional social* [Where are the girls? Everyday life and traits of low-income female youngsters from the perspective of social occupational therapy] (Master's thesis in Occupational Therapy, p. 101). São Carlos, São Paulo: Graduate Studies Program in Occupational Therapy, Universidade Federal de São Carlos.

Caria, T. H. (2003). A construção etnográfica do conhecimento em Ciências Sociais: reflexividades e fronteiras [The ethnographic construction of knowledge in social sciences: Reflexivity and borders]. In T. H. Caria (Eds.), *Experiências etnográficas em Ciências Sociais* [Ethnographic experiences in social sciences] (pp. 9–20). Porto: Afrontamento.

Castel, R. (1994). Da indigência à exclusão, a desfiliação. Precariedade do trabalho e vulnerabilidade relacional [From indigence to exclusion, disaffiliation. Precarious work and relational vulnerability]. In A. Lancetti (Eds.), *Saúdeloucura* [Health and madness] (Vol. 4., pp. 21–48). São Paulo: Hucitec.

Feltran, G. S. (2008). *Fronteiras de tensão: um estudo sobre política e violência nas periferias de São Paulo* [Tension frontiers: A study on politics and violence in the outskirts of Sao Paulo] (PhD dissertation in Social Sciences, p. 336). Campinas, São Paulo: Instituto de Filosofia e Ciências Humanas da Universidade Estadual de Campinas.

Feltran, G. S. (2010). Periferias, direito e diferença: notas de uma etnografia urbana [Peripheries, legislation, and difference: Notes on urban ethnography]. *Revista de Antropologia, 53*(2), 565–610.

Lopes, R. E., Borba, P. L. O., & Cappellaro, M. (2011). Acompanhamento Individual e articulação de recursos em Terapia Ocupacional Social: compartilhando uma experiência [Individual territorial follow-up and articulation of resources in social occupational therapy: Sharing an experience]. *O Mundo da Saúde, 35*, 233–238.

Lopes, R. E., & Garcia, D. B. (2004). *Problemas e perspectivas escolares no cotidiano dos meninos e meninas trabalhadores da UFSCar* [School problems and perspectives in the everyday life of young workers of UFSCar] [Relatório de Pesquisa – Research report]. Universidade Federal de São Carlos: Pró-Reitoria de Pesquisa e Pós-Graduação and Fundação de Amparo à Pesquisa do Estado de São Paulo – FAPESP.

Lopes, R. E., Malfitano, A. P. S., Silva, C. R., & Borba, P. L. O. (2014). Recursos e tecnologias em terapia ocupacional social [Resources and technologies in social occupational therapy: Actions with the poor youth in town]. *Cadernos de Terapia Ocupacional da UFSCar, 22*(3), 591–602. doi:10.4322/cto.2014.081

Pais, J. M. (1999). *Traços e riscos de vida. Uma abordagem qualitativa a modos de vida juvenis* [Life traits and risks – A qualitative approach to juvenile everyday living]. Lisboa: Âmbar.

Silva, C. R. (2007). Oficinas [Workshops]. In M. B. Park, M. B. R. S. Fernandes, & R. S. A. Carnicel (Eds.), *Palavras-chaves em educação não-formal* [Keywords in informal education] (pp. 213–214). Campinas: Setembro.

Trajber, N. K. A. (2010). *Oficinas de atividades como processos educativos e instrumento para o fortalecimento de jovens em situação de vulnerabilidade social* [Activity workshops as educational processes and instrument for the strengthening of youths under social vulnerability] (Master's thesis in Education). São Carlos, São Paulo: Graduate Studies Program in Education, Universidade Federal de São Carlos.

Weller, W. (2005). A presença feminina nas (sub)culturas juvenis: a arte de se tornar visível [The feminine presence in youth subcultures: The art of getting visible]. *Revista Estudos Feministas, 13*(1), 107–126.

24

Social Occupational Therapy, Gender, and Sexuality

Gustavo Artur Monzeli

In this chapter, I will briefly discuss some proposals for reflections and practices addressing the relationship between social occupational therapy and the various expressions of gender and sexuality, a theme to which I have given scholarly focus at the university levels of teaching, research, and extension activities. In Brazil, these interconnections accompany an extremely important contemporary moment for the occupational therapy field and, more specifically, for social occupational therapy. Since the Metuia Project was created in the late 1990s, social occupational therapy (Barros, Ghirardi, & Lopes, 2005; Barros, Ghirardi, Lopes, & Galheigo, 2011) has multiplied its forms of action, as well as its research, by dialoguing with related areas such as social assistance, culture, and public health. Social occupational therapy carries, as an important debate agenda, different ways of understanding the production of meanings that people construct for their own lives and the overcoming of their daily difficulties, within different social frameworks and configurations.

This expansion has provided Brazilian occupational therapists engaged with the social area with numerous possibilities in their role as social articulators (Galheigo, 1997). These professionals have been addressing classical themes in this area, such as social vulnerabilities produced by several factors and in many contexts and, above all, the possibility of approaching, at the levels of technical action and research, themes on which little knowledge and practice have been produced. Some of the main themes recently addressed in this context are associated with national and international migration flows, situations of traditional indigenous or *quilombola* communities, and actions conducted with individuals and groups not necessarily included in the spectrum of social vulnerability (Castel, 1995); the particular group my actions are directed toward consists of people who move between the norms of gender and sexuality.

Thanks to the possibilities opened up by the theoretical and methodological expansion of social occupational therapy, I was able to participate in the academic research context of this area through the Graduate Studies Program in Occupational Therapy of the Federal University of São Carlos (UFSCar).[1] Since my undergraduate studies, I have been mobilized by a flow of demands arising from practice in the field of teaching-research-extension in social occupational therapy (Lopes, Malfitano, Silva, Borba, & Hahn, 2012) and have embarked on a trajectory that relates both to the demands of university extension and to those of research. It is worth highlighting that in the broader context of occupational therapy, research matters arise mostly from practical demands; that is, it is the field of technical action of these professionals that generally raises the possibility of constructing reflections in the form of research, with all the potentialities and limitations inherent to this relationship.

My participation in the university extension activities developed by the Metuia-UFSCar Project enabled my insertion and action with demands associated with travestility[2] Contact with these young individuals, who described

[1]My graduate study at the Metuia-UFSCar Project was supervised by Professor Roseli Esquerdo Lopes (UFSCar) and secondarily by Professor Vítor Sérgio Ferreira (University of Lisbon, Portugal). The results of this research can be found in the master's thesis entitled *At Home, on the Road, or at School Is So Much Gossip: Social Areas of Young Transvestites*, developed with funding from the Sao Paulo Research Foundation (FAPESP)—process no. 2011/03536-3— and the support of the Institute of Social Sciences, University of Lisbon, Portugal (ICS-UL).

[2]This term was coined by Peres (2005), and it refers to the variety of identity processes undergone by transvestites to constitute themselves as "females" and, in addition, not only to mark their heterogeneity but also to replace the suffix "-ism," which refers to pathologies.

themselves as transvestites and whom I accompanied for approximately 4 years, began when they were enrolled in a public school in the municipality of Sao Carlos (in the countryside of the state of Sao Paulo, Brazil) at a time when conflicts began to occur due to the fact that some of them decided to attend school wearing clothes and accessories identified as feminine, such as lipstick, nail polish, bracelets, and so forth. As the use of these accessories by these young people increased, there was a proportional increase in school staff intervention aimed at minimizing the visibility of what was perceived as problems caused by their presence in the school environment.

I then began to wonder to what extent these institutional places differed from the "street corners,"[3] places where they regularly spent time and worked, with respect to daily exposure to insults and violence. At the same time, I was faced with many ambiguities in the relationships and spaces that they, as well as I, frequented. The street corner that exposes and insults is the same one that welcomes and pleases; the institution that should welcome and educate is the same one that exposes and insults. Thus, I began a process of constructing/deconstructing meanings that were internal and external to my own body, my own desire, and my own beliefs. As an occupational therapist of an institution, would I be welcoming in a violent way those individuals, bodies, and desires that manage their masculinities and femininities? Would I be contributing to the resignification of these institutional spaces? Or would I just be helping to domesticate these bodies, conforming them to the institution's norms? These and other reflections began to mobilize me to rethink my technical action and reassess the institutions themselves as a reference for certain demands. These interventional experiences as an occupational therapist and, later, in the activities of academic research led me to discuss the need to redefine a theoretical repertoire, because the questions that arose from this field experience problematized different "troublesome" and "pleasant" situations. In this context, I developed an ethnographic experience with these young transvestites that provided me with problematization and transit between the guidelines for occupational therapy and, especially, for social occupational therapy (Monzeli, 2013; Monzeli, Ferreira, & Lopes, 2015).

The perception that the themes of gender and sexuality can be established as demands for the area of occupational therapy is extremely important, because there are interconnections between possibilities of micro-individual and macro-social understanding at the levels of subjectivity

and social rights, respectively. The premise of sex-gender-sexuality asserts that a particular sex indicates a specific (and only one possible) gender, and this gender, in turn, induces a specific desire that is also invariable. According to this logic, it is assumed that sex is natural, and naturalness is understood as a given; the same applies to gender and sexuality. This discussion is headed by many authors of the so-called queer theory,[4] who focus on the social knowledge and practices that organize society and the sexualization of bodies, desires, and identities from the heterosexuality/homosexuality binomial (Miskolci, 2009).

Berenice Bento (2006) notes that the main assumptions of queer studies are the understanding of sexuality as a historical device of power (Foucault, 1979), the performative character of gender identities (Butler, 1990), the subversive scope of performances and sexuality beyond the gender norms, and the body as a bio-power manufactured by precise technologies (Bento, 2006). Certain bodies and individuals escape the sex-gender-sexuality coherence line. Transvestites are a good example of how these seemingly mathematical and immutable combinations are actually questionable and uncertain constructs. An individual genetically identified as XY who abdicates all the privileges rendered by the fact of being male and transforms his male body, through techniques, into a female body is certainly an example of a body that has escaped and does not care. Or rather, according to Butler, they exemplify bodies that do care: care about being known, described, explained, and identified, as well as classified, divided, regulated, and disciplined. In this sense, discourses laden with the authority of science are produced, along with religious, legislative, familial, and pedagogical discourses, among others.

The categories of gender and sexuality have long become potential differentiators in Brazilian society, as in the historical construction of the very notion of citizenship, such as the conquest of political and social rights for women or the history of constant violence and participation restrictions to which lesbians, gays, transvestites, and

---

[3]Reference to spaces of street prostitution.

[4]Foreign authors include Judith Butler, Beatriz Preciado, and Eve Kosofsky Sedgwick, inspired by Michel Foucault, in addition to the Brazilian authors Guacira Lopes Louro, Richard Miskolci, Berenice Bento, Leandro Colling, and Larissa Pelúcio, among others. "Queer" is an old term that originally held negative, offensive connotations for those who broke standards of gender and sexuality (Miskolci, 2009). "Queer" studies address not only homosexuality but also the construction of the homosexuality/heterosexuality binomial, in which heterosexuality will reveal itself both as a producer of homosexuality and as a parasitic structure of the perverse side (Bento, 2006, p. 81).

transsexuals have been subjected. A previous study (Monzeli & Lopes, 2012) emphasizes the lack of training and the curricular gap regarding the theme of sexuality in the daily practice of occupational therapists, noting that on the few occasions when these professionals engage with this issue, they start from a conception of sexuality related to people with some type of disability. Thus, sexuality is understood as an activity of the daily life of individuals that, as with any other activity, needs to be professionally included in the habilitation/rehabilitation process.

Furthermore, in the practice of occupational therapy, there has been insufficient debate problematizing the link between sex, gender, sexuality, and subjectivity. Most of the analyses conducted by professionals start from the conception of sexuality as something naturally given, eventually reiterating the premise of sex-gender-sexuality (Monzeli & Lopes, 2013). In this context, something that seems so private, such as sexuality, presents countless interfaces and interconnections with the macro-social reality, which quite often is not realized.

Regarding gender, for occupational therapists, it is important to expand understanding beyond the mere representation of the roles to be played by bodies of men and women under the hegemony of heteronormativity that is, first and foremost, a permanently open complexity (Melo, 2016). Other studies have indicated that gender discussions have no place in the curricular frameworks of occupational therapy undergraduate courses in Brazilian public universities. Aspects such as social issues, public policies, public health, legislation, and corporeity are found; however, individuals who escape gender intelligibility are not considered in the discussion (Leite & Lopes, 2017).

In the specific context of social occupational therapy, there is a need to understand to what extent differences in gender and sexuality evidence the limits and possibilities of articulation for each individual within their spaces of circulation and belonging. They also problematize the different levels of acceptance and/or denial of institutions and their territories in relation to their bodies, subjectivities, and identities (Monzeli, 2013; Monzeli et al., 2015). Professionals working under the perspective of social occupational therapy can produce professional actions that consider the identity productions of individuals and collectives that transcend the norms established for gender and sexuality. The contribution of occupational therapists should consider the multiplicity of forms of expression of these categories and act to overcome the violence and restrictions of rights that these populations experience in their everyday activities and in their occupations. In this context, social occupational therapy is responsible for analyzing the dynamics between individuals and collectives that transcend the norms of gender and sexuality and the

restriction of access to social rights and engagement in the activities and occupations that these populations aim to enjoy.

If social occupational therapy establishes the struggle for a fairer society for all as its task, I reiterate and add that our theoretical and methodological options and actions should seek and guide the expansion of life and the valuing of different ways of living permitted by a legal framework parameterized by human and social rights obtained historically through many struggles. Thus, the themes of gender and sexuality arise as a field of action for occupational therapy beyond the rehabilitation of individuals with disabilities. The understanding that gender and sexuality are social categories enables us to consider the production of social practices and technologies that aim to minimize the effects of constant stigmatization and violence that certain social groups are subjected to, mainly through understanding the experiences of people who transcend the binary expressions of male/female and homosexuality/heterosexuality. In these cases, it is important to analyze how human activities and occupations of individuals and collectives, their daily lives, and their ways of life are permeated by expressions of gender and sexuality. Moreover, it is necessary to understand how the social participation and social rights of these populations are limited and violated because they do not fit into the logic of a gender/sexuality binary division. It is also important to realize that differences in gender and sexuality cannot be displaced and detached from other categories such as ethnicity, nationality, social class, regionality, generation, and so forth that connect and are associated with limited social participation and the restriction of rights.

REFERENCES

Barros, D. D., Ghirardi, M. I. G., & Lopes, R. E. (2005). Social occupational therapy: A socio-historical perspective. In F. A. Kronenberg (Ed.), *Occupational therapy without borders: Learning from the spirit of survivors* (pp. 140–151). London: Elsevier Science/Churchill Livingstone.

Barros, D. D., Ghirardi, M. I. G., Lopes, R. E., & Galheigo, S. M. (2011). Brazilian experiences in social occupational therapy. In F. Kronenberg, N. Pollard, & D. Sakellariou (Eds.), *Occupational therapy without borders: Towards an ecology of occupation-based practices* (pp. 209–215). Edinburgh: Elsevier.

Bento, B. (2006). *A reinvenção do corpo: sexualidade e gênero na experiência transsexual* [The reinvention of the body: Sexuality and gender in the transsexual experience]. Rio de Janeiro: Garamond.

Butler, J. (1990). *Gender trouble: Feminism and the subversion of identity*. New York, NY: Routledge.

Castel, R. (1995). *Les métamorphoses de la question sociale. Une chronique du salariat*. Paris: Fayard.

Foucault, M. (1979). *The history of sexuality* (Vol. 1): *An introduction*. London: Allen Lane.

Galheigo, S. M. (1997). Da adaptação psicossocial à construção do coletivo: a cidadania enquanto eixo [From the psychosocial adaptation to the construction of the collective: The citizenship as axis]. *Revista de Ciências Médicas – PUCCAMP, Campinas, 6*(2/3), 105–108.

Leite, J. D., Jr., & Lopes, R. E. (2017). Travestility, transsexuality and demands for occupational therapists training. *Cadernos Brasileiros de Terapia Ocupacional São Carlos, 25*(3), 481–496.

Lopes, R. E., Malfitano, A. P. S., Silva, C. R., Borba, P. L. De O., & Hahn, M. S. (2012). Occupational therapy professional education and research in the social field. *World Federation of Occupational Therapists Bulletin, 66*, 52–57.

Melo, K. M. M. (2016). Terapia Ocupacional Social, pessoas trans e Teoria Queer: (re)pensando concepções normativas baseadas no gênero e na sexualidade [Occupational social therapy, trans people and queer theory: (Re) thinking normative conceptions based on gender and sexuality]. *Cadernos de Terapia Ocupacional da UFSCar, 24*, 215–223.

Miskolci, R. (2009). A teoria queer e a sociologia: o desafio de uma analítica da normalização [Queer theory and sociology: The challenge of an analytic of normalization]. *Sociologias, Porto Alegre, 21*, 150–182.

Monzeli, G. A. (2013). *Em casa, na pista ou na escola é tanto babado: espaços de sociabildiade de jovens travestis* [At home, on the dance floor or at school, it is so much trouble: Spaces of sociability of young transvestites]. São Carlos: Dissertação de Mestrado, Programa de Pós-graduação em Terapia Ocupacional, Universidade Federal de São Carlos.

Monzeli, G. A., Ferreira, V. S., & Lopes, R. E. (2015). Among protection, exposure and conditioned admissions: Travestilities and sociability spaces. *Cadernos Brasileiros de Terapia Ocupacional, São Carlos, 23*(3), 451–462.

Monzeli, G. A., & Lopes, R. E. (2012). Terapia ocupacional e sexualidade: uma revisão nos periódicos nacionais e internacionais da área [Occupational therapy and sexuality: A review in the national and international periodicals of the area]. *Revista de Terapia Ocupacional da Universidade de São Paulo, 23*(3), 237–244.

Peres,, W. S. (2005). *Subjetividade das travestis brasileiras: da vulnerabilidade da estigmatização à construção da cidadania* [Subjectivity of Brazilian transvestites: from the vulnerability of stigmatization to the construction of citizenship]. Tese de Doutorado. Rio de Janeiro, Programa de Pós- Graduação em Saúde Coletiva, Universidade Estadual do Rio de Janeiro, 2005.

25

Activity Workshops: Exploring the Use of Digital Media by Brazilian Youths

Rafael Garcia Barreiro

The advancement of the Internet and digital technologies has transformed the relationships between social groups. We understand the Internet from a sociotechnical perspective (Fuchs, 2008) from which society invents, designs, and changes the functioning of its information technology (IT) and communication based on human actions. We characterize technology by contextualizing it within the framework of a social structure, considering our understanding of a capitalist society and the economic aspects involved in this structure as determining factors. With the popularization of the Internet, systems have been created that allow not only access to information but also the interaction of people through so-called digital social networks (DSNs) (Santana, Melo-Solarte, Neris, Miranda, & Baranauskas, 2009). With the advent of the Web 2.0, the traditional ways of communicating, working, informing, moving about, and other everyday habits have changed as a result of technological innovations. This is exemplified by the creation of several digital platforms, such as Facebook, Instagram, and YouTube, which not only disseminate content and information but also provide the foundation of cultural practices based on technological devices. According to Di Felice (2008), these platforms are presented by their makers as vectors of interaction between social groups, catalyzed by the dissemination of connection and access to high-speed and mobile Internet, offering new resources for the construction of identities in communication spaces transformed into interaction spaces. In this context, we observe that the younger generations show greater aptitude in the handling of these technologies, incorporating them into their routines, cultural practices, value systems, and social representations (Sampaio, 2006). Margulis and Urresti (1998) cite generational differences as a factor in the adoption (or nonadoption) of new cultural codes related to socialization; these evolving codes present new ways of perceiving the world, as well as changing habits, skills, and interests that separate new generations from

older ones. We understand youths as a plural social group, composed of historical dimensions and social processes that go beyond the biological rhythm and situations common to human life (Mannheim, 1982). Youths are not homogenous but have an array of cultural forms that unfold from the interaction of characteristics such as social class, gender, and age, as well as from the incorporated memory and institutions present in this population segment (Bourdieu, 1983).

The experience reported herein is part of an approach to contemporary youth based on the framework of social occupational therapy. Social occupational therapists seek to address the potentialities of individuals through their everyday activities by proposing resources and intervention strategies addressing social demands and seeking to articulate citizenship and social rights. It is performed within public policies in community spaces and situations of social vulnerability and disaffiliation, focusing particularly on the processes of personal and social disruption (Lopes & Malfitano, 2017). Social occupational therapy's intervention with urban youths focuses on contemporary lifestyles, and this includes the technological resources accessed by individuals, which present new forms of sociability through contemporary social transformations. In this context, this chapter aims to present the experience of the author with activity workshops, Brazilian youths, and social occupational therapy. The activity workshops were part of the exploratory stage of my doctoral research, in which I investigated the relationship of youths with virtual environments and their impact on their everyday lives and ways of life. These workshops were used to establish a dialogue between youths about their understanding of the Internet, the digital media they make use of, and how they view digital influencers. In the field of communication, digital influencers are defined as content producers who use independent digital media channels to influence both the online and offline behavior of a particular social group (Woods, 2005).

Activity workshops were conducted in a public school and three cultural centers based on actions of the Metuia Network – Social Occupational Therapy (Barros, Lopes, Galheigo, & Galvani, 2005) at the University of Brasilia (UnB) and the Federal University of Sao Carlos (UFSCar). Six workshops were held, with an average of 12 participants, offering free-use graphic materials such as paint, paper, colored pencils, magazine clippings, and images from the Internet. The following group dynamics were adopted: initially, an activity was performed so that the participants could introduce themselves by choosing a word or phrase that symbolized the young person by means of a hashtag.[1] The purpose of this activity was to engage with the language established on the Internet by hashtags, terms derived from the concept of folksonomy that allow Internet users to share information through their broad semantic organization, enabling intentional (or not), collective, collaborative organization via the web (Santos, 2013). The second activity consisted in constructing a profile based on the interests assigned in DSNs. In this activity, the participants received a card divided into two columns, named "like" and "dislike," approaching once again the language of digital platforms. Several images taken from the Internet, magazines, and art materials were made available so that the youths could freely develop personal profiles using what interested or did not interest them in digital platforms. At the end of each workshop, a discussion was held with the participants eliciting their points of view based on the contents they access in DSNs, and a joint analysis of the most-cited topics was conducted.

The strategy of the activity workshops is based on the development of activities through Brazilian occupational therapy, associated with significant action that activates creativity and enables cultural expression, constructing a field of sharing and interaction for the individuals involved (Jurdi, Brunello, & Honda, 2004). In the field of research, Silva (2013) points out that these activities are resources over which occupational therapy researchers must have comprehensive domain, with capacity to "structure, format, adapt, apply, and even perform the analyses and interpretations necessary of the results obtained, enabling more appropriate consideration of the individuals and their contexts and expressions, incorporated into the demands of research" (Silva, 2013, p. 464).

From the perspective of social occupational therapy, activities can be understood as a mediating resource to approach, follow up, and apprehend individual or collective demands, allowing the interpretation and apprehension of the social reality through creative components (Barros, Ghirardi, & Lopes, 2005). The activity workshops, as methodological procedures for data collection in research, provide occupational therapy researchers with the understanding that the experiences and productions of occupational-therapeutic practice can offer rich data about the realities, subjectivities, and objectivities of the individuals involved in the process and, therefore, assist with construction of knowledge (Pereira & Malfitano, 2014). The activity workshops allowed the meanings attributed by youths to digital platforms to be made explicit, as the activities offered opportunities to express reflections and experiences obtained in virtual environments. The youths were able to expose how digital platforms are embedded in their everyday lives, highlighting the languages, cultures, and contents disseminated in these environments. Figure 25.1 shows some profiles made by the participants as examples of what was produced during these workshops.

The language of memes, which are shared and multiplied in DSNs through copy/imitation, was commonly found in the profiles (Recuero, 2007). On the Internet, memes have become a cybernetic culture of communication, sharing "imaginary and textual language, of humorous tone" on digital platforms (Souza, 2014, p. 163). Memes have gained the status of cultural activators, which originate processes of shared construction of meanings for the users who access this type of communication action (Jenkins, 2006). Thus, the processes of network interaction have formulated, for the new generations, a specific communication language of images and electronic texts, among other formats, spread on the Internet. This language can be considered an avant-garde element that has been incorporated into society as a whole, which has participated in the creation of specific cultural codes that establish digital communication networks (Souza & Gobbi, 2014). Thus, memes are understood as an element of communication, present in the everyday life of youths in the contemporary world.

In their profiles, the youths also showed their musical preferences and the singers and bands that they follow on digital platforms, specifically video clips on YouTube. This demonstrates the transformation that the music market has undergone by appropriating digital platforms for the dissemination and promotion of musical artists through video clips that, until then, had only been available through television programs directed to that market niche (Caroso, 2010). It is understood that, in music, dissemination of this content occurs primarily through digital platforms, which is how youths now access and consume this content.

Political issues were discussed in the activity workshops, and various politicians received a "dislike" in the young

---

[1] Hashtags are words or phrases preceded by the pound/number sign (#) that create hyperlinks that group the produced content (images, videos, publications) to other content that also uses the tagged term (Antunes, 2017).

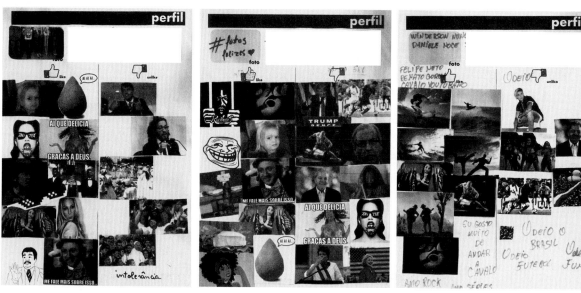

Fig. 25.1 Examples of profiles made by young people in activity workshops

people's profiles. It is worth noting that "politics" herein refers to the political situation at the national and global levels, represented by politicians and social movements. In this context, youths inserted in DSNs can be recognized as aligned with a certain political position by the algorithms, in some cases contradictory, since in virtual environments, exposure to mathematical algorithms highlights customization of the profiles based on the interests demonstrated by users in the networks (Pariser, 2012). Castro (2008) states that in Brazil and in globalized countries, consumer culture leads young people (and the population in general) to "privatization of the experience" (p. 255), in which experiences are guided by the individual values of well-being, security, and comfort. The phenomenon of political aversion in the DSNs expressed by the young people in the activity workshops suggests that networks produce the privatization of the political experience. This privatization is linked to virtual technologies that intensify personification according to a commercial bias and particularly alienates the socially deprived youths from the political arena of debate. It should be emphasized that this reflection is being made under the parameters of this experience and acknowledges successful experiences in the youth political fronts mobilized by DSNs.

FINAL REMARKS

The activity workshops enabled greater engagement with the youths, creating "potential spaces of experimentation and learning, conceiving each participant as active in the process of constructing subjectivity, a being of the praxis, action and reflection" (Lopes, Malfitano, Silva, & Borba, 2014, p. 595). This fact demonstrates that the model under which the activities were conducted allowed the more comprehensive interpretation that a specific individual needs, but this was also due to the collective nature of the activities, creating a possible space for sociability and exchanges that can transcend the workshop environment and involve other living spaces of these youths (Lopes, Borba, Trajber, Silva, & Cuel, 2011). The activity workshops prioritized individual freedom of expression, within a democratic context in which exchanges between the participants were realized, configuring a space of plurality where different identity issues could be collectively discussed.

The methodology used provided elements that supported the proposed discussion on DSNs and the experiences of young people in and with them. The activity workshops have demonstrated that the practical action of occupational therapy in general and, in this case, specifically of social occupational therapy, can contribute knowledge that enriches our understanding of the everyday lives, occupations, habits, and ways of living of the participating individuals.

Discussions of technological advancement and the relationships of individuals with digital platforms indicate the relevance of this theme to the current field of knowledge in occupational therapy, which needs to reflect on the modifications to everyday life caused by this incorporation of technological devices; these changes impact the work of occupational therapists insofar as they need to under-stand the different ways of life of individuals in their personal and historical moments, including those of youths. Within the scope of social occupational therapy, this understanding is essential for professional action articulated with its context, in search of fostering inclusion and social participation.

REFERENCES

Antunes, B. F. (2017). #tbt e o problema da instantaneidade e do imediatismo do Instagram [#tbt and Instagram's instantaneousness and immediacy problem] (pp. 1–13). *Anais do 40° Congresso Brasileiro de Ciências da Comunicação.*

Barros, D. D., Ghirardi, M. I., & Lopes, R. E. (2005). Social occupational therapy: A socio-historical perspective. In F. Kronenberg, S. S. Algado, & N. Pollard (Eds.), *Occupational therapy without borders: Learning from the spirit of survivors* (pp. 140–151). Londres: Elsevier Science – Churchill Livingstone.

Barros, D. D., Lopes, R. E., Galheigo, S. M., & Galvani, D. (2005). The Metuia Project in Brazil: Ideas and actions that bind us together. In F. Kronenberg, S. S. Algado, & N. Pollard (Eds.), *Occupational therapy without borders: Learning from the spirit of survivors* (pp. 402–413). Londres: Elsivier Science – Churchill Livingstone.

Bourdieu, P. (1983). A "juventude" é apenas uma palavra [Youth is just a word]. In P. Bourdieu (Ed.), *Questões de sociologia* [Sociology issues] (pp.112–121). Rio de Janeiro: Marco Zero.

Caroso, L. (2010). *Etnomusicologia no ciberespaço: processos criativos e de disseminação em videoclipes amadores* [Ethnomusicology in cyberspace: Creative and dissemination processes in amateur music videos] (Programa de Pós-Graduação em Música) (p. 214). Salvador: Universidade Federal da Bahia.

Castro, L. R. (2008). Participação política e juventude: do mal-estar à responsabilização frente ao destino comum [Political participation and youth: From malaise to accountability to common destiny]. *Revista de Sociologia e Politica [Journal of Sociology and Politics],* 16(30), 253–268.

Di Felice, M. (2008). *Do Público para as redes – a comunicação digital e as novas formas de participação social* [From the public to the networks - Digital communication and new forms of social participation]. São Caetano do Sul: Difusão.

Fuchs, C. (2008). *Internet society.* New York, NY: Routledge.

Jenkins, H. (2006). *Convergence culture: Where old and new media collide.* New York, NY: NYU Press.

Jurdi, A. P., Brunello, M. B., & Honda, M. (2004). Terapia ocupacional e propostas de intervenção na rede pública de ensino [Occupational therapy and intervention proposals in the public school system]. *Revista de Terapia Ocupacional da Universidade de São Paulo,* 15(1), 26–32.

Lopes, R. E., Borba, P. L., Trajber, N. K., Silva, C. R., & Cuel, B. T. (2011). Oficina de atividades com jovens da escola pública: tecnologias sociais entre educação e terapia ocupacional [Workshop on youth activities of the public school: Social technologies between education and occupational therapy]. *Interface,* 15(36), 277–288.

Lopes, R. E., & Malfitano, A. P. (2017). Social occupational therapy, Citizenship, rights and policies: Connecting the voices of collectives and individuals. In D. Sakellariou & N. Pollard (Eds.), *Occupational therapies without borders: Integrating justice with practice.* Edinburgh: Elsevier.

Lopes, R. E., Malfitano, A. S., Silva, C. R., & Borba, P. L. (2014). Recursos e tecnologias em Terapia Ocupacional Social: ações com jovens pobres na cidade [Resources and technologies in occupational social therapy: Actions with poor young people in the city]. *Cadernos de Terapia Ocupacional da UFSCar,* 22(3), 591–602.

Mannheim, K. (1982). Os problemas das gerações [The problems of the generations]. In K. Mannheim (Ed.), *Sociologia* [Sociology] (pp. 66–95). São Paulo, Brasil: Ática.

Margulis, M., & Urresti, M. (1998). La juventude és mas que uma palabra [Youth is more than a word]. In M. Margulis (Ed.), *La juventude és mas que uma palavra: ensayos sobre cultura y juventude* [Youth is more than a word: Essays on culture and youth] (pp. 3–12). Buenos Aires: Biblos.

Pariser, E. (2012). *O Filtro invisível: o que a internet está escondendo de você* [The invisible filter: What the internet is hiding from you]. São Paulo: Zahar.

Pereira, P. E., & Malfitano, A. S. (2014). Olhos de ver, ouvidos de ouvir, mãos de fazer: oficinas de atividades em Terapia Ocupacional como método de coleta de dados [Eyes to see, ears to hear, hands to do: Workshops of activities in occupational therapy as a method of data collection]. *Interface,* 18(49), 415–422.

Recuero, R. D. (2007). Memes em weblogs: proposta de uma taxonomia [Memes in weblogs: Proposal of a taxonomy]. *Revista FAMECOS,* 14(32), 23–31.

Sampaio, J. (2006). A sociedade em rede e a economia do conhecimento – Portugal numa perspectiva global [The network society and the knowledge economy – Portugal in a global perspective]. In M. Castells & G. Cardoso (Eds.), *A sociedade em rede: do conhecimento á acção política* [The network society: from knowledge to political action] (pp. 419–426). Belém: Casa da Moeda.

Santana, V. F., Melo-Solarte, D. S., Neris, V. P., Miranda, L. C., & Baranauskas, M. C. (2009). Redes Sociais Online: Desafios e Possibilidades para o Contexto Brasileiro [Online social networks: Challenges and possibilities for the Brazilian context]. In *XXXVI Seminário Integrado de Software e Hardware/XXIX Congresso da Sociedade Brasileira de Computação. XXX Congresso da Sociedade Brasileira de Computação – Programas e Resumos* (pp. 339–353).

Santos, H. P. (2013). Etiquetagem e folksonomia: o usuário e sua motivação para organizar e compartilhar informação na Web 2.0 [Labeling and folksonomy: The user and their motivation to organize and share information in Web 2.0]. *Perspectivas em Ciências da Informação [Perspectives in Information Science],* 18(2), 91–104.

Silva, C. R. (2013). As atividades como recurso para pesquisa [Activities as a resource for research]. *Cadernos de Terapia Ocupacional da UFSCar, 21*(3), 461–470.

Souza, H. D. (2014). Memes(?) do Facebook: reflexões sobre esse fenômeno de comunicação na cultura ciber [Facebook Memes (?): Reflections on this phenomenon of communication in cyber culture]. *Temática, 10*(7), 156–174.

Souza, J. F., & Gobbi, M. C. (2014). Geração digital: uma reflexão sobre as relações da "juventude digital" e os campos da comunicação e da cultura [Digital generation: A reflection on the relations of "digital youth" and the fields of communication and culture]. *Revista Geminis, 5*(2), 129–145.

Woods, J. (2005). Digital influencers: Do business communicators dare overlook the power of blogs. *Communication World, San Francisco, 22*(1), 26–30.

26

Under and Between Trees: Social Occupational Therapy in a Public Square

Marina Jorge da Silva

Castro Alves Square belongs to the people
just like the sky belongs to the planes
a new frevo,[1] I want a new frevo
everyone in the square
and a lot of dull people in the ballroom
Put out your elbows and open your way
Grab my hair so as not to get lost and end up alone
Time goes by, but with courage I'll make it
It is here in this square that everything is going to happen
A new frevo

Caetano Veloso

Since 2005, when its work with urban low-income youth was proposed, the Metuia/UFSCar Project has been developing collective actions aimed at promoting spaces for life-sharing and social activities (Lopes et al., 2008) among residents on the outskirts of Sao Carlos, a municipality in the interior of the state of Sao Paulo, Brazil. Comprising neighborhoods characterized by poverty, this region is known for its high instances of violence and drug trafficking and for its precarious infrastructure, such as its limited access to social services (Rosa, 2008). For nearly fifteen years, the Metuia/Federal University of São Carlos (UFSCar) Project team has been developing projects in partnership with the community and public service providers in this region, and has accumulated data and experiences related to the territory and its residents (Lopes, Malfitano, Silva, & Borba, 2014). The accumulated data made it possible to understand the youths who live in São Carlos and how they make use of the available spaces. Usage of public spaces varies depending on several factors, such as gender and access to employment (or lack of it), as well as the legality or illegality of their jobs.

Social occupational therapy actions developed by the Metuia/UFSCar Project in this neighborhood have occurred in different spaces, such as a public school, a leisure and social space called the "youth center," and the Community Station (ECO)—a social assistance service (Lopes et al., 2014). The diversity of the projects conducted called for the professional team to circulate widely throughout the territory, although it must be understood that many young people remained unknown because they did not access the services available at the project sites. Based on a previous community project, conducted by the Metuia/UFSCar team in a public square (Silva & Souza, 2016), we chose to return to the Sao Carlos neighborhood. Older residents reported the importance of this square to the organization of the neighborhood's social life because of both its geographical location and the region's developmental history, since the square is a space around which the first dwellings were built in the 1970s (Rosa, 2008). Thus, we decided there was a role for occupational therapy in this public square, working with a group of young people who did not attend school or spaces of leisure such as the youth center or the ECO. Our team observed that the square was used as a space of recreation (particularly for children), as a meeting place for people from the neighborhood on weekend nights, for barbecues and social gatherings, and as an informal work space, with the selling of savory snacks and illegal drugs. Many youths work in the illegal drug trade in this square.

---

[1]A dance and musical style originating from Recife, state of Pernambuco, Brazil, traditionally associated with Brazilian Carnival. The word *frevo* is said to come from *frever*, a variant of the Portuguese word *ferver* (to boil). It is said that the sound of the *frevo* makes listeners and dancers feel as if they are boiling on the ground. The word *frevo* is used for both the *frevo* music and the *frevo* dance.

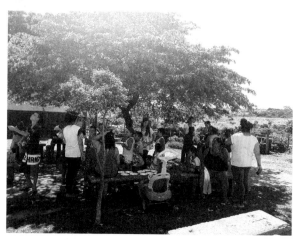

Fig. 26.1 The square: a meeting point and space of intervention. (Source: Metuia/UFSCar collection.)

The team then decided to hold weekly workshops in the square, which were open to anyone nearby. We began the workshops on "activities, dynamics, and projects"—the Metuia Workshops, as they became known—which utilized drama, art and play, and experiences of group dynamics to complete various projects. The workshops were designed to explore the notions of citizenship, rights and duties, and democratic participation (Lopes et al., 2014). The workshops were proposed as a mediating resource to uncover the identified needs of the community and strengthening of individuals and collectives to whom their action is directed (Lopes et al., 2014). See Figure 26.1.

What follows is a brief report on the experience of seven workshops held in this square. The purpose of the workshops was to map the public spaces known and used by youths in the neighborhood and the city. Based on this experience, we seek to reflect on the use of public spaces, such as squares, as important places of intervention for social engagement, where social and personal support networks are formed and maintained, with occupational therapists as possible mediators of this process.

MAPPING SPACES AND THEIR USES (OPPORTUNITIES AND EXPERIMENTATION)

The restricted circulation of many youths not only led the Metuia/UFSCar Project team to carry out the proposed intervention in the square but also drew attention to the need for further research on the (limited) circulation of these youths around their city and its impact on their lives. We consider public space as a synthesis of multiple political and symbolic dimensions (Arendt, 2005), as "the space where social and political life occurs" (Medeiros, 2013,

p. 44). As a project team, we understood that public spaces hold significant importance in the lives of these individuals, collectives, and social groups, including as a place and means of exercising citizenship (Hermany & Maschio, 2008). Considering the relevance of this debate to social occupational therapy, which considers citizenship and rights to be the basis practice (Galheigo, 1997; Lopes, 1999; Lopes & Malfitano, 2017), we attempted to understand how those youths understood the public space. After three conversation circles, it was uncovered that the youths did not relate this theme to their lives, nor did they associate their social-historical, economic, or cultural reality with their use of public spaces.

According to Milton Santos (2017), the territory—or the space where people live and engage—is determinant of their opportunities in life. With this premise, we proceeded to map, together with the youths, the public spaces known and used by them in their neighborhood and city. In the shadow of one of the few trees in the square, 3-hour workshops were held weekly for approximately 2 months (7 weeks), with an average of five participants per meeting.

In the first two encounters, we worked with the youths on the local, spatial, and geographical recognition, using a simple map of the area that contained the names of the streets of the neighborhood, the names of the surrounding neighborhoods, and the names of local public spaces and devices, such as schools, health services, and leisure spaces (parks, squares, etc.). In the following two meetings, with a simple map of the entire city (Figure 26.2), we sought to list the public spaces identified by them throughout the municipality. In continuity with the mapping proposal, the last three meetings were directed at the identification of uses for all of the public spaces identified.

Each stage of the workshops brought different elements of reflection and understanding. The mapping of the public spaces in the neighborhood and its surroundings revealed the youths' vast knowledge of the region, in contrast to their knowledge of public spaces in other areas of the city. Despite a certain competitiveness between the participating youths, who challenged themselves to list the largest number of known spaces, they had great difficulty in performing aspects of this task. Thus, numerous private spaces were quickly listed, such as homes of relatives and friends and churches, but their recognition of public spaces was quite limited.

These findings are in alignment with Pereira and Malfitano's (2014), who discussed the circulation of some youths from the same region of the city and highlighted the lack of access and decreased engagement among low-income youths in the city and their confinement to spaces of social exchange within their own neighborhood or its surroundings. Their limited circulation means those

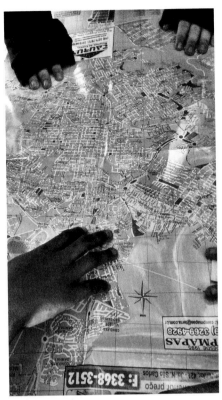

Fig. 26.2 Mapping spaces known and used by the youths. Source: Metuia/UFSCar collection.

youths are unable to experience other life-sharing and social events occurring in the city. Therefore, it is necessary to learn about the relationships that are established *with* and *in* the territory, such as the networks of support and solidarity, as well as the interconnections of this territory with the other spaces in the city.

During the course of this project, it was impressive to note the large number of squares that were successively mapped. Perhaps because this activity was conducted in a square, identification of similar spaces was encouraged, as was perhaps the recognition of these spaces as synonymous with public and collective spaces. Furthermore, it was interesting to observe that many of the spaces listed throughout the city had been visited/used by the Metuia/UFSCar Project team in the previous months and years, by social projects whose activities occur in the neighborhood (usually recreational activities offered by religious entities to children and youths during after-school hours), or even by public services related to education and/or health care, especially mental health care, or offering assistance to young offenders.

Therefore, access to public spaces, life sharing, and social engagement are considered opportunities that need

to be created, planned for, and experienced, and they might be part of the social occupational therapist's work. Although some authors present the possibility of life sharing as something that is innate to certain spaces (Alex, 2008), in our understanding, these spaces can (and should) be promoted as places that foster encounters and life sharing, collective conversations, and actions that transcend the individual and encourage collective engagement, culminating in the construction of common/collective agendas. In addition to this, there is an understanding that by studying locations such as a square, researchers can uncover important information about the local community, which can give insight into the everyday lives of the individuals who access it, as well as uncover the production of values and social exchanges (Malfitano & Bianchi, 2013).

FINAL REMARKS

As spaces of social integration and engagement, public squares have become central in the configuration of urban spaces and public life (Alex, 2008). In our opinion, the main characteristic of squares as important public spaces is their openness and the access they allow different individuals and groups. Through social occupational therapy actions, young residents in the neighborhood utilize the square as a space for life sharing and social engagement but also recognize the potential of other public spaces they could use.

This experience illustrates possibilities for an emerging field of practice. The intervention in the public square encourages occupational therapists to work within a local context without necessarily being restricted by institutional frameworks. It therefore encourages reflection on the validity and necessity of theorizing about collective life in the public space, which is an important aspect of the lives of the individuals whom social occupational therapists assist.

Facilitating social engagement and collective action is a key outcome of social occupational therapy. Therefore, discussing (with a view of fostering) usage of public spaces in the territory and in different socially meaningful spaces is of great relevance. From this point of view, the mapping activity not only facilitated greater knowledge of the reality of the individuals' lives but also encouraged the awareness of other spaces in the city and offered insight into other spaces in the neighborhood and their uses. Work in this area is especially important, as with the support of several professionals, young people can sometimes require permission to enter certain spaces, and access to public spaces is the first step toward fostering citizenship and democracy, with the latter presupposing political participation.

Thus, we advocate the need to discuss public spaces as one of the areas of action and reflection for social occupational therapists and as a possible strategy for communitarian work with young people. In our experience, public spaces are a promising area that enables collective encounters, experiences, and practices with different groups and generations.

ACKNOWLEDGMENTS

The author is especially grateful to Ana Paula Serrata Malfitano and Marina Leandrini de Oliveira for their direct contribution to the writing of this manuscript. I am also grateful to Roseli Esquerdo Lopes and Lívia Celegati Pan of the Metuia/UFSCar Project team for their partnership and co-construction of the project reported in this chapter. The reflections expressed were only possible thanks to the combined efforts of the Metuia Network (Social Occupation Therapy) and UFSCar, in our joint and supportive construction at work.

REFERENCES

Alex, S. (2008). *Projeto da Praça: Convívio e exclusão no espaço público* [Square project: Conviviality and exclusion in the public space] (2nd ed.). São Paulo: Editora SENAC.

Arendt, H. (2005). *A condição humana* [The human condition] (10th ed.). Rio de Janeiro: Forense Universitária.

Galheigo, S. M. (1997). Da adaptação psicossocial à construção do coletivo: a cidadamia enquanto eixo [From psychosocial adaptation to construction of a collective society citizenship as basis]. *Revista de Ciências Médicas - PUCCAMP, 6*(2/3), 105–108.

Hermany, R., & Maschio, D. (2008). Cidadania e espaço público constitucional: Uma abordagem a partir da esfera pública [Citizenship and constitutional public space: An approach from the public sphere]. *Âmbito Jurídico, 58*, 1–4.

Lopes, R. E. (1999). *Cidadania, políticas públicas e terapia ocupacional, no contexto das ações de saúde mental e saúde da pessoa portadora de deficiência, no Município de São Paulo* [Citizenship, public policies and occupational therapy, in the context of the actions of mental health and health of the person with disability, in the city of São Paulo]. Campinas, SP, Brasil: Tese de doutorado, Universidade Estadual de Campinas.

Lopes, R. E., Adorno, R. de C. F., Malfitano, A. P. S., Takeiti, B. A., Silva, C. R., & Borba, P. L. de O. (2008). Juventude pobre, violência e cidadania [Poor youth, violence and citizenship]. *Saúde e Sociedade, 17*(3), 63–76.

Lopes, R. E., & Malfitano, A. P. S. (2017). Social occupational therapy, citizenship, rights and policies: Connecting the voices of collectives and individuals. In D. Sakellariou & N. Pollard (Eds.), *Occupational therapies without borders: Integrating justice with practice.* Edinburgh: Elsevier.

Lopes, R. E., Malfitano, A. P. S., Silva, C. R., & Borba, P. L. O. (2014). Recursos e tecnologias em Terapia Ocupacional: ações com jovens pobres na cidade [Resources and technologies in social occupational therapy: Actions with the poor youth in town]. *Cadernos De Terapia Ocupacional Da UFSCar, 22*(3), 591–602.

Malfitano, A. P. S., & Bianchi, P. C. (2013). Terapia ocupacional e atuação em contextos de vulnerabilidade social: distinções e proximidades entre a área social e o campo de atenção básica em saúde [Occupational therapy and action in social vulnerability contexts: Proximities and distinctions between the social field and the primary health care area]. *Cadernos De Terapia Ocupacional Da UFSCar, 21*(3), 563–574.

Medeiros, A. P. G. (2013). Políticas públicas de produção e gestão de espaços públicos na cidade do Rio de Janeiro [Public policies for production and management of public spaces in the city of Rio de Janeiro]. *Cadernos de Pós-Graduação em Arquitetura e Urbanismo (Mackenzie. Online), 12*(1), 39–56.

Pereira, P. E., & Malfitano, A. P. S. (2014). Atrás da Cortina de Fumaça: Jovens da Periferia e a Temática das Drogas [Behind the smokescreen: Youths from the periphery and the drugs issue]. *Saúde & Transformação Social, 5*(1), 27–35.

Rosa, T. T. (2008). *Fronteiras em disputa na produção da cidade: a trajetória do "Gonzaga" de favela a bairro de periferia* [Borders under dispute in the urban space production: The trajectory of the "Gonzaga," from slums to outskirt neighborhood] (Dissertação de Mestrado). Campinas, São Paulo, Brasil: Instituto Filosofia e Ciências Humanas, Universidade Estadual de Campinas.

Santos, M. (2017). The return of the territory. In L. Melgaço & C. Prouse (Eds.), *A pioneer in critical geography from the global South* (pp. 25–32). New York: Springer.

Silva, C. D., & Souza, L. B. (2016). O plantio que virou plantação: germinar relações para semear vínculos. In R. E. Lopes & A. P. S. Malfitano (Eds.), *Terapia Ocupacional Social: desenhos teóricos e contornos práticos* [Social occupational therapy: Theoretical designs and practical outlines] (pp. 365–370). São Carlos: EdUFSCar.

27

The Planting Has Become a Plantation: Germinating Relationships to Sow Ties

Carolina Donato da Silva and Letícia Brandão de Souza

In this chapter, we present an experience associated with the Metuia Project of the Occupational Therapy Department of the Federal University of Sao Carlos (UFSCar). The experience reported in this chapter is part of "ArticulAÇÃO com Jovens no Território do Jardim Gonzaga" ("Articulation with Youths in the Jardim Gonzaga Territory"), a university extension project that has been conducted by the Metuia team in a territory located on the outskirts of the municipality of Sao Carlos, state of Sao Paulo, Brazil. It was identified that the peripheral neighborhoods of the municipality lack infrastructure and offer limited access to public network facilities for adolescents. Therefore, the project aimed to establish ways to approach, understand, and collaboratively develop social technologies for action involving socially vulnerable youths (Lopes et al., 2008; Lopes, Malfitano, Silva, & Borba, 2014).

> problematized, from a social historical point of view, are ways of facing the violence that afflicts teenagers and children of urban areas in Brazil. Violence is a complex phenomenon of great importance in many different communities. The vulnerability of those young people, as demonstrated by a number of indexes, has reached unacceptable highs in Brazil, and so far, public policies have proven to be inadequate, insufficient, and fragmented (Lopes et al., 2008, p. 73).

In general, the project aims to gain an understanding of disadvantaged youth in the territory, specifically their realities of everyday life, and the professions involved in developing proposals to offer alternatives to their daily lives. Most of these actions, coordinated by Professor Roseli Esquerdo Lopes, have been presented and discussed at events and publications in the areas of occupational therapy and education.

Thanks to the work of the Metuia/UFSCar team at a local youth center, workshops on "activities, dynamics, and projects"—the so-called Metuia Workshops—were offered mostly in the youth center. However, these workshops sometimes occurred in the streets, which facilitated knowledge and understanding about the territory through the eyes of the young people who lived there. From our constant dialogue with these youths, we became aware that a square located right in the center of this neighborhood was, for several reasons, used as a place for garbage disposal but also as a meeting point for the residents. It was one of the few spaces in the neighborhood with benches and some trees. In conversations with the people who used the square, it was evident that, in general, the population would like the place to be better cared for, but they did not know exactly how to make this happen. During a workshop in the square, one of the participating children proposed the idea that some trees could be planted there because their shadows would make it more conducive to play and conversations. While the children and adolescents participating in the intervention analyzed the space, imagining how it would be after the implementation of that proposal, the waste and rubble present were no longer considered part of the landscape. It was then proposed that among the set of activities conducted with the youths who participated in the Metuia Workshops at the youth center, one would be the cleaning of the square, aiming to transform a place that was, until then, mostly used for waste disposal and drug dealing rather than being a place of well-being (Silva, Souza, Lopes, & Malfitano, 2013).

According to Silva (2007), workshops provide space where groups of people can develop proposals and ideas for action to foster shared learning. Valuing each individual is emphasized in the process, as well as the dynamic nature of the relational experiences between participants, space, materials, memory, and sensations—in short, everything that is being done during this experience. With the "Cleaning of the Square" workshop, we intended, at first, to prepare the space to plant some seedlings, without imagining that it would become a much larger plantation. During the cleaning of the square, in the discussions with the young people present, we reflected on the importance of providing education to the population regarding public spaces and the importance of such spaces as part of the daily life of the community. These conversations were mainly directed at the promotion of public spaces that could provide leisure, entertainment, and shared living, which are very scarce in the region, with the existing squares badly or not maintained.

After the cleaning and planting in the square, which was completed by the youths and other residents of the neighborhood, it was proposed that the collective and continuous maintenance of the square would be organized by the children in the neighborhood as well (Figure 27.1). As we developed the project in collaboration with the public, we found that this developed partnerships in line with the original objectives but also fostered and expanded the project. One of these partnerships was with an association of neighborhood residents called "Friends of the Square," which had already been organized to take better care of the square. This was a natural collaboration because of our shared goal. Thereafter, meetings were held at the Reference Center for Social Assistance with the Friends of the Square, who made contact with the Municipal Coordination of Environment, Municipal Secretary of Citizenship and Social Assistance, Municipal Public Services Secretary, Jardim Gonzaga Community Station, Nascente Community Bank, and the project Experiences in Diversified Leisure Activities.

The coming together of actors with common interests enabled the planting, together with the neighborhood residents—adults, children, and adolescents—of 20 seedlings and the "sowing" of improvement, strengthening the use of the square as a space of shared living, leisure, meeting, and

play. During the planting activities, we observed the coordination of participants in enabling ways to decide collectively where each seedling would be planted. Together they decided which houses would see the Yellow Ipe, which would have the fruit trees, and which would be planted in a strategic position to guarantee shade to the children, who would be able to play in the newly painted hopscotch grid within the newly cleaned square (Figure 27.2). The importance and need to take care of the space so that it could give back to the population informed every conversation effort and every aspect of the construction and planting.

An entirely new landscape was offered to the children with the discovery of the tools necessary to make the holes where the seedlings would be planted and with the attention and enthusiasm needed to manipulate the seedlings, carry them, and put them in the defined spot. All the children wanted to participate in each stage: digging the holes, transporting the seedlings, preparing them, putting them in place, and completing the watering. The adolescents, in turn, took a position of responsibility and leadership and were always ready to help the children and find solutions.

As the plantation germinated, other "offshoots" emerged: the square gained new colors with a graffiti workshop

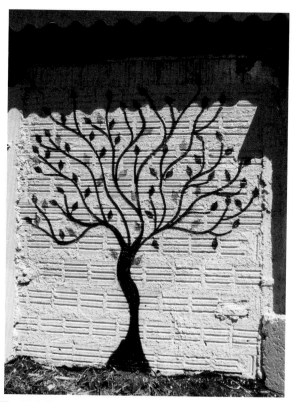

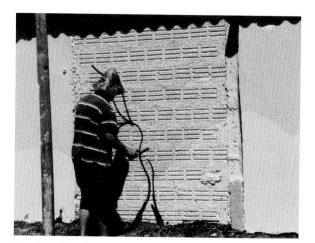

Fig. 27.1 Drawing the tree during planting

Fig. 27.2 The new tree on the wall

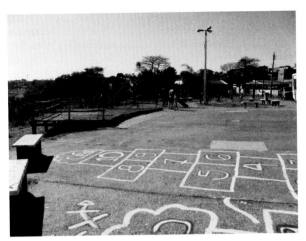

Fig. 27.3 How the place looks like after the project

organized by the residents and community workers (Figure 27.3). With the help of the youths, who were very interested in learning the graffiti technique, trees were painted on the walls, a hopscotch grid was drawn on the ground, and leaves were painted on all the tables and benches of the square. After the intervention, it was possible to observe that an understanding of the space had occurred through its occupation, and the community could appreciate the possibility of using the square in different ways than they had previously, considering that it was mainly a degraded space with limited use. The right to leisure in the territory is an extremely important issue for the community. This proposal encouraged reciprocal appreciation between the population and the project, an appreciation that authorizes, considers, and prioritizes the historical cultural context of each party and, with this, proposes changes that meet their own demands.

The use of contextualized and meaningful activity enabled closer contact with the youth in the neighborhood, from which it was possible to deepen the understanding of individual and collective needs. Likewise, it fostered greater contact and shared living between the participants and provided experimentation and the development of a pleasant space for socializing and exchange of experiences that could grow out of the physical space of the workshop and transcend the contexts of life, family, friends, and school. The projects also provided the benefit of practical and meaningful training for all the students and professionals involved.

This project has been designed and pursued by the Metuia/UFSCar team (Lopes et al., 2006, 2008, 2011; Lopes, Borba, & Monzeli, 2013; Lopes et al., 2014). Our intention has been to create new relationships for the development of projects that can be led by these young people, to foster

learning and teaching of each other, enabling their own initiative; developing the notion of social belonging, cooperation, and solidarity; and seeking to expand and strengthen their social support networks, all following the assumptions of occupational social therapy (Barros, Ghirardi, & Lopes, 1999, 2002). Our actions conducted at the youth center were aimed at promoting the participation of youths from the neighborhood, considering that they are highly exposed to daily situations of violence—declared or hidden—by organized crime or even by the state. This youth center is an institution that has succeeded in welcoming this population of youths, but it still offers few services that meet their specific situation and needs. The Metuia/UFSCar Workshop is one such example of meeting the community's needs. Thus, the benefit of social occupational therapy has been highlighted through this project by not only providing a desirable living space but also, throughout the process, empowering the people in the neighborhood through assurance of their rights, access to citizenship, and an understanding of future possibilities for life.

REFERENCES

Barros, D. D., Ghirardi, M. I. G., & Lopes, R. E. (1999). Terapia Ocupacional e Sociedade [Occupational therapy and society]. *Revista de Terapia Ocupacional da Universidade de São Paulo, 10*(2–3), 71–76.

Barros, D. D., Ghirardi, M. I. G., & Lopes, R. E. (2002). Terapia Ocupacional Social [Social occupational therapy]. *Revista de Terapia Ocupacional da Universidade de São Paulo, 13*(3), 95–103.

Lopes, R. E. (2006). Terapia ocupacional social e a infância e a juventude pobres: experiências do Núcleo UFSCar do Projeto METUIA [Social occupational therapy, poor childhood and youth: Experiences of the METUIA Project]. *Cadernos de Terapia Ocupacional da UFSCar, 14* (1), 5–14.

Lopes, R. E., et al. (2008). Juventude pobre, violência e cidadania [Poor youth, violence and citizenship]. *Saúde e Sociedade, 17*(3), 63–76.

Lopes, R. E., et al. (2011). Oficinas de atividades com jovens da escola pública: tecnologias sociais entre educação e terapia ocupacional [Workshops with public school youngsters: Social technologies between education and occupational therapy]. *Interface, 15*(36), 277–288.

Lopes, R. E., Borba, P. L. O., & Monzeli, G. A. (2013). Expressão livre de jovens por meio de Fanzine: recurso para a terapia ocupacional social [Youth free expression through Fanzine: A social occupational therapy resource]. *Saúde e Sociedade, 22*, 937–948.

Lopes, R. E., Malfitano, A. P. S., Silva, C. R., & Borba, P. L. O. (2014). Recursos e tecnologias em terapia ocupacional social: ações com jovens pobres na cidade [Resources and technology in social occupational therapy: Working with poor youngsters in the city]. *Cadernos de Terapia Ocupacional da UFSCar, 22,* 591–602.

Silva, C. R. (2007). Oficinas. In M. P. Brandini, R. F. Siero, & A. Carnicel (Eds.), *Palavras-chaves em educação não-formal* [Key-words in non-formal education] (pp. 213–214). Campinas: Setembro.

Silva, C. D., Souza, L. B., Lopes, R. E., & Malfitano, A. P. S. (2013). O plantio que virou plantação: germinar relações para semear vínculos [The planting became a plantation: Germinating relationships to sow bonds]. In *Proceedings of the 9th Congress of Higher Education Extension of the Federal University of São Carlos, Brazil*, 9; Scientific and Technological Day of the Federal University of São Carlos, Brazil, 10, São Carlos, SP. São Carlos: Universidade Federal de São Carlos – UFSCar. CD.

INDEX

Page numbers followed by "*b*", "*f*" and "*t*" indicate boxes, figures, and tables, respectively